Shaping Nursing Science and Improving Health

The Michigan Legacy

Shaké Ketefian

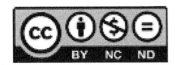
Published in the United States of America by
Michigan Publishing
Manufactured in the United States of America

ISBN 978-1-60785-393-0 (paper)
ISBN 978-1-60785-384-7 (e-book)

An imprint of Michigan Publishing, Maize Books serves the publishing needs of the University of
Michigan community by making high-quality scholarship widely available in print and online. It
represents a new model for authors seeking to share their work within and beyond the academy,
offering streamlined selection, production, and distribution processes. Maize Books is intended as a
complement to more formal modes of publication in a wide range of disciplinary areas.

http:/www.maizebooks.org

The search for truth is more important than its possession.

ALBERT EINSTEIN

Contents

Acknowledgments   xi

List of Contributors   xiii

Prologue   xix

Introduction   xxiii

Section I. Biobehavioral Health

Chapter 1. Biological Science: Getting at the Cause to Promote the Cure   3
Janean Holden

Chapter 2. Biobehavioral Research in Cardiovascular and Respiratory Nursing   15
Janet Larson

Chapter 3. Cognition and Nursing Science at the University of Michigan   35
Donna L. Algase

Chapter 4. Biobehavioral Research in Cancer Nursing   47
Laurel Northouse

Section II. Building a Healthy Nation Through Nursing Science

Chapter 5. Advancing the Science of Health Promotion for Children, Adolescents, and Their Families   65
Carol Loveland-Cherry and Nola J. Pender

Chapter 6. Promoting Worker Health and Safety   81
Sally L. Lusk

Chapter 7. Primary Care and Nurse-Managed Health Centers: Research Team 1998–2013   97
Joanne M. Pohl and Violet H. Barkauskas

Short Papers   97

    The Many Facets of Cardiovascular Health Disparities in Black Americans,
        Debra J. Barksdale   105

    The Effect of Cross-Cultural Provider-Patient Dyadic Relationships on
        Health Outcomes, Ramona A. Benkert   108

    Culturally Tailored, Community-Based Diabetes Prevention and
        Management Interventions, Deborah Vincent   111

Section III. Advancing the Health of Women Globally

Chapter 8. Three Decades of Research to Improve Women's Health   117
    Carolyn Sampselle

Short Papers   117

    Gender, Health, and Drugs of Abuse, Carol J. Boyd   126

    Improving Maternal and Newborn Health in Low-Resource Countries,
        Jody Lori   130

    Labor Care Practices for Optimal Health Outcomes for
        Childbearing Women, Lisa Kane Low   134

    Advocating Cultural and Gender-Sensitive Policies in Women's Health
        Through Research, Zxy-Yann Jane Lu   139

    Understanding, Mitigating, and Eliminating Lower Urinary Tract
        Symptoms, Janis Miller   141

    Prevention of Urinary Incontinence in Women, Carolyn Sampselle   145

    Effects of Posttraumatic Stress Disorder on Women's Health, Julia S. Seng   149

Section IV. Nursing and Health Care Systems

Chapter 9. Nursing Health Care Systems at the University of Michigan   157
    Richard W. Redman

Short Papers   157

    Highlights From a Program of Nursing Workforce Research,
        Carol S. Brewer   172

    A Workforce Policy to Highlight the Contribution of Nurses,
        Sung-Hyun Cho   176

    The Opportunity and Obligation to Improve Care Delivery,
        Christopher Friese   178

Nursing Research Shaping Health Policy, Ada Sue Hinshaw   181

From Policy/Politics to History to Image to Nursing Studies,
  Beatrice J. Kalisch   183

An Intellectual Journey, Shaké Ketefian   186

Rethinking Communication for Improved Patient Outcomes,
  Milisa Manojlovich   191

Care Quality, Safety, and Clinical and Organizational Outcomes,
  Richard W. Redman   194

Staff Nurse Fatigue and Patient Safety Research Program, Ann E. Rogers
  and Linda D. Scott   197

From Health Promotion and Risk Reduction to Health System
  Entrepreneurship and Innovation, Anne Snowdon   200

Research in Translation and Implementation Science, Marita G. Titler   203

A Shift From Being Clinician-Centric to Patient-Centric,
  Huey-Ming Tzeng   207

Chapter 10. Nursing Informatics at the University of Michigan School
of Nursing: A View of the Past, Perspectives on the Future   213
Patricia A. Abbott and Marcelline Harris

Short Papers   213

Building a Foundation for Nursing Informatics Science, Judy G. Ozbolt   217

Patient Care Quality and Safety Through Technology and Clinical
  Information, Dana Tschannen   221

Informatics: The Road Less Taken, Patricia A. Abbott   225

Clinical and Research Informatics: Joint Contributions to Research
  Infrastructure, Marcelline Harris   229

Health Science Analytics: Data- and Technology-Driven Approaches for
  Addressing Health Care Challenges, Advancing Well-Being, and
  Enhancing Nursing Education, Ivo D. Dinov   232

Section V. Nursing Leadership

Chapter 11. Innovation Leadership   245
Daniel J. Pesut

Chapter 12. Leadership as Scholarship   251
Joanne Disch, Linda R. Cronenwett, and Jane Barnsteiner

Chapter 13. Commentary on Leadership Papers   267
    Kathleen Potempa

Section VI. Short Papers Submitted for Chapters 1–6

Short Papers for Chapter 1   273

Cognitive and Behavioral Neuroscience Research, Hala Darwish   273

Untangling the Biology of Sickness Symptoms, Donna McCarthy   276

Discovering the Genetics of Diet Preference: Carbohydrates Versus Fats,
    Brenda K. (Smith) Richards   280

Short Papers for Chapter 2   283

Decision Making and Coronary Heart Disease,
    Cynthia Arslanian-Engoren   284

Dyspnea Assessment and Treatment at the End of Life,
    Margaret L. Campbell   287

Innovative Therapies for Heart Failure and Circulatory Support,
    Jesus M. Casida   291

Improving Health Outcomes for People With COPD, Nancy Kline Leidy   293

Investigating Cardiovascular Risk in a Conflict Zone, Samar Noureddine 298

A Program of Research to Improve Memory in Heart Failure,
    Susan J. Pressler   301

Challenges in Contemporary Pediatric Pain Management,
    Terri Voepel-Lewis   304

Short Papers for Chapter 3   307

A Journey With Nursing Science: Australia to Michigan and Back Again,
    Elizabeth R. A. Beattie   307

Improving Quality of Life: Culturally Sensitive Nursing Interventions
    Using the Concept of Familiarity in Korean Elders With Dementia,
    Gwi-Ryung Son Hong   311

Theory-Based Nonpharmacological Interventions for Persons Living
    With Dementia, Ann Kolanowski   314

Cognitive Representations Assessment to Guide Medication Taking and
    Dietary Interventions to Improve Blood Pressure in Diverse Women,
    Margaret Scisney-Matlock   316

Managing Behavioral and Psychological Symptoms of Elders
    With Dementia, Jun-Ah Song   320

Care of Chronically Mentally Ill and Late-Stage Dementia Patients:
    A Scientific Journey Embedded Within Philosophy of Science,
    Ann L. Whall   323

Depression and Stress: Research to Practice and Practice to Research,
    Reg A. Williams and Bonnie M. Hagerty   326

Short Papers for Chapter 4   329

    Cognitive Dysfunction in Breast Cancer, Bernadine Cimprich   329

    The Case for Nurse-Delivered Health Behavior Interventions,
        Sonia A. Duffy   333

    Measuring and Managing Chronic Pain in Cancer Survivors,
        Ellen M. Lavoie Smith   336

Short Papers for Chapter 5   339

    Event History Calendars: A Clinical Intervention Innovation,
        Kristy K. Martyn   339

    Promoting Physical Activity of Children and Adolescents in
        Diverse Populations, Lorraine B. Robbins   341

    Reducing Sexual Risk Among Mexican and Latino Adolescents,
        Antonia M. Villarruel   344

    Critically Ill Children and Their Families, JoAnne M. Youngblut 348

Short Papers for Chapter 6   352

    Reducing Auditory Problems Due to Harmful Noise and
        Chemical Exposure, OiSaeng Hong   352

    Occupational Health: Hearing Health Behavior Research and
        Public Health Informatics, Madeleine J. Kerr   356

    Cultivating Hearing Health Among Farm Operators,
        Marjorie McCullagh   359

Acknowledgments

A project of this magnitude cannot be accomplished without a team effort, and I was fortunate that many colleagues participated in the conception and preparation of this volume.

First, gratitude is expressed to the 125th Anniversary Committee formed by Dean Kathleen Potempa to prepare materials for the various celebratory events from 2015 through 2017. The members were graduate students Brian Kaminski and Amanda Schuh; community representative Susan Nenadic; alumni representative Janet Tarolli; staff members Mary Beth Lewis and Jaime Meyers; and present or past faculty members Esther Bay, Sally Lusk, Milisa Manojlovich, Marjorie McCullagh, and Richard Redman. I would also like to extend a special gratitude to my committee cochair, Linda Strodtman, for her steady support and insightful suggestions.

During the conception and design of the book, colleagues Milisa Manojlovich and Richard Redman formed a subcommittee and generously advised me at important decision points via in-person meetings or electronically; I thank them.

Debt of gratitude to the many individuals, past and present faculty members and PhD alumni, who submitted short papers; these formed the foundation for the chapter authors and discussants who had the challenging task of synthesizing papers with different types of content, though they may have had a common starting place. These authors did a yeoman's job.

Our two external reviewers, Margaret Reynolds and Suzanne Brouse, who are alumnae of different programs of the school, graciously agreed to serve in this role and provided their comments to the authors; the process was collegial and immensely helpful to the authors and editors alike.

Dean Kathleen Potempa has been supportive throughout the process, providing overall guidance and facilitation, as well as the resources to bring this vision into reality. Along with Dean Potempa, two other deans before her share the responsibility and kudos for nurturing and shepherding the science represented here: Dean Rhetaugh G. Dumas, who sadly is not with us to share the moment, and Dean Ada Sue Hinshaw, who joined the project as a contributor and gave us her support. I thank all three deans for their leadership.

SHAKÉ KETEFIAN
Editor
July 2016

Contributors

Patricia A. Abbott, PhD, RN, FAAN, FACMI. Associate Professor; Director of the Hillman Scholars in Nursing Innovation Program, University of Michigan, School of Nursing.

Donna L. Algase, PhD, RN, FAAN, FGSA, F-NGNA. Josephine M. Sana Collegiate Professor of Nursing Emerita, University of Michigan; Associate Dean for Research and Evaluation (ret.), University of Toledo, College of Nursing.

Cynthia Arslanian-Engoren, PhD, RN, ACNS-BC, FAHA, FAAN. Associate Professor; Director of Faculty Affairs and Faculty Development, University of Michigan, School of Nursing.

Violet Barkauskas, PhD, RN, FAAN. Associate Professor Emerita, University of Michigan, School of Nursing.

Debra Barksdale, PhD, RN, FNP-BC, ANP-BC, CNE, FAANP, FAAN. Associate Dean of Academic Programs, Virginia Commonwealth University School of Nursing, Richmond, Virginia.

Jane Barnsteiner, PhD, RN, FAAN. Professor Emerita, University of Pennsylvania, School of Nursing.

Debra Barton, PhD RN, AOCN, FAAN. Mary Lou Willard French Professor of Nursing, University of Michigan.

Elizabeth R. A. Beattie, PhD, RN, FGSA, FAAN. Professor of Aging and Dementia Care, Queensland University of Technology, Australia.

Ramona A. Benkert, PhD, RN. Associate Dean for Academic and Clinical Affairs; Associate Professor, Wayne State University, College of Nursing, Detroit, MI.

Carol J. Boyd, PhD, RN, FAAN. Deborah J. Oakley Collegiate Professor of Nursing; Professor of Women's Studies; Research Professor, Addiction Research Center, Department of Psychiatry, University of Michigan.

Carol S. Brewer, PhD, RN, FAAN. University of Buffalo Distinguished Professor Emerita, State University of New York at Buffalo, School of Nursing.

Margaret Campbell, PhD, RN, FPCN. Professor, Wayne State University, College of Nursing, Detroit, Michigan.

Jesus Casida, PhD, RN. Assistant Professor, University of Michigan, School of Nursing.

Sung-Hyun Cho, PhD, RN. Professor, Seoul National University, College of Nursing, Seoul, Korea.

Bernadine Cimprich, PhD, RN, FAAN. Associate Professor Emerita, University of Michigan, School of Nursing.

Linda R. Cronenwett, PhD, RN, FAAN. Dean Emerita and Professor, University of North Carolina at Chapel Hill, School of Nursing; Codirector, Robert Wood Johnson Foundation Executive Nurse Fellows Program.

Hala Darwish, PhD, RN. Associate Professor, Managing Director, Abou Haidar Neuroscience Institute, Nehme and Therese Tohme Multiple Sclerosis Center, American University of Beirut, Hariri School of Nursing, Beirut, Lebanon.

Ivo D. Dinov, PhD. Associate Professor, Department of Health Behavior and Biological Sciences; Director of Statistics Online Computational Resource, University of Michigan, School of Nursing.

Joanne Disch, PhD, RN, FAAN. Professor ad Honorem, University of Minnesota, School of Nursing.

Sonia A. Duffy, PhD, RN, FAAN. Mildred E. Newton Endowed Chair, Ohio State University, College of Nursing; Research Investigator, Ann Arbor Veterans Affairs Center for Clinical Management Research.

Christopher Friese, PhD, RN, FAAN. Professor, University of Michigan, School of Nursing.

Bonnie M. Hagerty, PhD, RN, Associate Professor; Associate Dean of Undergraduate Studies, University of Michigan, School of Nursing.

Marcelline Harris, PhD, RN. Associate Professor, University of Michigan, School of Nursing.

Ada Sue Hinshaw, PhD, RN, FAAN. Dean Emerita, University of Michigan, School of Nursing; Dean Emerita, Daniel K. Inouye Graduate School of Nursing, Uniformed Services University of the Health Sciences, Bethesda, Maryland.

Janean Holden, PhD, RN, FAAN. Barbara A. Therrien Collegiate Professor of Nursing, Associate Dean for Research, University of Michigan, School of Nursing.

OiSaeng Hong, PhD, RN, FAAN. Professor; Director of Occupational and Environmental Health Nursing, University of California, San Francisco; Northern California Center of Occupational and Environmental Health.

Gwi-Ryung Son Hong, PhD, RN. Professor, Hanyang University, College of Nursing, Korea.

Beatrice J. Kalisch, PhD, RN, FAAN. Professor Emerita; Titus Distinguished Professor of Nursing (Emerita), University of Michigan, School of Nursing.

Maria Katapodi, PhD, RN, FAAN. Professor of Nursing Science, Faculty of Medicine, University of Basel, Switzerland.

Shaké Ketefian, EdD, RN, FAAN. Professor Emerita, University of Michigan, School of Nursing.

Madeleine Kerr, PhD, RN. Associate Professor, University of Minnesota, School of Nursing.

Eileen Kintner, PhD, RN, FAAN. Associate Professor, University of Texas at Austin, School of Nursing.

Ann Kolanowski, PhD, RN, FAAN. Elouise Ross Eberly Professor of Nursing, Pennsylvania State University, College of Nursing.

Janet Larson, PhD, RN, FAAN. Shaké Ketefian Collegiate Professor of Nursing; Chair, Department of Health Behavior and Biological Sciences, University of Michigan, School of Nursing.

Nancy Kline Leidy, PhD, RN. Senior Vice President, Scientific Affairs, Evidera, Bethesda, Maryland.

Jody Lori, PhD, RN, FAAN. Associate Professor, Department of Health Behavior and Biological Sciences; Associate Dean of Global Affairs, University of Michigan, School of Nursing.

Carol Loveland-Cherry, PhD, RN, FAAN. Professor Emerita, University of Michigan, School of Nursing.

Lisa Kane Low, PhD, RN, FAAN. Associate Professor of Nursing and Women's Studies; Associate Dean, Practice and Professional Graduate Programs, University of Michigan, School, of Nursing.

Zxy-Yann Jane Lu, PhD, RN. Professor, National Yang-Ming University, Institute of Community Health Nursing, Taipei, Taiwan.

Sally L. Lusk, PhD, RN, FAAN, FAAOHN. Professor Emerita, University of Michigan, School of Nursing.

Milisa Manojlovich, PhD, RN. Associate Professor, University of Michigan, School of Nursing.

Kristy Kiel Martyn, PhD, RN, FAAN, CPNP-PC. Professor; Independence Chair in Nursing, Assistant Dean for Clinical Advancement, Emory University, Nell Hodgson Woodruff School of Nursing, Atlanta, Georgia.

Donna McCarthy, PhD, RN, FAAN. Professor and Interim Dean, Marquette University, College of Nursing.

Marjorie McCullagh, PhD, RN, APRN-BC, COHN-S, FAAOHN, FAAN. Professor, University of Michigan, School of Nursing.

Janis Miller, PhD, RN, FAAN, Professor of Nursing; Research Professor, Department of Obstetrics and Gynecology, University of Michigan.

Laurel Northouse, PhD, RN, FAAN. Professor Emerita, University of Michigan, School of Nursing.

Samar Noureddine, PhD, RN, FAHA, FAAN. Professor, Assistant Director for Academic Affairs, American University of Beirut, Hariri School of Nursing, Beirut, Lebanon.

Judy G. Ozbolt, PhD, RN, FAAN. Consultant in Health and Biomedical Informatics; Visiting Professor, University of Maryland.

Nola Pender, PhD, RN, FAAN. Professor Emerita, University of Michigan; Distinguished Professor, Loyola University, Chicago.

Daniel J. Pesut, PhD, RN, PMHCNS-BC, FAAN. Professor of Nursing, Population Health and Systems Cooperative Unit; Director of Katherine Densford International Center for Nursing Leadership; University of Minnesota, School of Nursing, Minneapolis.

Joanne Pohl, PhD, RN, ANP-BC, FAAN, FAANP. Professor Emerita, University of Michigan, School of Nursing.

Kathleen Potempa, PhD, RN, FAAN. Dean and Professor, University of Michigan, School of Nursing.

Susan J. Pressler, PhD, RN, FAAN, FAHA. Professor, Sally Reahard Endowed Chair; Director, Center for Enhancing Quality of Life in Chronic Illness, Indiana University, School of Nursing, Indianapolis.

Richard W. Redman, PhD, RN. Ada Sue Hinshaw Collegiate Professor of Nursing Emeritus, University of Michigan, School of Nursing.

Brenda K. (Smith) Richards, PhD, RN. Associate Professor, Pennington Biomedical Research Center. Louisiana State University, Baton Rouge.

Lorraine B. Robbins, PhD, RN, FAAN, FNP-BC. Associate Professor, Michigan State University, College of Nursing, Lansing.

Ann E. Rogers, PhD, RN, FAAN, FAASM. Professor and Edith F. Honeycutt Chair in Nursing; Director of the Graduate Program, Emory University, Nell Hodgson Woodruff School of Nursing, Atlanta, Georgia.

Caroline Sampselle, PhD, RN, FAAN. Carolyne Davis Collegiate Professor of Nursing Emerita; Professor Emerita of Women's Studies, and Obstetrics and Gynecology, University of Michigan.

Margaret Scisney-Matlock, PhD, RN, FAAN. Professor Emerita, University of Michigan, School of Nursing.

Linda D. Scott, PhD, RN, NEA-BC, FAAN. Dean, University of Wisconsin-Madison, School of Nursing.

Julia S. Seng, PhD, RN, CNM, FAAN. Professor of Nursing, Obstetrics, and Gynecology and Women's Studies, University of Michigan.

Ellen Lavoie Smith, PhD, RN, APN-BC, AOCN, FAAN. Associate Professor; Director of the PhD Program, University of Michigan, School of Nursing.

Anne Snowdon, PhD, RN. Professor; Chair, International Center for Health Innovation, Richard Ivey School of Business, University of Windsor, Windsor, Canada.

Jun-ah Song, PhD, RN. Professor, Korea University, College of Nursing, Seoul, Korea.

Marita G. Titler, PhD, RN, FAAN. Professor, Rhetaugh G. Dumas Endowed Chair; Chair, Department of Systems, Populations and Leadership, University of Michigan, School of Nursing.

Dana Tschannen, PhD, RN. Clinical Associate Professor; Vice Chair for Academic Affairs; Director of the Post-Master's DNP Program, University of Michigan, School of Nursing.

Huey-Ming Tzeng, PhD, RN, FAAN. Dean and Professor, Tennessee Technological University, Whitson-Hester School of Nursing, Cookesville, Tennessee.

Antonia Villarruel, PhD, RN, FAAN. Professor and Margaret Bond Simon Dean of Nursing; Director, WHO Collaborating Center for Nursing and Midwifery Leadership, University of Pennsylvania, School of Nursing; Senior Fellow, Leonard Davis Institute of Health Economics.

Deborah Vincent, PhD, RN, FAANP. President of Deborah Vincent Consulting.

Terri Voepel-Lewis, PhD, RN. Associate Research Scientist, Department of Anesthesiology, University of Michigan, Medical School.

Ann Whall, PhD, RN, FGSA, FAAN. Professor Emerita, University of Michigan, School of Nursing; Maggie Allesee Endowed Professor in Gerontological Nursing Research, Oakland University, Rochester, Michigan.

Reg A. Williams, PhD, RN, FAAN. Professor Emeritus, University of Michigan, School of Nursing and Department of Psychiatry, Medical School.

Joanne Youngblut, PhD, RN, FAAN. Dr. Herbert and Nicole Wertheim Professor in Prevention and Family Health, Nicole Wertheim College of Nursing and Health Sciences, Florida International University, Miami.

Prologue

The University of Michigan's School of Nursing celebrates its 125th year in 2016. We began as a training school for nurses in 1891 and later became a collegiate program in 1941. We celebrate many achievements and a global impact. But this volume addresses a particular focus, that of the University of Michigan School of Nursing's early and impressive leadership, which is to say, the development and impact of research on the discipline of nursing since the launch of the Doctor of Philosophy program in 1975.

Historical archives of the School of Nursing show a memo dated January 30, 1973, from the research faculty to the graduate faculty recommending the launch of a doctoral program in clinical nursing research. In that document, the research faculty note: "We are proposing that we train nurses to be sophisticated researchers. We think that there is a demonstrated need for extensive clinical research in nursing. Nursing practice must be founded on a solid knowledge base that says that certain interventions have predictable outcomes for certain kinds of people in certain settings" (University of Michigan, School of Nursing, 1973). This framework set the course for both efficacy studies in clinical research and the much later focus on implementation and effectiveness science approaches that aim to determine the "predictability of outcomes" in "certain settings." The clinical nursing research directive was established at a time when most of the researchers in the discipline were not nurses. The School of Nursing was one of the pioneers in undertaking clinical nursing research, which would ultimately become the major focus of the national nursing research community.

The School of Nursing was one of the first programs in the country to launch a Doctor of Philosophy program, approved by the Rackham Graduate School on November 27, 1974, and the Regents of the University of Michigan in March 1975 (University of Michigan, Board of Regents, 1975). The proposal for the PhD occurred during a time when many schools of nursing were launching Doctor of Nursing (DN) or Doctor of Nursing Science (DNSc) programs as alternatives to the traditional research degree, the PhD. The University of Michigan's School of Nursing PhD program launched in Fall 1975, and our first graduate, Marcia DeCann Andersen, graduated in Spring 1978. In 1981, to expand and strengthen the doctoral program as well as facilitate faculty in their research agendas,

President Harold Shapiro recruited Dr. Rhetaugh Dumas, then deputy director of the National Institute of Mental Health, to be dean of the School of Nursing and to build a research-intensive environment. She established a research infrastructure with an associate dean for research, a research office with staff, and research awards for faculty. She also recruited the first endowed chair for a recognized nurse researcher. Since then, the number of endowed professorships has been increased to encourage and facilitate research within our faculty.

The chapters of this volume are organized into sections representing the overall thrust of our faculty and alumni work since the inception of the Doctor of Philosophy. The major themes of this work include biobehavioral studies, health promotion and risk reduction, women's health, nursing and health care systems, and nursing leadership. A current underlying all the research is the global context in which our faculty and students consider the health care issues of interest. Biobehavioral research focuses on the interface and interaction of human biological and behavioral systems that influence health and illness. The human responses that underlie both the maintenance of health and the occurrence and management of diseases were an early emphasis of the school's research program. The authors of Chapters 1 through 4 provide illustrations of basic research, including using animal models, as well as research in humans as individuals and as groups. Focus on cancer, cardiopulmonary disease, and cognitive functioning were prevailing concerns as the faculty and students grappled with contemporary issues in managing these rapidly escalating chronic conditions.

Health promotion and risk reduction have been a prevailing priority for the faculty since the beginning of our research enterprise. The emphasis crosses the life-span from children and adolescents to older adults. Nola Pender, internationally renowned for her development of the health promotion model (Pender, 1982) has been a major influencer on several cohorts of faculty and students. Sally Lusk led our emphasis on occupational health and has had sustained influence over decades of occupational health research. Another major thread has been an enduring focus on primary care. As the role of nurse practitioners expanded across the country, our faculty and students developed the research base related to models and practice in primary care.

Women's health and health care has also been a major thrust since the early days of the school's research. From basic research to pelvic floor functioning and child birth issues, to issues encountered later in life, the women's health faculty has built a body of knowledge related to women's reproductive health and psychosocial health as well. Many studies have developed methods to reduce complications at birth and have also evaluated new models of mother/infant care in other countries and continents.

Another area of research has been women's and adolescent girl's mental health. Research on the effects of posttraumatic stress experienced early in life on later parenting has resulted in an international collaboration among women's health researchers in

England, Australia, and our school. Other faculty members have investigated the factors related to drug use and abuse in adolescents and adults—an area of emphasis that also has international collaborators.

With the appointment in 1977 of Lillian Simms as director of Nursing Health Services Administration, a lineage of health services research was initiated. The program attracted Kellogg funding and groups of international students to the new master's program. Originally a small group of investigators, the program in health services research expanded with key faculty recruitments of individuals with interests in leadership, systems, health care quality and safety, and interprofessional communications. Faculty recruitment expanded areas of emphasis to keep the school at the cutting edge of health care evolution. A major thread of the research has also been methodologies, such as implementation and effectiveness science, to understand the effect of interventions on individuals, groups, and systems. Most recently, the expansion into clinical informatics, health informatics, and the use of "big data" to understand population health and systems is setting the pace for future research and discovery. Finally, the impact PhD graduates have had on national leadership and the evolution of the field is illustrated in Chapters 11 and 12.

Faculty members have been highly successful in obtaining funding and resources for their research programs. The primary sources have been through the competitive programs of the federal government, such as the institutes and centers of the National Institutes of Health and the Agency for Healthcare Research and Quality. Faculty members have been very creative in obtaining funding for their research through foundations and other non-governmental sources.

The chapters in this volume represent the work of only a small group of our PhD faculty and alumni. The goal of this publication is to provide a glimpse of the impact of our collective research and the concomitant development of our programs of research at the School through the stories of our faculty members and the lineages that they created through their students, building on the early research foundations. "Impact" is the word we use to describe the evolving and growing body of knowledge created by our first research faculty, expanded by their students and continued in a trajectory that today stand as substantial bodies of evidence driving science and care in the United States and around the globe.

I thank the University of Michigan School of Nursing 125th Anniversary Committee for the inception of this volume and the dedication of its editor, Dr. Shaké Ketefian, and the many authors who contributed. Understanding our history is a necessary foundation to launching the future. It is our hope at the School of Nursing that this volume inspires others to boldly advance the science that will transform the future of health care.

References

Pender, N. J. (1982, revised 1996). *Health promotion in nursing practice*. Norwalk, CT: Appleton-Century-Crofts.

University of Michigan, Board of Regents. (1975). March meeting, 1975. In *Proceedings of the Board of Regents (1972–1975)* (p. 1259). http:/quod.lib.umich.edu/u/umregproc/acw7513.1972.001/1303?view=pdf

University of Michigan, School of Nursing. (1973, January 30). [Memorandum, research faculty to graduate faculty]. Bentley Historical Library (Box 34, Swain, Research Area Faculty, 1973–1974, School of Nursing [University of Michigan] records 1891–2010 [ongoing]), Ann Arbor, MI.

KATHLEEN POTEMPA, *Dean and Professor*
ADA SUE HINSHAW, *Dean Emerita*
June 2016

Introduction

Since its inception in 1975, the University of Michigan PhD program in clinical nursing research, as one of the first doctoral programs nationally, has taken seriously its task of preparing leaders for the discipline and the nation. The educational experiences, mentorship approaches, and program elements offered have varied over the 40 years since its inception, but the overarching goal of leadership preparation has not.

Historical beginnings. In order to provide context for the subject matter this book deals with, some historical background might be helpful. During the 1960s and 1970s, a number of universities were offering what were then called "nurse scientist" programs. These were approved and funded by Congress to educate nurses at the doctoral level in different disciplines, especially in social science and basic science fields, as it was thought that having a cadre of nurses in these fields would enable these individuals to bring to bear creativity and relevant ideas from those disciplines as they worked to develop nursing science. At the University of Michigan the faculty, university administration, and Regents had the foresight to embark on a new PhD program in nursing. This era corresponded with a period when nursing nationally was heavily reliant on contributions from other disciplines.

From those beginnings, the scientific evolution in nursing has been rapid and spectacular. There was a huge influx of nursing doctoral programs nationally, starting in the 1980s, which continued in subsequent decades, to the present 135 research-focused doctoral programs. The number of nurses enrolled in doctoral and postdoctoral study, and who are engaged in research, has increased, along with the number of journals in nursing and institutions offering an increasing number of specialties at the graduate level in advanced practice. All this was facilitated by the establishment of the Center for Nursing Research at the National Institutes of Health (NIH) and its subsequent conversion into institute status (National Institute of Nursing Research [NINR]).

The creativity and intellectual ferment of those years was heady indeed. The University of Michigan faculty, by the mid-1980s, was comprised mainly of doctorally prepared nurses (mostly recent graduates) who decided to grow the discipline while taking advantage of the science that was available. The faculty took an organized approach to how it wished to frame the emerging nursing science and translate it into curricular and research programming. Careful consideration was given to research priorities of the NINR and major nursing organizations and the topical areas being funded by the NIH/NINR. While analyzing the national priority areas, the faculty also considered the research being conducted by individual faculty members. A list emerged from those analyses that guided faculty and student research; doctoral seminars were taught in the areas identified as they were developed. Over time, as research assumed a cumulative feature, the seminars were refined and updated, while research experiences and faculty mentorship became more focused.

As a result of this process, four scientific areas emerged: biobehavioral phenomena, health promotion/risk reduction, women's health, and nursing and health care systems. This book is thus organized into the same four sections, with relevant subtopics comprising the chapters of the book. We have added a section on leadership, given its centrality to what the PhD program aims to achieve, whether it is leadership in research/scholarship, education, policy, or other important domains in society. The areas identified in this manner to guide the PhD program were subsequently adopted by the School of Nursing for its "scientific and intellectual thrusts," in the words of the then-dean Rhetaugh Dumas; the areas became concentrations in the PhD program. The school thus pivoted to a greater emphasis on research than was the case prior to the launch of the PhD program. As research became programmatic, the school developed a postdoctoral program, and over time, the NIH/NINR funded several Institutional National Research Service Awards (T32s) for support of doctoral students and postdoctoral fellows (these were in addition to any individual awards students and fellows were receiving).

Approach to choosing topics and authors for inclusion. We note that there was important research within the School of Nursing prior to the establishment of the PhD program. We established several parameters for inclusion in this commemorative volume: (a) the research was conducted following the launch of the PhD program; (b) the research has been integrated in the academic and research fabric of the PhD program—that is, it has become part of the program's curriculum and has attracted teams of faculty, postdoctoral fellows, and doctoral students who engage in research in the area; and (c) the research has been programmatic in nature and has matured over many years of investigation, yielding noteworthy results. Having said these, no attempt was made to be exhaustive. As a starting point, we sent letters to all PhD graduates, inviting them to share with us their curriculum vitae, which less than half did. We then used the literature to explore the work of alumni and used faculty members, current and retired, as resources to compile a list of individuals who were invited to contribute short papers describing their research program, with emphasis on results and its contribution to nursing science. The majority who were invited agreed to participate. All chapter authors and short paper contributors are recognized authorities in the subject areas they write about. The chapter authors are current faculty or those retired recently who have been or continue to be central to the development of the topics covered in the volume.

The science presented in this volume is a distillation of what the University of Michigan's nursing faculty and PhD nursing alumni produced over a 30-year period and provides an assessment of the impact of the collective body of work. This project is being presented at the juncture of several important milestones in the life of the school:

- the bicentennial of the University of Michigan and the start of its third century
- the 125th anniversary of the founding of the School of Nursing, through many of its structural and organizational evolutions
- the 40th Anniversary of the establishment of the PhD program
- the first-ever building built exclusively to house the School of Nursing in its long and distinguished history

As nursing doctoral education faced a turning point 30 years ago, at present, there is clearly a ferment in nursing doctoral education circles nationally. While the final shape of the next phase of development is not entirely clear, new ideas are being proposed. We do know that there will be changes, and it is therefore timely to take stock of the science of the past 30 years, evaluate the yield, and assess areas that form the foundation for the next steps in scientific endeavors, whether these efforts are in the form of replications, testing hypotheses in different populations or settings, translational research, or other strategies.

Impact of international scholars on our science and vice versa. During the past 30 years, a major influence on nursing science has been the work of international scholars. Several developments within the School of Nursing created a hospitable climate. First was the formation of the International Network for Doctoral Education in Nursing (http://www.nursing.jhu.edu/exccellence/inden/) in the late 1990s, which was housed, administered, and led within our School during its formative years. Another happy event was the approval of the World Health Organization Collaborating Center for research and clinical training. These two events served to facilitate our international work and relationships with multiple colleagues from many countries and allowed us to engage in extensive faculty and student exchanges in educational and research activities. Over the years, the PhD program has attracted an impressive number of international students who are making major contributions to nursing, nursing education, and research all over the world. The level of understanding between and among nurse scientists and educators improved with regard to cultural aspects of care along with the need for science to be responsive to cultural differences. In addition, those international students and visiting scholars at the doctoral and postdoctoral levels who studied in the United States and returned to their home countries have continued their research and have pursued collaborative work with their faculties in the United States and other fellow students from the United States and elsewhere. Indeed, the University of Michigan School of Nursing has been a major seeding ground for nursing science that has flourished in other parts of the world.

Concurrent with these developments, the number of countries offering nursing doctoral study and the number of scientific journals available has increased in many countries, providing venues for the increasing volume of nursing research being produced by nurse scientists. These developments collectively have meant that nursing science, regardless of where it is produced, is readily accessible to anyone, with an increasing number of databases and digital outlets. As more and more nurse scientists produce their own science in their own countries, dealing with health problems of their own populations, there is more confidence in the relevance of science they are using. This is a major shift in the attitude of scientists worldwide, where, due to low material resources and constrained human resources, they historically tended to rely on research done in resource-rich countries, a situation that raised concerns about the relevance of the science to the specific needs of populations and settings other than where the research may have been conducted.

More than 10 years ago, when an international colleague and I wrote and edited a book on international doctoral education, we likened nursing doctoral education to a kaleidoscope: "Viewed from a worldwide perspective, nursing doctoral education is . . . like a rich and complex kaleidoscope, with many differences and variations, always evolving and undergoing change through evolution rather than revolution. It is this kaleidoscope that we aim to capture" (S. Ketefian & H. P. McKenna. [2005]. *Doctoral education in nursing: International perspective.* New York: Routledge, p. xvi.). At that time, we had the process of doctoral education in mind. I submit that the parallel to kaleidoscope is no less true today, but this time what we present is the substance of nursing doctoral education, its scientific content, rather than the process.

Organization of the volume. We have designed this commemorative volume with an eye to involving as many of the primary scientists as possible. More than 70 individuals participated in writing and providing information on their research and scholarship; they provided short papers on their works that enabled chapter authors to prepare their chapters summarizing the different research on the same general topic. Most of the topics covered here have contributors representing several countries. We have thus chosen to integrate the international works and perspectives into the relevant scientific areas rather than present them separately.

All individuals contributing to this volume—as chapter authors or as writers of short papers or commentators—have been active scientists over the course of their careers. In Chapters 1 through 6, chapter authors rely on short papers or other materials submitted by scientists who have had programs of research on the topic and draw on common elements across studies in synthesizing the works and commenting on trends and the future. The briefs for these chapters are placed in Section VI of the book. These chapter authors have incorporated their own research into the chapter, as it was determined that separate briefs on their work were not necessary. In Chapters 7 through 10, while short paper authors present works on the same topic, it was felt that there was not sufficient commonality; rather, chapter authors describe the contributions of the various scientists in the context of existing science. In the case of these chapters, the short papers immediately follow the chapter. In all, there are a total of 54 short papers. In addition, a number of scientists provided material on their research without a brief, which were incorporated into the chapters. These individuals are included in the list of contributors. Chapters 11 through 13 represent scholarship on leadership, presented by four of our PhD alumni, followed by commentary provided by Dean Kathleen Potempa.

SHAKÉ KETEFIAN
Editor
Ann Arbor, Michigan
July 2016

SECTION I

Biobehavioral Health

CHAPTER 1

_____

Biological Science

Getting at the Cause to Promote the Cure

Janean Holden, PhD, RN, FAAN

The University of Michigan School of Nursing (UMSN) has a long history of producing nurse scientists skilled in the investigation of biological processes. Biological and biopsychological investigation is a critical, though often undervalued, aspect of nursing research. Most biological studies examine the physiological underpinnings or mechanisms of health or disease processes, which necessitate looking at parts of the person, rather than the whole person all at once. Mechanism questions often require measurements of cellular or subcellular responses, utilize experimental design with a control group for tight control of variables, and often involve animal models. Animal models, including whole animal models, tissue models, and cell culture, have been part of scientific investigation for centuries and have led to the development of many therapies that have translated to humans.

A Word on Animal Models

Before discussing the biological research of some of our UMSN graduates, it might be of value to consider animal model use, an area that still is controversial in the minds of some nurse researchers, despite the fact that the National Institute of Nursing Research has funded animal work for decades. Although there is still criticism by some nurse scientists who view research using animals as not "nursing research," and although there has been criticism recently about the inability to translate some findings from animal studies to humans, one must question the criticism and the lack of appreciation for this type of research. Past and continued success of animal work in predicting human outcomes cannot be ignored. An Internet search on the topic of animal therapies produces a plethora of sites. Treatments for breast cancer, Parkinson's disease, Alzheimer's disease, clot retrieval in stroke patients, the biochemical processes of schizophrenia, further development of the artificial heart, further development of organ transplantation, development of a vaccination against tuberculosis, and identification of treatments for autism are just a few of the areas in which current research uses animal models (UCLA, 2008).

Implicit in the use of a model of human functioning is the idea that the model allows investigation into realms of activity that cannot be ethically done in humans. For example, it would be unethical to test a new drug on a human before it is tested in an animal model. It would likewise be ludicrous (not to mention criminal) to ask the typical college sophomore, so frequently the subject in many human studies, to allow his or her brain to be taken and sectioned to determine which cells engage in modulating pain in the spinal cord. Until, if ever, we can use computer-generated models to effectively predict all aspects of human functioning, animal models still remain the best alternative to ignoring or censuring research questions that deal with mechanisms of human functioning.

Why then might some animal work not translate well to the human condition? The brief answer is that successful use of an animal model depends on at least two factors: proper choice of the model and proper experimental design (Festing, 2006, 2009; Holden, 2011). An animal model is selected because it is thought to respond in a manner similar to humans. The choice might be made based on specific evidence that such a response between model and human will occur, which usually leads to meaningful results. Or the choice might be assumed from a biological similarity between the model and the human, which could produce either useful results or disastrous ones (Blackburn-Munro, 2004). A good example of this latter choice can be seen in the long-held belief that male and female rats have the same physiology, a belief tied directly to the fallacy that male and female human physiology is the same.

The second aspect of animal modeling is related to the experimental design. If a model does not prove useful for translation to humans, the model may not be valid. Alternatively, if the study design is flawed or too few animals are used in the name of animal protection, it is unwise to discard the use of all animal models. As with all science, rigorous evaluation of each study should be done.

Correlating with the idea that basic science is important to nursing are the recommendations that have recently emerged regarding PhD training in nursing. These ideas include the proposition that nursing PhD students, and perhaps all nursing students, need more preparation and training in "omics" in their core curriculum because these are seen as critical emerging areas of health science research (Henly et al., 2015). Omics areas include genomics; transcriptomics to understand RNA mechanisms; proteomics, or the role of proteins expressed from genes; epigenomics, the study of genetic responses to both the internal and the external environment; exposomics, which measures the exposure over time of environmental factors on health; metabolomics to examine the small molecules in a biological sample that originate from either the internal or the external environment; and microbiomics, or the study of genetic material from microscopic organisms that inhabit the human body (Conley et al., 2015). Implied in these areas of research is the use of animal as well as human models and the further implication that doctoral students then need some exposure to aspects of animal work, even if they never cross the threshold of an animal lab again in their careers.

Contributions of UMSN-Trained Biological Researchers

Presented below are highlights of the contributions of four UMSN graduates who use animal models in their science, including areas of "omics." These graduates cover a wide range of topics, but all have a single theme in common: examining mechanisms of a major physiological problem. It is important to note that rarely do basic science findings translate directly into a change in patient care. Basic science is a foundational study, and much of the information presented below will have to go through a series of clinical trials before therapies can be developed. However, the foundational work is a necessary first step in the process. All four of the contributions below provide insights into how human functioning can be improved and outline the ways in which UMSN-trained nurse scientists are impacting the body of knowledge.

Hala Darwish—Cognitive Function: The Neurobiology of Learning and Memory

The cognitive aspects of learning and memory are critical to normal functioning, and this area of study is of great interest clinically because natural aging, disease, or injury may negatively affect the ability to learn and remember. With the increase in the aging population in the United States, the effects of traumatic brain injury in returning veterans, and the concern for head injury in athletes of all ages, the topic of cognitive impairment is timely.

While investigating the effect of traumatic brain injury on the cognitive functions of learning and memory, Dr. Hala Darwish used a rat model to discover that even mild to moderate brain injury can lead to persistent cognitive deficits for as long as 35 days postinjury, that the injury impairs synaptic function in the brain, and importantly, that these deficits might benefit from pharmacological and behavioral interventions, such as simvastatin and environmental enrichment (Darwish et al., 2012; Darwish, Mahmood, Schallert, Chopp, & Therrien, 2014; Hebda-Bauer, Pletsch, Darwish, & Fentress, 2010).

Darwish is currently collaborating on two traumatic brain injury studies. The first aims to develop a means of detecting traumatic brain injury biomarkers, a priority for the National Institutes of Health, as scientists attempt to identify specific molecules, both in humans and animals, that can be used to develop better therapeutic targets. The second will examine the effect of aspirin and the blood-clot inhibitor clopidogrel on neuronal damage after moderate brain injury.

In previous studies that investigated agents that can improve learning and memory, Darwish discovered that vitamin D supplementation lessens the age-related increase in proinflammatory levels and amyloid burden in the brain of aged animals. This finding indicates that vitamin D might be useful in alleviating the effects of aging on cognitive function (Briones & Darwish, 2012); further, this finding led to a translational study when Darwish realized that vitamin D deficiency is surprisingly prevalent among the Lebanese, her native country. She found that for both adults and older adults, lower serum 25 hydroxyvitamin D was associated with impaired cognitive performance (Darwish et al., 2015).

As managing director of the Abu Haidar Neuroscience Institute and the Multiple Sclerosis Center at the American University of Beirut Medical Center, it became evident to Darwish that multiple sclerosis (MS) is also affected by vitamin D levels (Knippenberg, Bol, Damoiseaux, Hupperts, & Smolders, 2011; Smolders, 2010) and has cognitive impairment sequelae (Deloire, Ruet, Hamel, Bonnet, & Brochet, 2010; Hildebrandt et al., 2006; Kiy et al., 2011). She and her colleagues have designed a clinical trial to collect cognitive data on a group of MS patients before and after vitamin D supplementation and have collected data on risk factors in MS patients (Mouhieddine et al., 2015).

Darwish's work is a strong example of how basic science findings can contribute to potential clinical therapeutics. Her career path demonstrates how an investigator can translate basic science findings to a human context and in so doing can contribute to a greater understanding of a major clinical problem.

Donna McCarthy—Symptom Science

Dr. McCarthy's program of research is based on the pathobiology of sickness symptoms. Using an animal model, she first studied the frequent association between fever and anorexia. Her findings indicate that fever does not contribute to loss of appetite, and both fever and appetite loss are mediated by a small protein produced by activated leukocytes, later identified by Dr. Matt Kluger and others as interleukin-1 (IL-1). These findings indicate that anorexia is part of the acute phase response to infection (McCarthy, Kluger, & Vander, 1985).

Subsequently, McCarthy sought to understand why influenza infection confers immunity to the virus, whereas infection with respiratory syncytial virus (RSV) does not. She found that leukocytes exposed to RSV produce an inhibitor of IL-1 that prevents activation of the immune response to the virus. There are now two known inhibitors of IL-1 activity—namely, IL-1 receptor antagonist and IL-1 soluble receptors (McCarthy, Domurat, Nichols, & Roberts, 1989).

McCarthy also used an animal model to study symptoms of cancer and cancer treatment, focusing first on anorexia and weight loss. She showed IL-1-induced appetite reduction is associated with increasing plasma levels of cholecystokinin that decrease emptying of the stomach contents. She also found that weight loss occurs in association with increased expression of IL-1 and other cytokines in animals with various tumors that did or did not induce weight loss and that it was not possible to increase food intake or total caloric intake of tumor-bearing rats. She and her team demonstrated that nutritional supplements only marginally improve food intake but do not prevent weight loss during radiotherapy.

These experiments show that anorexia is a regulated or defended response to tumor growth and is not due solely to the effects of cancer treatment (McCarthy, 1997, 2000, 2003; Murray, Schell, McCarthy, & Albertini, 1997).

Doctoral student Terry Lennie (who was a postdoctoral fellow at the University of Michigan) demonstrated that weight loss after traumatic injury is also a regulated response that is affected by preinjury body mass (Lennie, McCarthy, & Keesey, 1995). In another study, using a mouse model of cancer-related fatigue, doctoral student Sadeeka Al-Majid demonstrated that loss of muscle mass could be prevented with resistance exercise (Al-Majid & McCarthy, 2001) and that anti-inflammatory drugs could reduce muscle wasting in tumor-bearing mice (McCarthy, Whitney, Hitt, & Al-Majid, 2004).

McCarthy also found that myocardial muscle is affected by tumor growth, which produces a decline in systolic function associated with reduced exercise tolerance of tumor-bearing mice. Importantly, while treatment with a drug commonly used to treat heart failure did not improve voluntary exercise, it could improve myocardial function and preserve muscle mass in tumor-bearing mice (Xu et al., 2011).

As a result of her previous findings, McCarthy began exploring the occurrence of depression in her mouse model of cancer-related fatigue. She and her team found that depressionlike behaviors precede fatiguelike behaviors and that a drug that blocks cytokine production reduces depressionlike behaviors without affecting cytokine production, but it does not improve muscle mass or fatiguelike behaviors. Lastly, treatment with an anti-inflammatory drug improves depression- and fatiguelike behaviors and reduces cytokine production. These very exciting data support the prior work of others showing that treatment with anti-inflammatory drugs preserves body weight and prolongs the survival of patients with cancer cachexia (Lundholm, Daneryd, Körner, Hyltander, & Bosaeus, 2004). McCarthy is currently conducting experiments to determine if aerobic exercise will reduce muscle wasting and depressionlike behaviors in the mouse model of cancer-related fatigue (Norden et al., 2014, 2015).

Turning her focus to psychoneuroimmunology, the effects of the stress response on immune cell function, McCarthy found that different stressors such as noise, academic exam stress, pregnancy, and income factors, affect immune responses in rats and humans (Corwin et al., 2015; Corwin et al., 2015; Kang, Coe, & McCarthy, 1996; McCarthy, Ouimet, & Daun, 1992; Sribanditmongkol, Neal, Szalacha, & McCarthy, 2015).

McCarthy's work in humans and animals has provided significant insights into symptom science. The identification of specific molecules that affect immune responses, appetite, fatigue, and muscle wasting in cancer has led to potential interventions that can prevent or reduce the negative aspects of tumor growth and immune function.

Brenda K. (Smith) Richards—Macronutrient Selection and Total Energy Intake

The aim of Dr. Richards's basic science research program is to identify the genetic determinants of macronutrient selection and total energy intake. Eating behaviors involving appetites for fat-, carbohydrate-, or protein-rich foods are influenced by an array of molecular signals throughout the body, including those involved in neural and metabolic processes. Despite growing evidence for a strong genetic influence on food selection in children and adults, the specific genes that encode these molecular signals and contribute to macronutrient-specific appetites are virtually unknown. Using molecular genetic methods, it is possible to identify specific genes that contribute to individual differences in food preferences. To understand the processes that bring about macronutrient selection and to then ensure that those choices are healthy are critical factors for addressing the epidemics of obesity and diabetes.

Richards's early research discovered key evidence that macronutrient selection is a quantitative, or complex, genetic trait—that is, measurable in nature and having a continuous distribution (as opposed to a discrete trait)—that depends on the actions of numerous genes and the environment. First, she developed an experimental system for measuring food intake and macronutrient selection in mice, whereby animals compose their own diet while choosing among individual sources of fat, carbohydrate, and protein. Next, she evaluated a dozen mouse inbred strains and uncovered the continuous distribution of preferential fat intake, ranging from 26% to 83% of total energy (Smith, Andrews, & West, 2000). Complementary studies showed that the phenotype of fat-rich versus carbohydrate-rich diet preference in inbred strains generalizes across diet paradigms, indicating a robust model for investigation (e.g., Smith, Andrews, York, & West, 1999). Her findings established that macronutrient selection is a complex trait and thus amenable to genetic analysis and enabled her to identify a suitable model: two inbred strains that exhibit markedly different preferences for eating fats versus carbohydrates. This finding illustrates an important aspect of animal research, that of developing appropriate models to study a phenomenon.

Continuing this work, Richards and her team crossed two inbred strains of mice that had either high- or low-fat preference and evaluated their second-generation offspring (F2 animals) for macronutrient preference. They then conducted a genome-wide scan and found nine quantitative trait loci (QTL) in which a section of DNA (the locus, region within a genome, or genotype) was correlated with variation in the quantitative trait or phenotype (Smith Richards et al., 2002). They discovered loci for preferential fat intake on chromosomes 8, 18, and X; preferential carbohydrate intake on chromosomes 6, 17, and X; and kilocalorie intake (adjusted for body weight) on chromosomes 17 and 18. Another locus for kcal intake on chromosome 2 was body weight dependent. These results provide strong evidence for multiple genetic controls on total energy and macronutrient-specific intakes. Richards and her team selected the chromosome 17 QTL for further investigation and confirmed that this locus specified the original linked traits, using a congenic strain generated in her laboratory (Kumar et al., 2007). The genome of this congenic strain has a differential segment of chromosome 17 (QTL for preferential carbohydrate intake in the mapping study) from one inbred strain that is introgressed on the genetic background of the second, fat-preferring strain. The new congenic strain ate 27% more carbohydrate and 17% more total calories per body weight, yet equivalent fat calories, compared to the genetic background control, confirming that the differential segment contains a gene(s) that determines these traits (Kumar, DiCarlo, Volaufova, Zuberi, & Smith, 2010; Kumar et al., 2007). They then narrowed and precisely localized the responsible ~19 Mb interval through fine mapping (Gularte-Mérida et al., 2014). Notably, no genetic linkage for fat intake was detected, clearly emphasizing the carbohydrate-specific effects of this chromosome 17 locus. Current investigations are focused on candidates within the fine-mapped region. Richards and her team have characterized several highly plausible candidate genes (Gularte-Mérida et al., 2014; Kumar et al., 2008; Kumar & Smith Richards, 2008; Simon et al., 2015). Locating the DNA variation that controls preferential carbohydrate and total calorie intake in animals will clarify the contribution of human genetic variants to food intake and selection.

Richards's laboratory also investigates the role of fat oxidation in the metabolic control of fat intake and fat preference. She led research demonstrating that mice with a global, genetic inactivation of ACADS (short-chain acyl-CoA dehydrogenase), the enzyme responsible for the first step of mitochondrial beta-oxidation of four carbon straight-chain fatty acids, shift consumption away from fats and toward carbohydrates when choosing between macronutrient-rich diets. Yet these animals maintain total energy intake equivalent to that of wild type controls (Smith Richards, Belton, York, & Volaufova, 2004), suggesting a mechanism for precise metering of changes in available energy. This is the first report of an alteration in eating behavior associated with deficiencies in ACADS. Her further studies suggest that a specific molecule, AMP-kinase, is the cellular energy sensing mechanism linking impaired fat oxidation to fat avoidance in this model (Berthoud, Munzberg, Richards, & Morrison, 2012; Kruger, Kumar, Mynatt, Volaufova, & Richards, 2012).

The molecular mechanisms related to macronutrient selection and total energy intake, with their influence on eating and preferences, provide an essential understanding of how the body governs food intake and use. In light of the epidemic of obesity and obesity-related illness, such research is essential to understanding how health care providers approach weight management and eating disorders.

Janean E. Holden—Unraveling Hypothalamic Descending Pain Modulation

Over the past 50 years, there has been extensive study to define the mechanisms of the descending pain modulatory system. This innate system provides strong pain relief following an acute injury but lasts only briefly. Scientists have activated the system in animals through electrical and chemical stimulation of certain parts of the brain. A great deal of information has been elicited about the descending modulatory system in the spinal cord dorsal horn and in the brain stem, but very little is known about how the more complex higher brain centers participate. Holden's area of study explores the role of one of these higher centers, the hypothalamus, in acute pain and chronic, neuropathic pain. Acute pain warns of real or impending tissue damage and is usually treatable with opioids and non-steroidal anti-inflammatory drugs (NSAIDs). Neuropathic pain may or may not have an observable cause, rearranges the way the central nervous system processes painful impulses, and becomes the pathological problem. Neuropathic pain is more responsive to drugs such as selective serotonin and norepinephrine reuptake inhibitors (SNRIs), but these are effective only in about half the individuals taking them. Why this is so is of great interest to the National Institutes of Health, which issues challenge topics about pain itself, how acute pain becomes chronic, biomarkers of pain, and sex/gender differences (see http:/grants.nih .gov/grants/finding/challenge_award).

One of the major findings from Holden's research has been the idea that when the lateral hypothalamus (LH) is stimulated, analgesia occurs. Holden and colleagues have shown this effect in a rat model of acute pain and of neuropathic pain from sciatic nerve ligation (Holden & Naleway, 2001; Holden et al., 2014). They found male/female differences and stimulating-dose and pain-type differences. Importantly, while all rats responded to the highest stimulating dose, female rats with neuropathic pain had greater analgesia than male neuropathic rats. This finding of a sex difference in rats for pain modulation is important because the pain anatomy and physiology of rats is similar to that of humans and can successfully predict human responses. This information suggests that males and females process pain information differently in the brain and could direct future individualized therapies that may need to be adjusted to account for gender differences.

Holden and colleagues also showed that this analgesic effect occurs by direct projection to the spinal cord dorsal horn via the orexin-A neurotransmitter (Wardach, Wagner, Jeong, & Holden, 2016) and also indirectly through connections with the brain stem periaqueductal gray (Holden, Pizzi, & Jeong, 2009), the rostroventromedial medulla (Holden & Pizzi, 2008), and the noradrenergic A7 catecholamine cell group in the pons (Holden, Van Poppel, & Thomas, 2002). These three brain stem areas are known to reduce pain in the spinal cord dorsal horn. Taken together, it is clear that there are multiple ways that the descending pain modulatory system works, and so there are multiple sites that scientists can target to reduce pain.

Another major finding from Holden's work is that the neurotransmitter (i.e., norepinephrine) released in the spinal cord after LH stimulation produces analgesia at one type of receptor (α_2 adrenoceptors) in the spinal cord dorsal horn but an opposing increased pain response (hyperalgesia) when it binds to another receptor (α_1 adrenoceptors; Holden & Naleway, 2001). The net effect is analgesia that is attenuated by concurrent pain facilitation, or hyperalgesia. This finding is important because the idea of SNRIs, like the drug Cymbalta, is to keep norepinephrine in the synapse longer so it can bind to α_2 adrenoceptors to relieve pain, but norepinephrine binds equally to pain-promoting α_1 adrenoceptors. This finding may provide evidence as to why SNRIs are effective only in about 50% of the population, and this effectiveness may depend on the ratio of α_2 to α_1 adrenoceptors the individual has, which could eventually be a biomarker for a personalized approach to pain management.

The idea of opposing actions of norepinephrine receptor subtypes has led to further study. Holden and colleagues discovered that these hyperalgesic α_1 adrenoceptors are significantly more active in nerve-injured rats than in controls, and this activity occurs in the absence of LH stimulation (Wagner, Jeong, Banerjee, Yang, & Holden, 2016). They hypothesized that nerve damage may increase the number of α_1 adrenoceptors, which may then promote some of the symptoms seen in chronic pain. They also found that in both male and female rats, there is continual (tonic) release of norepinephrine in the nerve-injured model. So there is a constant release of norepinephrine that can then bind to an increased number of receptors that increase pain. However, Holden and colleagues found that there is a sex difference in the pathway that provides tonic norepinephrine release. In males, the LH innervates the pathway unilaterally, but in females, the LH provides bilateral innervation (Wagner et al., 2016). This finding is suggestive of a fundamental difference in how females process neuropathic pain as compared to males.

The value of these studies in contributing to our knowledge of pain is twofold. First, it is becoming clear that sex differences in hypothalamic activity exist and should be considered as therapeutics are developed for pain relief. Second, by defining the pathways through which the LH modifies pain and the neurotransmitters involved, scientists can identify sites that can be manipulated therapeutically in clinical pain conditions. Such therapies include not only deep brain stimulation and the development of drugs that target various areas along the pathway but also the development of noninvasive, nonpharmacological therapies inherently attractive to nurses, including research-based massage techniques or exercise regimens that affect hypothalamic output.

Summary

From the work presented above, it is clear that biologically trained nurse scientists are doing research that impacts health care in critical areas, including cognition, cancer symptomatology, eating behaviors and metabolism, and pain. The findings from this work have implications for translation to patients with head injury, multiple sclerosis, cancer, eating choices that contribute to obesity or diabetes, and chronic pain. It is essential that the University of Michigan School of Nursing continues to produce scientists with biological training who are prepared to lead the way in the next phase of PhD evolution. This preparation must include training in the "omics" of science—the areas of physiological functioning that are at the forefront for establishing individualized patient therapies. It is hoped that many more PhD programs will do similarly as qualified faculty researchers become available.

References

Al-Majid, S., & McCarthy, D. O. (2001). Resistance exercise training attenuates wasting of the EDL muscle in mice bearing the Colon-26 adenocarcinoma. *Biological Research for Nursing, 2,* 155–166.

Berthoud, H.-R., Munzberg, H., Richards, B. K., & Morrison, C. (2012). Neural and metabolic regulation of macronutrient intake and selection. *Proceedings of the Nutrition Society, 71*(3), 390–400.

Blackburn-Munro, G. (2004). Pain-like behaviours in animals—how human are they? *Trends in Pharmacological Sciences, 25*(6), 299–305.

Briones, T. L., & Darwish, H. (2012). Vitamin D mitigates age-related cognitive decline through the modulation of pro-inflammatory state and decrease in amyloid burden. *Journal of Neuroinflammation, 9*(1), 244–257.

Conley, Y. P., Heitkemper, M., McCarthy, D., Anderson, C. M., Corwin, E. J., Daack-Hirsch, S., . . . Voss, J. (2015). Educating future nursing scientists: Recommendations for integrating omics content in PhD programs. *Nursing Outlook, 63*(4), 417–427.

Corwin, E. J., Guo, Y., Pajer, K., Lowe, N., McCarthy, D., Schmiege, S., . . . Stafford, B. (2013). Immune dysregulation and glucocorticoid resistance in minority and low income pregnant women. *Psychoneuroendocrinology, 38*(9), 1786–1796.

Corwin, E. J., Pajer, K., Paul, S., Lowe, N., Weber, M., & McCarthy, D. O. (2015). Bidirectional psychoneuroimmune interactions in the early postpartum period influence risk of postpartum depression. *Brain and Behavior Immunology, 49,* 86–93.

Darwish, H., Mahmood, A., Schallert, T., Chopp, M., & Therrien, B. (2012). Mild traumatic brain injury (MTBI) leads to spatial learning deficits. *Brain Injury, 26*(2), 151–156.

Darwish, H., Mahmood, A., Schallert, T., Chopp, M., & Therrien, B. (2014). Simvastatin and environmental enrichment effect on recognition and temporal order memory after mild-to-moderate traumatic brain injury. *Brain Injury, 28*(2), 211–226.

Darwish, H., Zeinoun, P., Ghusn, P., Khoury, B., Tamim, H., & Khoury, S. J. (2015). Serum 25-hydroxyvitamin D predicts cognitive performance in adults. *Journal of Neuropsychiatry Diseases and Treatments, 25*(11), 2217–2123.

Deloire, M., Ruet, A., Hamel, D., Bonnet, M., & Brochet, B. (2010). Early cognitive impairment in multiple sclerosis predicts disability outcome several years later. *Multiple Sclerosis, 16*(5), 581–587.

Festing, M. F. W. (2006). Design and statistical methods in studies using animal models of development. *Institute for Laboratory Animal Research Journal, 47,* 5–14.

Festing, M. F. W. (2009). Improving the design and analysis of animal experiments: A personal odyssey. *Alternatives to Laboratory Animals, 37* (Suppl-2), 75–81.

Gularte-Mérida, R., DiCarlo, L. M., Robertson, G., Simon, J., Johnson, W. D., Kappen, C., . . . Richards, B. K. (2014). High-resolution mapping of a genetic locus regulating preferential carbohydrate intake, total kilocalories, and food volume on mouse chromosome 17. *PLOS ONE, 9*(10), e11042.

Hebda-Bauer, E. K., Pletsch, A., Darwish, H., & Fentress, H. (2010). Forebrain glucocorticoid receptor overexpression increases environmental reactivity and produces a stress-induced spatial discrimination deficit. *Neuroscience, 169*(2), 645–653.

Henly, S. J., McCarthy, D. O., Wyman, J. F., Heitkemper, M. M., Redeker, N. S., Titler, M. G., . . . Dunbar-Jacob, J. (2015). Emerging areas of science: Recommendations for nursing science education from the Council for the Advancement of Nursing Science Idea Festival. *Nursing Outlook, 63*(4), 398–407.

Hildebrandt, H., Hahn, H. K., Kraus, J. A., Schulte-Herbrüggen, A., Schwarze, B., & Schwendemann, G. (2006). Memory performance in multiple sclerosis patients correlates with central brain atrophy. *Multiple Sclerosis, 12*(4), 428–436.

Holden, J. E. (2011). Putting the bio in biobehavioral research: Animal models. *Western Journal of Nursing Research, 33*(8), 1017–1029.

Holden, J. E., & Naleway, E. (2001). Microinjection of carbachol in the lateral hypothalamus produces opposing effects on nociception mediated by α_1 and α_2 adrenoceptors. *Brain Research, 911*, 27–36.

Holden, J. E., & Pizzi, J. A. (2008). Lateral hypothalamic-induced antinociception is mediated by a substance P connection with the rostral ventromedial medulla. *Brain Research, 1214*, 40–49.

Holden, J. E., Pizzi, J. A., Jeong, Y. (2009). An NK1 receptor antagonist microinjected into the periaqueductal gray blocks lateral hypothalamic-induced antinociception in rats. *Neuroscience Letters, 453*, 115–119.

Holden, J. E., Van Poppel, A. Y., & Thomas, S. (2002). Antinociception from lateral hypothalamic stimulation is mediated by NK1 receptors in the A7 catecholamine cell group in the rat. *Brain Research, 953*,195–204.

Holden, J. E., Wang, E., Moes, J. R., Wagner, M., Maduko, A., & Jeong, Y. (2014). Differences in carbachol dose, pain condition and sex following lateral hypothalamic stimulation. *Neuroscience, 270*, 226–235.

Kang, D.-H., Coe, C. L., & McCarthy, D. O. (1996). Academic examinations significantly impact immune responses, but not lung function, in healthy and well-managed asthmatic adolescents. *Brain, Behavior, and Immunity, 10*, 164–181.

Kiy, G., Lehmann, P., Hahn, H. K., Eling, P., Kastrup, A., & Hildebrandt, H. (2011). Decreased hippocampal volume, indirectly measured, is associated with depressive symptoms and consolidation deficits in multiple sclerosis. *Multiple Sclerosis Journal, 17*(9), 1088–1097.

Knippenberg, S., Bol, Y., Damoiseaux, J., Hupperts, R., & Smolders, J. (2011). Vitamin D status in patients with MS is negatively correlated with depression, but not with fatigue. *Acta Neurologica Scandinavica, 124*(3), 171–175.

Kruger, C., Kumar, K. G., Mynatt, R. L., Volaufova, J., & Richards, B. K. (2012). Brain transcriptional responses to high-fat diet in *Acads*-deficient mice reveal energy sensing pathways. *PLOS ONE, 7*(8), e41709.

Kumar, K. G., Byerley, L., Volaufova, J., Drucker, D. J., Churchill, G. A., Li, R., . . . Smith Richards, B. K. (2008). Genetic variation in *Glp1r* expression influences the rate of gastric emptying in mice. *American Journal of Physiology Regulatory Integrative and Comparative Physiology, 294*(2), R362–R371.

Kumar, K. G., DiCarlo, L. M., Volaufova, J., Zuberi, A. R., & Smith Richards, B. K. (2010). Increased physical activity co-segregates with higher intake of carbohydrate and total calories in subcongenic mice. *Mammalian Genome, 21*(1–2), 52–63.

Kumar, K. G., Poole, A. C., York, B., Volaufova, J., Zuberi, A., & Smith Richards, B. K. (2007). Quantitative trait loci for carbohydrate and total energy intake on mouse chromosome 17: Congenic strain confirmation and candidate gene analyses (*Glo1, Glp1r*). *American Journal of Physiology Regulatory Integrative and Comparative Physiology, 292*(1), R207–R216.

Kumar, K. G., & Smith Richards, B. K. (2008). Transcriptional profiling of Chromosome 17 QTL for carbohydrate and total calorie intake in a mouse congenic strain reveals candidate genes and pathways. *J Nutrigenetics and Nutrigenomics, 1*(4), 155–171.

Lennie, T. A., McCarthy, D. O., & Keesey, R. E. (1995). Relationship of body energy status and the metabolic response to injury. *American Journal of Physiology, 269*, R1024–R1031.

Lundholm, K., Daneryd, P., Körner, U., Hyltander, A., & Bosaeus, I. (2004). Evidence that long-term COX-treatment improves energy homeostasis and body composition in cancer patients with progressive cachexia. *International Journal of Oncology, 24*(3), 505–512.

McCarthy, D. O. (1997). Short-term regulation of energy intake is intact in hypophagic tumor-bearing rats. *Research in Nursing & Health, 20*, 425–429.

McCarthy, D. O. (2000). Cytokines and the anorexia of infection: Potential mechanisms and treatments. [Invited review]. *Biological Research for Nursing, 1*, 287–298.

McCarthy, D. O. (2003). Rethinking nutritional support for persons with cancer cachexia. *Biological Research for Nursing, 5*, 3–17.

McCarthy, D. O., Domurat, F. M., Nichols, J. E., & Roberts, N. J. (1989). Interleukin-1 inhibitor production by human mononuclear leukocytes and leukocyte subpopulations exposed to respiratory syncytial virus. *Journal of Leukocyte Biology, 46*(3), 189–198.

McCarthy, D. O., Kluger, M. J., & Vander, A. J. (1985). The role of interleukin-1 in the suppression of food intake during infection. *American Journal of Clinical Nutrition, 42,* 1179–1182.

McCarthy, D. O., Ouimet, M. E., & Daun, J. M. (1992). The effect of noise stress on leukocyte function in rats. *Research in Nursing & Health, 15,* 131–137.

McCarthy, D. O., Whitney, P., Hitt, A., & Al-Majid, S. (2004). Indomethacin and ibuprofen preserve gastrocnemius muscle mass in mice bearing the colon26 adenocarcinoma. *Research in Nursing & Health, 27,* 174–184.

Mouhieddine, T. H., Darwish, H., Fawaz, L., Yamout, B., Tamim, H., & Khoury, S. J. (2015). Risk factors for multiple sclerosis and associations with anti-EBV antibody titers. *Clinical Immunology, 158*(1), 59–66.

Murray, S., Schell, K., McCarthy, D. O., & Albertini, M. R. (1997). Tumor growth, weight loss, and cytokines in SCID mice. *Cancer Letters, 111,* 111–115.

Norden, D. M., Bicer, S., Clark, Y., Jing, R., Henry, C. J., Wold, L. E., . . . McCarthy, D. O. (2014). Tumor growth increases neuroinflammation, fatigue and depressive-like behavior prior to alterations in muscle function. *Brain, Behavior & Immunity, 43,* 76–85.

Norden, D. M., Devine, R., Bicer, S., Jing, R., Reiser, P. J., Wold, L. E., . . . McCarthy, D. O. (2015). Fluoxetine prevents the development of depressive-like behavior in a mouse model of cancer-related fatigue. *Physiology and Behavior, 140,* 230–235.

Simon, J., DiCarlo, L. M., Kruger, C., Johnson, W. D., Kappen, C., & Richards, B. K. (2015). Gene expression in salivary glands: Effects of diet and mouse chromosome 17 locus regulating macronutrient intake. *Physiological Reports, 3*(2), e12311.

Smith, B. K., Andrews, P. K., & West, D. B. (2000). Macronutrient self-selection in thirteen mouse strains. *American Journal of Physiology Regulatory Integrative and Comparative Physiology, 278*(4), R797–R805.

Smith, B. K., Andrews, P. K., York, D. A., & West, D. B. (1999). Divergence in proportional fat intake in AKR/J and SWR/J mice endures across diet paradigms. *American Journal of Physiology Regulatory Integrative and Comparative Physiology, 277*(3), R776–R785.

Smith Richards, B. K., Belton, B. N., Poole, A. C., Mancuso, J. J., Churchill, G. A., Li, R., . . . York, B. (2002). QTL analysis of self-selected macronutrient diet intake: Fat, carbohydrate, and total kilocalories. *Physiological Genomics, 11* (3), 205–217.

Smith Richards, B. K., Belton, B. N., York, B., & Volaufova, J. (2004). Mice bearing *Acads* mutation display altered postingestive but not 5-s orosensory response to dietary fat. *American Journal of Physiology Regulatory Integrative and Comparative Physiology, 286*(2), R311–R319.

Smolders, J. (2010). Vitamin D and multiple sclerosis: Correlation, causality, and controversy. *Autoimmune Diseases,* October 5, 2011, 629538.

Sribanditmongkol, S., Neal, J. L., Szalacha, L. A., & McCarthy, D. O. (2015). Effect of perceived stress on cytokine production in healthy college students. *Western Journal of Nursing Research, 37,* 481–493.

UCLA, Office of Media Relations. (2008). *Animal research generates new treatments, benefits society* [Press Release]. Retrieved from http://newsroom.ucla.edu/stories/animal-generates-new-treatments-45057

Wagner, M. A., Jeong, Y., Banerjee, T., Yang, J., & Holden, J. E. (2016). Sex differences in hypothalamic-mediated tonic norepinephrine release for thermal hyperalgesia in rats. *Neuroscience, 324,* 420–429. PMID: 27001177

Wardach, J., Wagner, M., Jeong, Y., & Holden, J. E. (2016). Lateral hypothalamic stimulation reduces thermal hyperalgesia through spinally descending orexin-A neurons in neuropathic pain. *Western Journal of Nursing Research, 38,* 292–307. PMID: 26475681

Xu, H., Crawford, D., Hutchinson, K. R., Youtz, D. J., Lucchesi, P. A., Velten, M., . . . Wold, L. E. (2011). Myocardial dysfunction in an animal model of cancer cachexia. *Life Sciences, 88,* 406–410.

CHAPTER 2

Biobehavioral Research in Cardiovascular and Respiratory Nursing

Janet Larson, PhD, RN, FAAN

Biobehavioral nurse researchers at the University of Michigan addressed issues related to the care of people with cardiovascular and respiratory disease. They advanced the measurement of clinical phenomena, symptom science, self-management, and health-promoting behaviors for people with chronic disease. This chapter highlights key contributions of PhD program graduates and members of the faculty.

Cardiovascular Nursing

Five researchers from the faculty and PhD graduates of the School of Nursing conducted clinical studies to advance cardiovascular nursing. Investigators studying cardiovascular disease focused on symptom management and the effects of symptoms on self-management. Dr. Jesus M. Casida (faculty member) studied clinical factors that influence outcomes after cardiac surgery and self-care of people with an implanted left-ventricular assist device. Dr. Terri Voepel-Lewis (recent PhD graduate) developed methods for assessing complex clinical phenomena in children during and after surgery. Dr. Susan J. Pressler (recent faculty member) studied cognitive function in people with heart failure. Investigators also focused on health-seeking behaviors, factors that influence self-care decisions, and care provider decisions that influence health risk. Dr. Samar Noureddine (PhD graduate) studied cognitive and psychosocial predictors of health behaviors in Lebanon. Dr. Cynthia Arslanian-Engoren (PhD graduate and faculty member) studied nurses' cardiac triage decisions and women's coronary heart disease risk perceptions.

Symptom and Self-Management in Cardiac Surgery Patients

Dr. Casida worked to advance the science that underpins the management of critically ill patients, specifically those requiring cardiac surgery and advanced heart failure therapies by implantation of a left-ventricular assist device (LVAD)—a type of a mechanical heart. In his work with cardiac surgery, he and his team examined the role of sleep pattern disturbances and inflammatory response from cardiopulmonary bypass machines (i.e., heart-lung machines used during cardiac surgery). They found significant relationships among sleep pattern disturbances (e.g., sleep fragmentation), stress (cortisol), and inflammatory markers (C-reactive protein [C-RP] and white blood cell counts); correlation coefficients ranged from r values of .50 to .82, all p values < .05 (Casida, Davis, Shpakoff, & Yarandi, 2014).

These findings led to the use of guided imagery to reduce stress. Casida pilot-tested (randomized controlled trial [RCT]) the integration of a self-administered (or nurse-assisted) guided imagery program in very busy intensive care and step-down units. He found that this intervention was feasible and acceptable by patients and staff nurses as demonstrated by a protocol compliance rate of 85% to 100% during postoperative nights 1 through 4. Notable findings included a significant reduction in pain and anxiety levels and narcotic analgesic consumption among guided imagery users (n = 20) versus nonusers (n = 20), p < .05. Although the between-group differences were not significant, he found an improvement in the guided imagery users' sleep patterns (i.e., lower sleep-onset latency) and sleep quality, as well as a reduction in stress (cortisol) and inflammation (C-RP) over time (postoperative nights/days 1 through 4), p < .05 (Casida et al., 2013). He is currently developing a larger RCT to expand this pilot work to further investigate the effects of guided imagery on sleep patterns and cardiac surgical outcomes (physical function, complications, hospitalization days, health status, and mortality).

Since sleep pattern disturbance is highly prevalent in heart failure, Casida extended this work to patients with *advanced/end-stage* heart failure requiring LVADs. He found that patients' sleep was severely disrupted (e.g., high sleep fragmentation index) before LVAD and continued up to 6 months after implantation of the LVAD. This finding was accompanied by patterns of excessive daytime sleepiness before and after LVAD (Casida, Davis, Brewer, Smith, & Yarandi, 2011). The severity of the sleep pattern disturbances, poor sleep quality, and daytime sleepiness among LVAD patients was associated with poor quality of life; correlation coefficients ranged from r = .66 to .84, all p values < .05 (Casida, Brewer, Smith, & Davis, 2012). In addition to sleep disturbances, patients also experienced high levels of fatigue, anxiety, and depression within 1 month before and up to 6 months after implantation of the LVAD (Casida & Parker, 2012). He recently completed a longitudinal study on cognition and self-care capabilities in patients with LVADs. Preliminary analysis showed a significant relationship between executive function (a domain of cognition) and LVAD pump flow (r = .72, p < .05), and patients' ability to care for themselves improved significantly from baseline (preimplant) to 6 months post-LVAD implant, p < .05 (Casida et al., ongoing analysis).

The symptom (e.g., sleep pattern disturbances, anxiety, depression) and self-management science for people with LVAD is in its formative stage of development. Further research is needed to definitively establish the impact of distressing symptoms on patients' self-efficacy for and adherence to the LVAD home care regimen (Casida, Wu,

Harden, Chern, & Carie, 2015) and to establish evidence-based interventions to improve symptoms and self-management.

Impact. Dr. Casida's work on sleep promotion and inflammation reduction in cardiac surgery and his work on symptoms (sleep, anxiety, depression, cognition, etc.) and self-management science in patients with LVADs have advanced the science (Casida et al., 2015; Casida, Peters, & Magnan, 2009). His work has laid the groundwork for improving self-management in patients who are tethered to a life-sustaining technology or an implantable artificial organ.

Managing Pain and Sedation in Children Before and After Surgery

Dr. Voepel-Lewis works with an interdisciplinary team of researchers to develop and improve methods of assessment that are needed for the care of children during and following surgery, including cardiac surgery. Voepel-Lewis and collaborators conducted several prospective studies to improve pain measurement and develop and test measures to assess sedation and perioperative risk in children, including, most recently, sleep disordered breathing (Tait, Voepel-Lewis, Christensen, & O'Brien, 2013; Voepel-Lewis, Malviya, Merkel, & Tait, 2003; Voepel-Lewis, Malviya, Prochaska, & Tait, 2000). The results of this work led to national and international clinical use of their pain measures in hospital and ambulatory settings and provided sensitive measures that have facilitated innumerable prospective clinical trials both institutionally and nationally. Additionally, providers and pain experts at large pediatric hospital settings found these instruments to have greater clinical utility compared with other pain assessment instruments. Her recent work, which is grounded in decision theory, prospectively examined parents' complex analgesic decisions and explored factors that influence their responsiveness to varying pain and analgesic adverse-effect signals. Her ongoing studies have examined and tested several of the hypothesized relationships among knowledge, preferences, patient education, and parents' decisions to treat their children's pain, using both hypothetical and real postdischarge decisions. The most recent findings showed that many parents lack a critical understanding of serious analgesic-related adverse events and that strong parent preferences for pain relief interfere with analgesic knowledge and decision making, potentially leading to poor or unsafe opioid decisions (Voepel-Lewis, Zikmund-Fisher, Smith, Zyzanski, & Tait, 2015). This work has enabled her to identify specific knowledge deficits that contribute to unsafe use and that might lead to poor pain outcomes in children.

Despite rigorous efforts to manage pain in children, many experience poor postoperative pain control and might go on to have recurrent or persistent pain and analgesic use for years, even into adulthood. Voepel-Lewis and collaborators identified significant numbers of children who experience poor responses to routine, intensive analgesic management strategies (Voepel-Lewis et al., 2013). Though some risk factors might explain, in part, postoperative and chronic pain experiences, the transition from acute to chronic pain remains poorly understood. Importantly, symptom patterns consistent with aberrant pain processing in the nervous system (i.e., central sensitization or pain vulnerability) are often present in adults and children with chronic pain and have been described in adults who recalled their onset of chronic pain in childhood.

Currently, Voepel-Lewis is focused on two major, but related, areas: (a) assessing and improving parents' knowledge and decision making to safely and effectively manage their children's pain in the home setting, and (b) testing the hypothesized role that centralized pain sensitivity plays in the postoperative pain experience in children.

Impact. Dr. Voepel-Lewis's work has been important because, historically, valid, reliable, and sensitive outcome measures have been lacking in the pediatric setting. Her research led to widespread use of her pain measures and sedation instrument both clinically and as an outcome measure in clinical studies, thereby improving the quality of pain assessment and the safety of sedation practices.

Cognitive Decline as a Symptom of Heart Failure

Dr. Pressler's program of research focuses on quality of life for people with heart failure (HF). In her early work, she demonstrated that health-related quality of life is diminished in HF because of two hallmark symptoms: dyspnea and fatigue. In three separate studies, she and her research team found that cognitive dysfunction was a common HF-related symptom. In one study, 40% of patients with HF reported cognitive dysfunction (Bennett, Baker, & Huster, 1998). In another study, patients with poorer cognitive function had significantly more hospitalizations at 6 months after baseline (Bennett, Pressler, Hays, Firestine, & Huster, 1997). In a focus group study investigating self-care strategies used to manage HF, patients (n = 23) and family members (n = 18) identified cognitive dysfunction (e.g., poor concentration, memory loss) as the third most common symptom after dyspnea and fatigue (Bennett, Cordes, Westmoreland, Castro, & Donnelly, 2000). These studies highlighted the burden of cognitive losses experienced by patients with HF, and from this, Pressler conducted a larger study to explore factors that contribute to and/or explain cognitive deficits: "Cognitive Deficits in Chronic Heart Failure" (THINK Study). This research was supported by the National Institute of Nursing Research, and Pressler et al.'s (2010) findings supported the need for intervention studies to prevent or delay memory loss, thereby reducing mortality and improving health-related quality of life in HF.

Pressler conducted two intervention studies called MEMOIR and MEMOIR-2 (Pressler et al., 2011; Pressler et al., 2015) to evaluate the efficacy of a novel computerized cognitive training program: Brain Fitness, developed by PositScience. Brain Fitness was developed based on scientific principles of neuroplasticity. Forty hours of training with Brain Fitness is proposed to improve the biological process of neuroplasticity and thereby improve memory. Efficacy of computerized cognitive training with Brain Fitness was demonstrated among healthy older adults, but it was not known if the intervention program would be efficacious in improving cognitive outcomes among HF patients who have or are at risk for cognitive dysfunction. MEMOIR and MEMOIR-2 evaluated the efficacy of computerized cognitive training with Brain Fitness in improving memory and secondary outcomes of working memory, processing speed, executive function, and health care resource use. In MEMOIR-2, Pressler added outcome variables of serum brain-derived neurotropic factor (BDNF), mobility, depressive symptoms, and health-related quality of life and examined the BDNF gene as a potential variable that might explain response to outcomes.

In MEMOIR and MEMOIR-2, HF patients were randomized to Brain Fitness or a health education intervention. Both interventions were delivered in patients' homes over 8 weeks to minimize the travel burden for patients and caregivers. In addition, a home-based intervention can be more easily "scaled up" to larger groups of HF patients. Both studies included a nurse enhancement to monitor intervention adherence and assess HF-related symptoms that might interfere with adherence. In MEMOIR, advanced practice nurses made weekly home visits to patients in both groups for 8 weeks during intervention delivery. In MEMOIR-2, advanced practice nurses made weekly telephone calls to patients in both groups for 8 weeks during intervention delivery. Data were collected at baseline and at 8 and 12 weeks after baseline.

In MEMOIR (Pressler et al., 2011), 40 HF patients were enrolled and randomized; 34 patients completed the study. Pressler found a significant interaction effect: Patients in the Brain Fitness group improved more than the control group on delayed recall memory ($p = .032$) at 12 weeks. Patients in both groups demonstrated a significant time effect with improved recall ($p < .001$) and delayed recall ($p = .015$) memory, psychomotor speed ($p = .029$), and instrumental activities of daily living ($p = .006$) over the 12 weeks of the study. Health care resource use was 49% higher for patients in the control group compared with the computerized cognitive training group, but this difference did not reach significance (Pressler et al., 2013).

In MEMOIR-2 (Pressler et al., 2015), 30 HF patients were enrolled and randomized; 27 patients completed the study. In a linear mixed models analysis, Pressler found that compared with patients in the active control group, patients in the cognitive training Brain Fitness group had significantly increased serum BDNF (brain-derived neurotropic factor) ($p = .011$) and improved working memory ($p = .046$) over time. Further analyses of this study are ongoing at the time of this writing.

MEMOIR was the first study to evaluate efficacy of a computerized cognitive training intervention in HF patients, and MEMOIR-2 was the first to examine BDNF as a variable that might influence outcomes in cognitive training studies. These studies have documented that HF patients can and do benefit from nurse-enhanced computerized cognitive training with Brain Fitness. Pressler and her team continue to test interventions to improve memory, understand mechanisms that underlie the memory improvements, and enhance quality of life of HF patients.

Impact. Dr. Pressler's work highlighted the importance of cognitive dysfunction in HF patients. National clinical practice guidelines now recommend assessment of cognitive function in HF patients.

Health Behaviors That Impact Cardiovascular Risk

Dr. Noureddine's research focuses on health-seeking behaviors, which she defines as "behaviors that people engage in to prevent illness, promote and/or restore their health," and their modification to reduce health risk. She focuses on cognitive and psychosocial predictors of health behaviors, as these are amenable to intervention by nurses in both healthy and chronically ill populations. In her dissertation, she examined cognitive and psychological predictors of healthy eating in a community sample of middle-age adults in the United States, and results showed strong associations between the behavior, self-efficacy, and perceived health risk. As she moved back to her native Lebanon, it became clear that cardiovascular disease (CVD) was prevalent and the leading cause of morbidity and mortality, so she focused on secondary prevention of CVD. The first step was investigating health-seeking behaviors of patients with acute coronary syndrome. The findings were similar to those reported from Western countries for variables such as the nature of symptoms and their perceived threat, but some were unique to the Lebanese culture—namely, the strong involvement of the family in patients' lives. One finding worth noting was that the mean time from symptom onset to arrival at the emergency hospital was 4.5 hours, longer than is reported in the United States, and it did not differ by whether the event was the first or a recurrent one.

To further explore this, Noureddine conducted a survey of beliefs and perceptions about heart disease and responses to acute symptoms. The findings suggested adequate knowledge of the main symptoms and the main causes of heart disease but inconsistent perceptions about the measures to treat and control it. The response to an acute cardiac event was not adequate when the symptoms were not typical of heart disease, with participants choosing self-help measures rather than seeking health care in response to a heart attack. These findings led to a clinical study that used a mixed method design to explore the decision-making process that underlies the response of cardiac patients to symptoms of acute myocardial infarction (MI) and related factors. The qualitative component addressed the experience of the cardiac event with emphasis on cognitive and emotional aspects, and the quantitative component assessed knowledge of symptoms of MI and the appropriate response to them. Results suggested that there is a need for raising awareness about heart disease. Since again in this study the family was shown to have a key role in the decision to seek care for acute coronary events, a community rather than individual intervention might be more appropriate. Another relevant finding was the inappropriate reaction of some general practitioners (GPs) to patients who seek their advice when having a heart attack, as these physicians were asking patients to do blood tests and electrocardiograms and return back to them, adding to the delay in emergency care; this suggests that GPs need more training in how to detect and manage heart attacks.

In all studies, Noureddine found a high rate of tobacco smoking among patients with CVD, regardless of whether their cardiac event was new or recurrent (prevalence rates 40%–60%). Smoking status is significant not only because it increases cardiovascular risk but also because smokers tend to attribute their cardiac symptoms to the lungs, thus further delaying their seeking emergency care. This led to a longitudinal study on smoking patterns of patients admitted with acute coronary syndrome or for elective coronary revascularization (percutaneous intervention and open heart surgery). This ongoing study is investigating smoking cessation, relapse rates, and related factors following discharge from the hospital. Preliminary findings suggest that patients prefer an individual counseling type of intervention and that only a few are aware of pharmacotherapy for smoking cessation. So a multidisciplinary team including psychiatrists, addiction experts, and public health professionals will be sought for planning an intervention study.

At present, there is no national policy in Lebanon on cardiopulmonary resuscitation and the poor survival rate of OHCA patients. Noureddine has completed a national online survey of physicians on resuscitation practices for OHCA patients in emergency departments in Lebanon. The results showed that the most important factors in the physicians' decision to initiate or continue resuscitation were the presence of pulse on arrival, the underlying cardiac rhythm, the physician's ethical duty to resuscitate, and the time from the arrest to resuscitation. The physicians reported frequent resuscitation in medically futile situations. The most frequently reported challenges during resuscitation decisions were related to the victim's family and lack of policy. These results are being used by a group from the American University of Beirut Faculty of Medicine, on which Noureddine serves and which is charged with developing national guidelines for resuscitation of those experiencing out-of-hospital cardiac arrest (OHCA). Representative samples of Noureddine's research are described in the following publications: Noureddine (2009); Noureddine et al. (2006); Noureddine, Arevian, Adra, and Puzantian (2008); Noureddine, Froelicher, Sibai, and Dakik (2010); Noureddine, Massouh, and Froelicher (2013); Noureddine and Stein (2009).

Impact. Dr. Noureddine's research has inspired development of patient education materials. Patient education materials on heart disease are being developed for use in an affiliated medical center. Materials were developed targeting women, and sessions were provided using the video and educational pamphlet in some primary health care centers. Patient education materials will be provided to nurses working in primary health care centers so they can teach their clients behavioral strategies aimed at cardiovascular risk reduction. This initiative was implemented by the Order of Nurses in Lebanon in collaboration with the Ministry of Public Health. As a member of the global leadership nursing forum of the Preventive Cardiology Nursing Association, Noureddine was involved in the preparation of a tool kit for community nurses for use in teaching patients cardiovascular risk reduction strategies through behavior change.

Influences on Clinical Decisions by Nurses and Self-Care Decisions by Individuals With Cardiac Disease

As a nurse scientist with decision-making expertise, Dr. Arslanian-Engoren's program of research focuses on the cardiac triage decisions of emergency department triage nurses and the self-care decisions of women to reduce their risk of coronary heart disease. She developed and tested an intervention that included a decision aid to improve emergency department nurses' cardiac triage decisions for women who present with symptoms of an acute myocardial infarction and developed an instrument to measure emergency department nurses' cardiac triage decisions.

Emergency department nurses' cardiac triage decisions. Her research revealed (a) age and gender differences in nurses' cardiac triage decisions (Arslanian-Engoren, 2000), (b) the inability of nurses' triage decisions to predict admission diagnosis for acute coronary syndromes (Arslanian-Engoren, 2004), (c) a mismatch between symptoms experienced by women who have a myocardial infarction and those used by nurses to triage women for suspected acute coronary syndromes (Arslanian-Engoren, 2009), and (d) that goals of practice for nurses do not always align with acute myocardial infarction guidelines (Arslanian-Engoren, Eagle, Hagerty, & Reits, 2011). As part of this work, she examined the prediction rules of emergency department nurses for persons with suspected acute coronary syndromes and showed that nurses use different prediction rules for triaging male and female vignette patients with acute coronary syndromes (Arslanian-Engoren & Engoren, 2007).

To improve nurses' cardiac triage decisions, she led an interdisciplinary research team that developed and tested the effectiveness of a multifocused intervention (education, vignettes, decision aid) that showed improvements in nurses' knowledge of women's myocardial infarction presentation, adherence to American College of Cardiology and American Heart Association myocardial infarction practice guidelines and in patient outcomes (e.g., likelihood of obtaining a timely electrocardiogram). Results were sustained 3 months after the intervention and resulted in practice changes (Arslanian-Engoren, Hagerty, & Eagle, 2010).

Arslanian-Engoren continues to lead this area of science with the development and testing of an instrument to measure emergency department nurses' cardiac triage decisions (Arslanian-Engoren & Hagerty, 2013). This is the first published instrument to quantify the decision-making processes of emergency nurses who triage men and women entering the emergency department for complaints suggestive of myocardial infarction. Factor analysis of the theoretically derived, empirically based 30-item instrument revealed three factors—patient presentation, unbiased nurse reasoning process, and nurse action—with good internal consistency and sample adequacy. This instrument has the potential to improve patient safety and outcomes related to early identification and treatment of myocardial infarction. Further evaluation is planned.

Self-care decisions to reduce the risk of coronary heart disease. As the overall goal of Arslanian-Engoren's program of research is to reduce coronary heart disease in women, she also examined women's coronary heart disease risk perceptions. Building on her earlier studies—which include rural and urban women's knowledge and risk perceptions for coronary heart disease, treatment-seeking decisions of women with myocardial infarction, and gender and age differences in acute coronary syndromes symptoms—she examined women's coronary heart disease risk factors and screening and physiological and anatomical bases for sex differences in acute coronary syndromes. She has found that social support helped women engage in heart-healthy behaviors to reduce their risk for coronary heart disease and stroke (Arslanian-Engoren, Eastwood, De Jong, & Berra, 2015).

Cognitive dysfunction in older adults with acute heart failure. Arslanian-Engoren recently extended her work to study cognitive dysfunction in older adults hospitalized for acute decompensated heart failure (Arslanian-Engoren et al., 2014). This work showed that more and worse acute heart failure symptoms were associated with cognitive dysfunction. She is currently testing the use of cognitive training to improve cognitive functioning.

Impact. Dr. Arslanian-Engoren was one of the first to show that female patients presenting with possible cardiac symptoms face gender inequities in nurses' triage decisions, placing them at risk for life-threatening delays in acute cardiac treatment.

Respiratory Nursing

Three researchers, comprising faculty and PhD program graduates at the School of Nursing, studied symptoms and functioning in people with respiratory disease. The researchers' time at the institution did not overlap, but their work clearly does and they are well acquainted with each other's work through professional interactions at the national level. Dr. Margaret L. Campbell's work focused on symptoms in palliative care, Dr. Nancy Kline Leidy developed and tested multiple self-reported measures of clinical phenomena for people with respiratory disease, and Dr. Janet L. Larson designed and tested exercise interventions to improve symptoms and functioning for people with chronic obstructive pulmonary disease (COPD).

Respiratory Distress at the End of Life

Dr. Campbell's research focuses on increasing the evidence base for assessing and treating dyspnea among patients at the end of life. *Dyspnea* is a subjective experience of breathing discomfort that can only be known from a person's *self-report*. Eliciting a patient's dyspnea self-report is the gold standard for assessment, yet decreased consciousness typifies the last phase of a terminal illness, leaving many patients unable to provide a dyspnea self-report (Campbell, Templin, & Walch, 2009). Campbell posited that *respiratory distress* is the *observed* corollary to dyspnea, based on the person's display of physical behaviors (Campbell, Templin, & Walch, 2010), and she established the behaviors associated with respiratory distress across cognitive states (Campbell, 2007). From this, she developed a Respiratory Distress Observation Scale (RDOS) and conducted a series of studies to establish its reliability and validity (Campbell, 2008; Campbell et al., 2010).

Oxygen is a routine intervention applied to patients with respiratory distress. From clinical work, Campbell hypothesized that patients near death, who often have decreased consciousness, could have oxygen withdrawn. She randomly provided oxygen, medical air, and no flow via nasal cannula in 10-minute intervals and ascertained that most patients do not need oxygen when near death (Campbell, Yarandi, & Dove-Medows, 2013). Clinical practice changes are suggested from these findings.

Patients near death often have small amounts of retained pharyngeal secretions that resonate and make noise, sometimes referred to as "death rattle." A number of studies have been done to determine if there is distress among patients with death rattle (Wee, Coleman, Hillier, & Holgate, 2006a, 2006b; Wee, Coleman, Hillier, & Holgate, 2008) and to determine which antisecretory medications are most effective at reducing death rattle. However, no one had established whether patients experience distress from death rattle. Campbell conducted the first study to establish that there is no difference in respiratory distress when patients with and without death rattle are compared. This study indicates that death rattle is a normal sound, and antisecretory agents that might produce adverse effects are not indicated (Campbell & Yarandi, 2013). Clinical users of the RDOS have requested distress cut-point identification, and Campbell continues to work with the instrument to generate evidence that facilitates the interpretation of RDOS data. She recently created a layperson's version of the RDOS for use in the home hospice setting, and she is conducting ongoing research to determine its utility in the home setting.

Critically ill patients who are undergoing terminal ventilator withdrawal are often unable to self-report dyspnea but are at high risk for experiencing respiratory distress if the withdrawal is not well-conducted. Campbell developed a nurse-led, RDOS-guided algorithmic approach to this common palliative care process in intensive care units. She completed a pilot study and established feasibility, acceptability, and proof of concept that the algorithm is superior to usual care in ensuring patient comfort (Campbell, Yarandi, & Mendez, 2015). This work is ongoing.

Future research is needed to determine the incidence, prevalence, and trajectory of respiratory distress among patients referred for hospice care. Previous studies of dyspnea prevalence drop patients when they can no longer self-report, so it is not known if respiratory distress accelerates, remains unchanged, or abates as death nears.

Impact. Dr. Campbell's RDOS has facilitated the study of dyspnea at the end of life when subjects are not fully conscious. Since publication, the RDOS has been embraced by palliative care providers for clinical use to standardize patient assessment. The RDOS has been translated into Dutch, French, and Chinese by investigators around the world.

Developing Patient-Reported Outcomes for Use With Lung Disease

Dr. Leidy is an internationally recognized expert in the development of patient-reported outcome (PRO) measures, and she has developed multiple PRO measures focusing on symptoms experienced by people with lung disease. Her contributions include the development of instruments that measure functional performance and acute exacerbations of COPD, assess COPD symptoms, and screen for COPD.

Functional status. As one of the first Intramural Fellows at the National Institute of Nursing Research (NINR), Leidy immersed herself in research to understand and operationalize functional outcomes in patients with COPD. This work led to the development of the Functional Performance Inventory (FPI), a PRO measure (Leidy, 1999). The analytical framework, qualitative insight, and the FPI and FPI Short Form (SF) have been used internationally to better understand functional performance in people with COPD, including validation of a new physical activity measurement approach involving monitoring and patient self-report developed by the European Medicines Initiative (EMI) PRO-ACTIVE program.

Acute exacerbations. Leidy addressed another important issue for the care of people with COPD: the measurement of acute exacerbations. Historically exacerbations were measured using health care resource utilization (HCRU; i.e., clinic visits, emergency visits, or hospitalization). Leidy and collaborators developed a symptom-based method of prospectively assessing exacerbations. The **EXA**cerbations of **C**hronic Pulmonary Disease **T**ool (EXACT®) is a 14-item daily diary designed to count and characterize symptom-defined exacerbations (frequency, severity, duration) and quantify the symptomatic experiences that accompany HCRU events (Leidy et al., 2011). The EXACT has been translated into more than 50 languages, used in more than 25 clinical trials and licensed to more than 50 academic investigators for clinical research. The EXACT was also the first PRO measure qualified by the FDA, an important milestone for patient-centered research and has been reviewed by the European Medicines Agency (EMA) under their novel methodologies qualification program. Results of studies to date offer insight into the natural history of exacerbations and the effects of treatment.

Leidy was a key participant in the EXACT-PRO Initiative, the first multisponsor consortium convened to develop a standardized outcome measure for use in drug development trials and clinical research, forming the basis for the C-PATH PRO Consortium the COPD Foundation Biomarker Qualification Consortium (CBQC) and other partnerships for advancing science through collaboration. The CBQC team, including Leidy, successfully completed an evidence package and FDA qualification for the use of fibrinogen as a prognostic biomarker for selecting COPD patients at high risk for exacerbations or all-cause mortality for inclusion in clinical trials, the fifth of only six biomarkers qualified by the FDA to date and another first for COPD.

Respiratory symptoms in stable disease. People with COPD experience respiratory symptoms even when in a stable clinical condition, and these symptoms are not only distressing but also a primary cause of functional limitations. Accurate assessment is important to clinical practice and research. Extending the EXACT-PRO Initiative, Leidy and colleagues developed and validated the Evaluating Respiratory Symptoms (E-RS) scale (Leidy et al., 2014). The E-RS scale has been reviewed by the EMA and is in the final stages of PRO qualification review by the FDA. Like the EXACT, it is being used in a number of international studies.

Assessing symptoms and impact in clinical practice. Assessing symptoms in clinical practice requires effective clinician-patient interaction to ensure the right information is gathered to inform decision making. Leidy and collaborators developed the COPD Assessment Test (CAT), a validated, standardized clinical tool, for this purpose (Jones et al., 2009). The brief 8-item measure is self-administered, with the information presented to the clinician in a format that allows the practitioner to quickly detect areas of greatest difficulty in need of further evaluation. The instrument is used in practices worldwide and often serves as a health outcome measure in clinical research, with more than 200 related publications to date.

Screening for COPD in primary care. The need for a simple yet precise screening strategy for identifying undiagnosed patients with clinically significant COPD in primary care settings was addressed through a novel multimethod empirical approach designed and led by Drs. Leidy, Fernando Martinez (Cornell University), and David Mannino (University of Kentucky). Funded by the National Institutes of Health, this project involved pulmonologists, primary care physicians, and nurses from across the United States and the participation of the COPD Foundation. A systematic analytical process uncovered a set of five simple questions and peak expiratory flow (PEF) thresholds capable of differentiating cases and controls with remarkable sensitivity and specificity. Results suggest that asking patients these five questions with selective use of PEF might be an effective and efficient clinical approach for identifying patients in primary care who are in need of further evaluation for clinically significant COPD.

Impact. The symptoms of lung disease are variable from day to day and challenging to assess in a systematic manner. Dr. Leidy's work has advanced research and practice by establishing precise and valid methods for measuring symptoms and functioning across different phases of lung disease. All of her PRO measures have been translated into multiple languages and are widely used in clinical research to document clinical phenomena. Some are used in the clinical setting.

Promoting Exercise and Physical Activity in COPD

Dr. Larson and her research team developed and tested interventions to promote exercise and physical activity in people with COPD with the long-term goal of increasing functional performance, reducing symptoms, and improving health. Much of her work was supported by grants from the National Institute of Nursing Research. Larson started this work at a time when it was thought that people with COPD could not benefit from exercise.

It is now recognized that some of the underlying shortness of breath is in part related to impairment of inspiratory muscle function, hence her early research focused on improving function of the inspiratory muscles and combining inspiratory muscle training with aerobic conditioning to reduce symptoms of shortness of breath. Larson designed and tested inspiratory muscle training interventions to improve functional strength of the inspiratory muscles with the goal of reducing dyspnea and enhancing functional performance. She demonstrated that it was possible to improve strength and endurance of the inspiratory muscles if reliable training loads were used, a problem that had plagued earlier research (Larson, Kim, Sharp, & Larson, 1988). Larson's research moved the science forward by developing and testing the first inspiratory muscle trainer that produced reliable training loads. She then demonstrated that high-intensity inspiratory muscle training improves dyspnea for people with very severe airflow obstruction (Covey et al., 2001). The improvements in dyspnea were both statistically significant and clinically meaningful, with patients reporting less dyspnea during activities of daily living. This was a new finding, and it was important because it suggested that people with the most severe symptoms of COPD were more likely to benefit from inspiratory muscle training, thereby allowing for the appropriate targeting of the intervention to people most likely to benefit.

Larson extended this research to examine the effects of bicycle training on functional capacity. Historically it had been thought that people with COPD could not train at sufficient intensity to improve maximum oxygen uptake, but in the late 1990s, it was demonstrated that supervised exercise training in the laboratory could produce a significant increase in maximum oxygen uptake, the gold-standard measure for functional capacity. Larson was the first to demonstrate that home-based exercise training could produce significant increases in maximum oxygen uptake (Larson et al., 1999). This finding was important because patients with COPD are frequently too fatigued to attend institutionally based exercise programs, making the home-based programs more attractive.

In a large randomized controlled trial, she examined the combined effects of upper-body resistance training and a self-efficacy-enhancing intervention to promote exercise adherence and to increase moderate-to-vigorous physical activity (MVPA). This study clearly demonstrated that patients could increase strength and lean arm mass, and some of the strength gains (24%) were retained for 1 year after the end of training. There was limited evidence that it improved dyspnea and no evidence that it improved overall functional performance (Covey et al., 2012). The self-efficacy-enhancing component of this intervention led to an increase in light physical activity (LPA) but no change in MVPA (Larson, Covey, Kapella, Alex, & McAuley, 2014). The increase in physical activity was not sustained over the 1 year of follow-up. The short-term gain was promising and led to further development of the self-efficacy-enhancing intervention to focus on long-term improvements in physical activity.

People with COPD are very inactive (Park, Richardson, Holleman, & Larson, 2013)—more inactive than most people with chronic disease—and recent evidence suggests that substantial health benefits can be accrued by decreasing sedentary time and increasing LPA. Larson's ongoing work focuses on the development and testing of an intervention designed to increase LPA and to sustain the increase in LPA over time.

Future research in this area should focus on increasing physical activity and decreasing sedentary time. Many people with COPD cannot maintain increases in MVPA, so focusing on increasing LPA is promising and has the potential to improve health and functioning.

Impact. Dr. Larson's research has influenced practice, and her threshold loaded training device is now used in pulmonary rehabilitation programs throughout the country. Her work and the work of others clearly demonstrate that people with COPD will benefit by exercising and increasing their physical activity.

Synthesis

Biobehavioral nurse researchers at the School of Nursing have advanced the science of symptom assessment and self-management as it relates to the care of people with cardiovascular and respiratory disease. They explored factors that influence symptoms and designed and tested innovative interventions to improve symptoms with the ultimate goal of improving health and functioning.

Developed measures that advance clinical science. Three researchers advanced symptom science by developing new measures of symptoms. They addressed very complex symptoms that are challenging to assess in the clinical and research setting. Dr. Voepel-Lewis established reliable and valid measures of pain and sedation in children before and after surgery. This is important because it filled a gap in the field and facilitated the systematic management of children before and after surgery. Dr. Campbell developed a proxy measure of dyspnea to be used at the end of life when people are not fully conscious. This is significant because it enables researchers and clinicians to evaluate the effects of interventions designed to promote breathing comfort at the end of life. Dr. Larson developed multiple PRO measures of complex phenomena experienced by people with lung disease. She developed measures for common problems such as functional performance in COPD, symptoms of an acute exacerbation of COPD, symptoms of stable COPD, and screening for COPD. These instruments are widely used in clinical research and pharmacological studies. They have advanced the field by enabling researchers and clinicians to measure important clinical phenomena in a systematic manner and to determine the effects of interventions using reliable and valid measures.

All of the above instruments were developed in a rigorous manner, and their reliability and validity were examined in multiple studies prior to establishing the final version of each measure. The measures are multidimensional, enabling them to capture the full breadth of the clinical phenomena. High-quality measures such as these make a lasting contribution to clinical knowledge. They will be used by many researchers long into the future.

Addressed complex symptoms. Biobehavioral researchers studied complex symptoms that interact with each other to influence health outcomes. They examined symptoms from an experiential and objective perspective, and they examined factors that contribute to symptoms, thereby identifying potential targets for intervention. Two researchers examined symptoms that contribute to the burden of cardiovascular disease including dyspnea, fatigue, sleep disturbance, and cognitive dysfunction. One researcher studied dyspnea at the end of life. Two of the researchers included biomarkers to better understand underlying factors that contribute to specific symptoms. This is cutting-edge work, and in recent years it has been recognized that the concurrent measurement of self-reported symptoms and biomarkers is important for fully understanding the clinical phenomena.

Effect of symptoms on self-management. It has long been recognized that symptoms of chronic disease can influence quality of life, but the recent work of biobehavioral researchers focuses on the effects of symptoms on self-management. Cognitive decline is recognized as an important symptom of chronic cardiovascular and respiratory disease. One researcher focused much of her recent work on improving cognitive function in people with chronic heart failure with the goal of ultimately improving self-management skills and quality of life. Two other researchers have begun to explore this challenging area for people undergoing LVAD therapy and people with acute heart failure. This is an important clinical area because people are living longer with multiple complex conditions that require substantial self-management skills. People are expected to carry out self-management regimens that are challenging even with the best of cognitive skills and can be overwhelming for people with declining cognitive function. This line of research is in its infancy, but it is promising and has the potential to make a difference in the lives of people living with chronic disease.

Health-promoting behavior in chronic disease. Biobehavioral researchers recognize the importance of a healthy lifestyle, health-promoting behaviors, and specific knowledge to promote optimal outcomes for people with cardiovascular and respiratory disease. Two investigators examined factors that support heart-healthy behaviors to reduce the risk of acute cardiovascular disease and improve the chances of a positive outcome if an acute event does occur. Another researcher examined the behavior of nurses in the emergency department to identify factors that influence treatment decisions during an acute event. This body of research highlights the importance of unique factors such as gender and culture in dealing with health behaviors. It emphasizes the importance of knowledge for promoting optimal decision making for both patients and nurses.

People with cardiovascular and respiratory disease live very sedentary lives, and increasing exercise has been a long-standing clinical goal for both populations. One researcher has addressed this issue by conducting a series of exercise and physical activity interventions in people with COPD; the results were promising but transient because people could not maintain the exercises on a long-term basis. More recently it has been recognized that increasing daily physical activity, even light physical activity, is more appropriate for people with chronic disease. So the ongoing challenge is to increase physical activity using strategies that can be maintained over long periods of time.

Long-term behavior change is a complex phenomenon and a well-established line of research that is often claimed by behavioral scientists. However, biobehavioral nurse researchers make a unique contribution to this field through their work with people who have chronic disease. Biobehavioral nurse researchers understand behavioral sciences and the experience of chronic disease. They bring the two together to design and test interventions that are appropriate for people with chronic disease. This is an important area of research given that people are living longer with multiple complex chronic diseases.

References

Arslanian-Engoren, C. (2000). Gender and age bias in triage decisions. *Journal of Emergency Nursing, 26*(2), 117–124.

Arslanian-Engoren, C. (2004). Do emergency nurses' triage decisions predict differences in admission or discharge diagnoses for acute coronary syndromes? *Journal of Cardiovascular Nursing, 19*(4), 280–286.

Arslanian-Engoren, C. (2009). Explicating nurses' cardiac triage decisions. *Journal of Cardiovascular Nursing, 24*(1), 50–57. doi:10.1097/01.JCN.0000317474.50424.4f

Arslanian-Engoren, C., Eagle, K. A., Hagerty, B., & Reits, S. (2011). Emergency department triage nurses' self-reported adherence with American College of Cardiology/American Heart Association myocardial infarction guidelines. *Journal of Cardiovascular Nursing, 26*(5), 408–413. doi:10.1097/JCN.0b013e3182076a98

Arslanian-Engoren, C., Eastwood, J. A., De Jong, M. J., & Berra, K. (2015). Participation in heart-healthy behaviors: A secondary analysis of the American Heart Association Go Red Heart Match data. *Journal of Cardiovascular Nursing, 30*(6), 479–483. doi:10.1097/jcn.0000000000000190

Arslanian-Engoren, C., & Engoren, M. (2007). Using a genetic algorithm to predict evaluation of acute coronary syndromes. *Nursing Research, 56*(2), 82–88. doi:10.1097/01.nnr.0000263965.16501.26

Arslanian-Engoren, C., Giordani, B. J., Algase, D., Schuh, A., Lee, C., & Moser, D. K. (2014). Cognitive dysfunction in older adults hospitalized for acute heart failure. *Journal of Cardiac Failure, 20*(9), 669–678. doi:10.1016/j.cardfail.2014.06.003

Arslanian-Engoren, C., & Hagerty, B. M. (2013). The development and testing of the nurses' cardiac triage instrument. *Research and Theory for Nursing Practice, 27*(1), 9–18.

Arslanian-Engoren, C., Hagerty, B., & Eagle, K. A. (2010). Evaluation of the ACT intervention to improve nurses' cardiac triage decisions. *Western Journal of Nursing Research, 32*(6), 713–729. doi:10.1177/0193945909359410

Bennett, S. J., Baker, S. L., & Huster, G. A. (1998). Quality of life in women with heart failure. *Health Care for Women International, 19*(3), 217–229. doi:10.1080/073993398246386

Bennett, S. J., Cordes, D. K., Westmoreland, G., Castro, R., & Donnelly, E. (2000). Self-care strategies for symptom management in patients with chronic heart failure. *Nursing Research, 49*(3), 139–145.

Bennett, S. J., Pressler, M. L., Hays, L., Firestine, L. A., & Huster, G. A. (1997). Psychosocial variables and hospitalization in persons with chronic heart failure. *Progress in Cardiovascular Nursing, 12*(4), 4–11.

Campbell, M. L. (2007). Fear and pulmonary stress behaviors to an asphyxial threat across cognitive states. *Research in Nursing and Health, 30*(6), 572–583. doi:10.1002/nur.20212

Campbell, M. L. (2008). Psychometric testing of a respiratory distress observation scale. *Journal of Palliative Medicine, 11*(1), 44–50. doi:10.1089/jpm.2007.0090

Campbell, M. L., Templin, T., & Walch, J. (2009). Patients who are near death are frequently unable to self-report dyspnea. *Journal of Palliative Medicine, 12*(10), 881–884. doi:10.1089/jpm.2009.0082

Campbell, M. L., Templin, T., & Walch, J. (2010). A Respiratory Distress Observation Scale for patients unable to self-report dyspnea. *Journal of Palliative Medicine, 13*(3), 285–290. doi:10.1089/jpm.2009.0229

Campbell, M. L., & Yarandi, H. N. (2013). Death rattle is not associated with patient respiratory distress: Is pharmacologic treatment indicated? *Journal of Palliative Medicine, 16*(10), 1255–1259. doi:10.1089/jpm.2013.0122

Campbell, M. L., Yarandi, H., & Dove-Medows, E. (2013). Oxygen is nonbeneficial for most patients who are near death. *Journal of Pain and Symptom Management, 45*(3), 517–523. doi:10.1016/j.jpainsymman.2012.02.012

Campbell, M. L., Yarandi, H. N., & Mendez, M. (2015). A two-group trial of a terminal ventilator withdrawal algorithm: Pilot testing. *Journal of Palliative Medicine, 18*(9), 781–785. doi:10.1089/jpm.2015.0111

Casida, J. M., Brewer, R. J., Smith, C., & Davis, J. E. (2012). An exploratory study of sleep quality, daytime function, and quality of life in patients with mechanical circulatory support. *International Journal of Artificial Organs, 35*(7), 531–537. doi:10.5301/ijao.5000109

Casida, J. M., Davis, J. E., Brewer, R. J., Smith, C., & Yarandi, H. (2011). Sleep and daytime sleepiness of patients with left ventricular assist devices: A longitudinal pilot study. *Progress in Transplantation, 21*(2), 131–136.

Casida, J. M., Davis, J. E., Shpakoff, L., & Yarandi, H. (2014). An exploratory study of the patients' sleep patterns and inflammatory response following cardiopulmonary bypass (CPB). *Journal of Clinical Nursing, 23*(15–16), 2332–2342. doi:10.1111/jocn.12515

Casida, J. M., & Parker, J. (2012). A preliminary investigation of symptom pattern and prevalence before and up to 6 months after implantation of a left ventricular assist device. *Journal of Artificial Organs, 15*(2), 211–214. doi:10.1007/s10047-011-0622-4

Casida, J. M., Peters, R. M., & Magnan, M. A. (2009). Self-care demands of persons living with an implantable left-ventricular assist device. *Research and Theory for Nursing Practice, 23*(4), 279–293.

Casida, J., Wu, H. S., Harden, J., Chern, J., & Carie, A. (2015). Development and initial evaluation of the psychometric properties of self-efficacy and adherence scales for patients with a left ventricular assist device. *Progress in Transplantation, 25*(2), 107–115. doi:10.7182/pit2015597

Casida, J. M., Yaremchuk, K. L., Shpakoff, L., Marrocco, A., Babicz, G., & Yarandi, H. (2013). The effects of guided imagery on sleep and inflammatory response in cardiac surgery: A pilot randomized controlled trial. *Journal of Cardiovascular Surgery, 54*(2), 269–279.

Covey, M. K., Larson, J. L., Wirtz, S. E., Berry, J. K., Pogue, N. J., Alex, C. G., & Patel, M. (2001). High-intensity inspiratory muscle training in patients with chronic obstructive pulmonary disease and severely reduced function. *Journal of Cardiopulmonary Rehabilitation and Prevention, 21*(4), 231–240.

Covey, M. K., McAuley, E., Kapella, M. C., Collins, E. G., Alex, C. G., Berbaum, M. L., & Larson, J. L. (2012). Upper-body resistance training and self-efficacy enhancement in COPD. *Journal of Pulmonary and Respiratory Medicine* (Suppl. 9), 001. doi:10.4172/2161-105x.s9-001

Jones, P. W., Harding, G., Berry, P., Wiklund, I., Chen, W. H., & Leidy, N. K. (2009). Development and first validation of the COPD Assessment Test. *European Respiratory Journal, 34*(3), 648–654. doi:10.1183/09031936.00102509

Larson, J. L., Covey, M. K., Kapella, M. C., Alex, C. G., & McAuley, E. (2014). Self-efficacy enhancing intervention increases light physical activity in people with chronic obstructive pulmonary disease. *International Journal of Chronic Obstructive Pulmonary Disease, 9*, 1081–1090. doi:10.2147/copd.s66846

Larson, J. L., Covey, M. K., Wirtz, S. E., Berry, J. K., Alex, C. G., Langbein, W. E., & Edwards, L. (1999). Cycle ergometer and inspiratory muscle training in chronic obstructive pulmonary disease. *American Journal of Respiratory and Critical Care Medicine, 160*(2), 500–507. doi:10.1164/ajrccm.160.2.9804067

Larson, J. L., Kim, M. J., Sharp, J. T., & Larson, D. A. (1988). Inspiratory muscle training with a pressure threshold breathing device in patients with chronic obstructive pulmonary disease. *American Review of Respiratory Disease, 138*(3), 689–696. doi:10.1164/ajrccm/138.3.689

Leidy, N. K. (1999). Psychometric properties of the functional performance inventory in patients with chronic obstructive pulmonary disease. *Nursing Research, 48*(1), 20–28.

Leidy, N. K., Murray, L. T., Monz, B. U., Nelsen, L., Goldman, M., Jones, P. W., . . . Sethi, S. (2014). Measuring respiratory symptoms of COPD: Performance of the EXACT-Respiratory Symptoms Tool (E-RS) in three clinical trials. *Respiratory Research, 15*, 124. doi:10.1186/s12931-014-0124-z

Leidy, N. K., Wilcox, T. K., Jones, P. W., Roberts, L., Powers, J. H., & Sethi, S. (2011). Standardizing measurement of chronic obstructive pulmonary disease exacerbations: Reliability and validity of a patient-reported diary. *American Journal of Respiratory and Critical Care Medicine, 183*(3), 323–329. doi:10.1164/rccm.201005-0762OC

Noureddine, S. (2009). Patterns of responses to cardiac events over time. *Journal of Cardiovascular Nursing, 24*(5), 390–397. doi:10.1097/JCN.0b013e3181ae4f0e

Noureddine, S., Adra, M., Arevian, M., Dumit, N. Y., Puzantian, H., Shehab, D., & Abchee, A. (2006). Delay in seeking health care for acute coronary syndromes in a Lebanese sample. *Journal of Transcultural Nursing, 17*(4), 341–348. doi:10.1177/1043659606291544

Noureddine, S., Arevian, M., Adra, M., & Puzantian, H. (2008). Response to signs and symptoms of acute coronary syndrome: Differences between Lebanese men and women. *American Journal of Critical Care, 17*(1), 26–35.

Noureddine, S., Froelicher, E. S., Sibai, A. M., & Dakik, H. (2010). Response to a cardiac event in relation to cardiac knowledge and risk perception in a Lebanese sample: A cross sectional survey. *International Journal of Nursing Studies, 47*(3), 332–341. doi:10.1016/j.ijnurstu.2009.07.002

Noureddine, S., Massouh, A., & Froelicher, E. S. (2013). Perceptions of heart disease in community-dwelling Lebanese. *European Journal of Cardiovascular Nursing, 12*(1), 56–63. doi:10.1177/1474515111430899

Noureddine, S., & Stein, K. (2009). Healthy-eater self-schema and dietary intake. *Western Journal of Nursing Research, 31*(2), 201–218. doi:10.1177/0193945908327157

Park, S. K., Richardson, C. R., Holleman, R. G., & Larson, J. L. (2013). Physical activity in people with COPD, using the National Health and Nutrition Evaluation Survey dataset (2003–2006). *Heart and Lung, 42*(4), 235–240. doi:10.1016/j.hrtlng.2013.04.005

Pressler, S. J., Martineau, A., Grossi, J., Giordani, B., Koelling, T. M., Ronis, D. L., . . . Smith, D. G. (2013). Healthcare resource use among heart failure patients in a randomized pilot study of a cognitive training intervention. *Heart and Lung, 42*(5), 332–338. doi:10.1016/j.hrtlng.2013.05.001

Pressler, S. J., Subramanian, U., Kareken, D., Perkins, S. M., Gradus-Pizlo, I., Sauve, M. J., . . . Shaw, R. M. (2010). Cognitive deficits and health-related quality of life in chronic heart failure. *Journal of Cardiovascular Nursing, 25*(3), 189–198. doi:10.1097/JCN.0b013e3181ca36fe

Pressler, S. J., Therrien, B., Riley, P. L., Chou, C. C., Ronis, D. L., Koelling, T. M., . . . Giordani, B. (2011). Nurse-enhanced memory intervention in heart failure: The MEMOIR study. *Journal of Cardiac Failure, 17*(10), 832–843. doi:10.1016/j.cardfail.2011.06.650

Pressler, S. J., Titler, M., Koelling, T. M., Riley, P. L., Jung, M., Hoyland-Domenico, L., . . . Giordani, B. (2015). Nurse-enhanced computerized cognitive training increases serum brain-derived neurotropic factor levels and improves working memory in heart failure. *Journal of Cardiac Failure, 21*(8), 630–641. doi:10.1016/j.cardfail.2015.05.004

Tait, A. R., Voepel-Lewis, T., Christensen, R., & O'Brien, L. M. (2013). The STBUR questionnaire for predicting perioperative respiratory adverse events in children at risk for sleep-disordered breathing. *Paediatric Anaesthesia, 23*(6), 510–516. doi:10.1111/pan.12155

Voepel-Lewis, T., Malviya, S., Merkel, S., & Tait, A. R. (2003). Behavioral pain assessment and the Face, Legs, Activity, Cry and Consolability instrument. *Expert Review of Pharmacoeconomics and Outcomes Research, 3*(3), 317–325. doi:10.1586/14737167.3.3.317

Voepel-Lewis, T., Malviya, S., Prochaska, G., & Tait, A. R. (2000). Sedation failures in children undergoing MRI and CT: Is temperament a factor? *Paediatric Anaesthesia, 10*(3), 319–323.

Voepel-Lewis, T., Wagner, D., Burke, C., Tait, A. R., Hemberg, J., Pechlivanidis, E., . . . Talsma, A. (2013). Early adjuvant use of nonopioids associated with reduced odds of serious postoperative opioid adverse events and need for rescue in children. *Paediatric Anaesthesia, 23*(2), 162–169. doi:10.1111/pan.12026

Voepel-Lewis, T., Zikmund-Fisher, B. J., Smith, E. L., Zyzanski, S., & Tait, A. R. (2015). Parents' preferences strongly influence their decisions to withhold prescribed opioids when faced with analgesic trade-off dilemmas for children: A prospective observational study. *International Journal of Nursing Studies, 52*(8), 1343–1353. doi:10.1016/j.ijnurstu.2015.05.003

Wee, B., Coleman, P., Hillier, R., & Holgate, S. (2008). Death rattle: Its impact on staff and volunteers in palliative care. *Palliative Medicine, 22*(2), 173–176. doi:10.1177/0269216307087146

Wee, B. L., Coleman, P. G., Hillier, R., & Holgate, S. H. (2006a). The sound of death rattle I: Are relatives distressed by hearing this sound? *Palliative Medicine, 20*(3), 171–175.

Wee, B. L., Coleman, P. G., Hillier, R., & Holgate, S. H. (2006b). The sound of death rattle II: How do relatives interpret the sound? *Palliative Medicine, 20*(3), 177–181.

CHAPTER 3

Cognition and Nursing Science at the University of Michigan

Donna L. Algase, PhD, RN, FAAN, F-GSA, F-NGNA

As a research focus within the doctoral program at the University of Michigan, School of Nursing (UMSN), cognition was the beneficiary of a then fortuitous combination of timing and talent. In this chapter, we provide programs of research bearing on cognition by the UMSN community of scholars, comprising of faculty and PhD alumni. Second, the body of work produced by its talented scientists in the area of cognition is organized and summarized to the extent possible by the materials made available to the author by involved individuals.

Timing and Context

The focus on cognition at UMSN and its doctoral program emerged during the 1990s, also known as the "decade of the brain," an initiative of the National Institutes of Health, the Institute of Mental Health, and the Library of Congress with the goal emphasizing the benefits of brain research. This led to an increase in federal and ancillary funding opportunities that came to benefit UMSN and other units of the university.

The university also afforded a number of related contextual factors favoring cognition as a focus within the UMSN doctoral program. Among them were the Michigan Alzheimer's Disease Research Center, part of a national federally funded network; the Geriatrics Center, an interdisciplinary collective within the medical school that hosted a wide range of clinical, educational, and training programs; and a significant cadre of collegial scientists in social, health, natural resources and environment, and neuroscience whose scientific interests complemented and augmented those of nursing faculty doing cognition-related research.

Within UMSN, that cluster of nursing faculty organized and developed structures and initiatives to support information sharing, mentoring, and collaboration among themselves and their students. These began loosely with community- and identity-building efforts, mainly in the form of a research interest group that brought like-minded faculty, students, and postdoctoral fellows together regularly to learn about each other's work and that of researchers in psychology, neuroscience, and other related fields.

A major step forward occurred in 1995 with the establishment of the Center for the Restoration and Enhancement of Cognitive Function (CERCF), funded internally following a school-wide competition at the initiative of then-dean Ada Sue Hinshaw. Under the leadership of Dr. Barbara Therrien, assisted by Drs. Bonnie Metzger and Donna Algase, the activities of the new center expanded well beyond those of the interest group. These included not only peer support for development of individual programs of research but also efforts to (a) formalize cognition-related, doctoral-level curricular content that undergirded these research programs; (b) secure funding for doctoral and postdoctoral training; and (c) foster clinical and community opportunities for practice and research partnerships.

As research programs matured and new funding opportunities emerged, the Center on Frail and Vulnerable Elders (COFVE) was conceived in 2002 with a population-based focus on cognition-related issues. Under the leadership of Algase, COFVE was established upon external review of a proposal presented to Dean Hinshaw by a subgroup of CERCF members. The primary research base for COFVE drew on the federally funded interactive research project grants of Algase and Dr. Ann Whall (along with Cornelia Beck of the University of Arkansas for Medical Sciences). Its funding base included a range of specialized graduate-level training grants from the John F. Hartford Foundation's Geriatric Nursing Initiative, which supported COFVE programs and projects related to research, policy, and mental health, and also the Division of Nursing of the Health Resources and Services Administration, which funded formal graduate-level curricula and community programming focused on dementia and frailty. COFVE also had contracts with the Michigan Department of Community Health to evaluate its home care program for nursing home–eligible individuals funded by the Center for Medicare and Medicaid Services.

Such was the timing—and context arising from it—that set the stage and served to support the development of cognition as an area of research and scholarship at UMSN from 1990 to 2006, the end of Dean Hinshaw's term of service. With new leadership at UMSN in 2006, research structures of the school soon were centralized and centers were dissolved. While many of the faculty whose efforts were instrumental in building and sustaining the thrust have since retired from UMSN and/or moved on to other settings, faculty brought aboard more recently in the trajectory of cognition-related research at UMSN continue to make contributions with this focus to the discipline of nursing.

Talent and Topics

The UMSN nursing faculty, doctoral students, and postdoctoral fellows who engaged in cognition-related research shared a common interest in theories and methods from departments of basic neuroscience, neurology, psychology, neuropsychology, natural resources and environment, and, often, aging. Thus a wide array of scholars from other schools and colleges across the university have served as collaborators, consultants, and/or coinvestigators on many of their projects. Consequently, the description and organization of the large body of work produced by UMSN scholars in this arena is neither simple nor straight-forward. Broadly, their work could be categorized as animal or human studies. Animal studies, which usually examine the effects of fundamental neural, biological, traumatic, or developmental mechanisms on basic cognitive or neural structures or processes, are sum-marized in Chapter 2 by Dr. Janean Holden. This chapter deals with human studies.

Focus. Overall, human studies conducted by faculty, students, and postdoctoral fellows spanned a wide range of topics dealing with cognition and various human and environmental conditions. This included studies on (a) how cognitive structures and/or processes were affected by biological and illness states, diagnosis or treatment of illness, or environmental factors and (b) how impaired cognition affected human behavior, func-tioning, or health. Over the course of developing various proposals for federal grants for training and for support of a center, several frameworks were developed by these faculty to encompass and describe their common field of endeavor. The most recent of these models as pertained to human studies, shown in Figure 3-a, was developed by Drs. Karen Stein, Donna Algase, Janean Holden, and Susan Pressler in a 2008 application for a P30 Center to the National Institute of Nursing Research. While all the work contained herein may not fit neatly within this framework, it does reflect the thinking of those scientists involved in work relating to cognition at UMSN at the time.

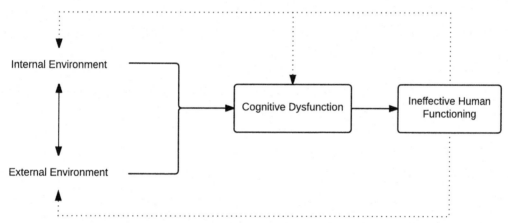

Figure 3-a. A general cognitive dysfunction framework.

Accordingly, the cognitive dysfunction framework is necessarily broad, encompassing both the basis of cognitive dysfunction, conceptualized as an individual's internal and/or external environment, and the outcomes of cognitive dysfunction, viewed as ineffective human functioning. Accordingly, a person's internal and external environments contribute directly to cognitive dysfunction that then directly results in ineffective human function-ing. In turn, ineffective human functioning feeds back to worsen cognitive dysfunction directly or indirectly through effects on internal and/or external environments. As a basis for intervention, the framework allows for (a) altering environmental inputs to reduce cognitive dysfunction, (b) compensating for irreversible cognitive dysfunction to reduce its effects on other areas of human functioning, and/or (c) mitigating effects of ineffective human functioning to prevent further cognitive decline. Internal and external environments can interact to affect one another and may have other direct and indirect effects on human functioning not depicted within the framework for simplicity's sake.

Cognitive dysfunction was understood as any impairment or defect in normal mental functioning, which was understood as the interplay of cognitive processes (e.g., memory) and structures (e.g., cognitive maps, schemas, representations) occurring at two interacting levels of processing: basic (perception, attention, memory, and language) and higher order (learning, problem solving, and decision making, collectively known as executive function). Basic processes support executive function. All cognitive processes depend on specific brain regions and neuroendocrine substrates, although regions and substrates may not yet be known; cognitive processes are integrated via interconnected neural network systems (structures), which are potentially modifiable as a function of neural plasticity (evident as growth or learning).

Cognitive dysfunction can arise in a process or a structure. Whether process oriented or structure oriented, dysfunction can vary in duration (acute, intermittent, chronic), modifiability (preventable, reversible, permanent), severity (mild to profound), and trajectory (self-limiting, sustained/stable, progressive). Cognitive dysfunction is based in both internal biological processes (genetic, pathological, and traumatic) and the quality and/or quantity of external environmental influences.

Ineffective human functioning, in the realms of behavior, self-care, and self-regulation, is the outcome of cognitive dysfunction within this framework. Outcomes are viewed as immediate, long-term, and/or cumulative effects of impaired mental processes or structures on human functioning within these three realms. With a cognitive dysfunction, a person might be less able to modulate behavior or to regulate or care for him- or herself; such outcomes, in turn, feed back to affect biological and environmental inputs and/or cognitive functioning itself.

Research Programs Focused on Cognitive Structures

Several faculty generated successful programs of research that focus on cognitive structures. An example of such work is that of Dr. Margaret Scisney-Matlock and colleagues, who utilized social cognitive theory in the context of hypertension (HTN) to clarify what (declarative knowledge) and how (procedural knowledge) people think (a cognitive representation) about disease/diagnosis and how these representations are linked to resulting health behaviors to manage HTN. Her objective was to build cognitive representations for the purposes of knowledge integration, appraisal, coping, adaptation, and continuous learning to sustain daily self-care regimes, with an emphasis on populations vulnerable to health disparities.

Scisney-Matlock's work builds systematically from a theory-based foundation to generate a valid and reliable measure to quantify multidimensional memories for (a) content (label, psychological, threat, control, and timeline) and (b) the structure of cognitive representations of hypertension (perception, preferences, and possibilities). Further, the control factors (intentions of behavior) of hypertension-related cognitive representations scales were hypothesized as sources for decisions guiding adherence/compliance with treatment recommendations for controlling essential HTN. This work was disseminated in papers describing the scales and their psychometric properties (e.g., Scisney-Matlock & Watkins, 2003), as well as in the bootstrapping methodology used to develop them (e.g., Scisney-Matlock & Beard, 1999).

Further methodological work on electronic monitoring of medication taking (MEMS) (Scisney-Matlock et al., 2000) and advances in ambulatory blood pressure monitoring and the delivery of tailored messages enabled Scisney-Matlock to design intervention work within Leventhal's self-regulation cognition theory to shape cognitive representations to lower blood pressure. Results of a federally funded project to test her resulting intervention, Managing Associated Perceptions, were impressive, showing significant blood pressure reductions and greater medication compliance in the experimental group (received tailored messages) as compared to the control group (received MEMS and ambulatory blood pressure monitoring only); African American women had better results than White American women. Published findings (e.g., Scisney-Matlock, Makos, Saunders, Jackson, & Steigerwalt, 2004) received broad media coverage, suggesting that reading framed, tailored messages aimed at providing critical knowledge to address medication-taking cognitive representation knowledge deficits might be a first step toward sustained compliance and improved blood pressure.

With funding from the National Institutes of Health (NIH), Scisney-Matlock's work was extended within Leventhal's theoretical perspective to include dietary life-style behaviors (Women's and Men's Hypertension Experiences and Emerging Lifestyles Intervention [WHEELS] program and the Dietary Approaches to Stop Hypertension [DASH] diet) were evaluated for consistency with the theory (e.g., Scisney-Matlock, Kachorek, McClerking, & Glazewski, 2006) and were widely acclaimed. In the final phase of her work, WHEELS-I and the Dash diet were evaluated for efficacy in a series of studies using a sophisticated web-based system for real-time delivery of messages to affect cognitive representations concerning dietary lifestyle and to evaluate adherence and blood pressure in a diverse population. The major findings of these studies demonstrated compelling evidence of the efficacy of the WHEELS-I program in reducing blood pressure, enhancing DASH diet adherence, and shaping DASH diet cognitive representations in women at the point of treatment. Results were published in an anthology (Scisney-Matlock et al., 2015).

Scisney-Matlock's body of work is foundational for clinical implementation of effective hypertension management for women from diverse backgrounds.

Another program of research with a structure-oriented approach to the study of cognition is that of Karen Stein and her protégés, whose work in the area of self-schemas built on the work of psychologist Hazel Markus. Generally, the body of work produced by this set of scholars examined how the content and organization of these cognitive structures (self-schemas), which contain information about how one thinks about oneself, operated to affect one's choices and behavior in relation to specific health problems, such as anorexia or addiction (e.g., Stein, Corte, Chen, Nuliyalu, & Wing, 2013).

A research program on sense of belonging and depression was developed by Drs. Bonnie Hagerty and Reg Williams. Sense of belonging—which is the experience of personal involvement in a system or environment so that persons feel (i.e., understand) themselves to be an integral part of that system or environment (Hagerty, Lynch-Sauer, Patusky, Bouwsema, & Collier, 1992)—can be viewed as a cognitive structure derived from perceptions and somewhat akin to a self-schema. Hagerty developed a conceptual model of the concept and a related measure (e.g., Hagerty et al., 1992). In collaborations with Williams on studies of students, sense of belonging (or lack of it) was found to be more important than social support, conflict, and loneliness in predicting depressive symptoms (Hagerty & Williams, 1999).

In a subsequent series of studies of naval recruits, funded by the Department of Defense, this research team determined the cut-off scores on the Sense of Belonging scale for those "at risk" for stress and depression, leading to an intervention study (BOOT STRAP, an acronym for Boot Camp Survival Training for Navy Recruits—A Prescription). Results of the randomized controlled trial showed that recruits "at risk" for stress and depression significantly increased their sense of belonging, experienced less loneliness, used more problem-solving coping skills, and decreased insecure attachment by the end of recruit training, providing evidence that BOOT STRAP improved recruit functioning, strengthened training performance, and helped reduce attrition (Williams et al., 2004).

In follow-up studies that compared divisions, rather than at-risk recruits, these researchers found that the recruits in the division receiving the intervention developed significantly greater group cohesion, greater problem-solving skills, and better perceived social support while reporting less anger than the control group. Cost-effective analysis showed a potential net savings to the Navy of more than $17 million if fully adopted (e.g., Williams et al., 2007). Subsequent policy changes to Navy training plans included helping recruits manage and cope with stressful conditions for the betterment of young men and women in the Navy. In further work, this cognitive behavioral therapeutic approach was converted into an online format called Stress Gym that was tested as a follow-up on participants of their earlier studies. Stress Gym was evaluated positively by the participants for its user interface, content, feasibility, and satisfaction; evaluation was not influenced by rank/status, sex, or previous deployment. Stress ratings also decreased significantly while using the program. Stress Gym was feasible to deploy, accepted by the intended end users, and demonstrated the intended goal of reducing stress. Stress Gym was subsequently modified for application to military nurses and wounded enlisted with similarly positive outcomes. This body of work received significant media attention and resulted in a book on then-current research in depression (Williams, Hagerty, & Ketefian, 2005). Further, it provided a number of students with research training and publication experience (e.g., Bay, Hagerty, Williams, Kirsch, & Gillespie, 2005).

Research Programs Focused on Cognitive Processes

Several faculty developed programs of research that focused on a cognitive process. One example of such work is that of Dr. Bernadine Cimprich, whose interest was the basic cognitive process of directed attention. Specifically, Cimprich was interested in the effects of chemotherapy in women undergoing breast cancer treatment and the use of natural environments to restore attentional deficits caused by chemotherapy. Her work is covered elsewhere in this publication.

Another process-oriented program of research was that of Penny Pierce, whose focus was on decision making, a higher-order cognitive process. Using qualitative methods, she elaborated on the decision-making processes employed by women facing breast cancer treatment decisions (Pierce, 1993).

Effects of Cognitive Dysfunction on Human Functioning

Other faculty conducted work related to the impact of cognitive dysfunction on human behavior and functioning. The bulk of this research was focused on elders with dementia and conducted independently and interactively by Drs. Ann Whall and Donna Algase, along with a host of doctoral students (notably Drs. Elizabeth Beattie, Cynthia Beel-Bates, Yi-Chen Chiu, Hyo-Jung Kim, Junah Song, and Lan Yao), and postdoctoral fellows, notably Drs. Kathleen Colling, Gwi-Ryung Son Hong, and Ann Kolanowski, who themselves established related independent programs of research and scholarship.

Whall's independent work in this area concerned tardive dyskinesia (TD), a complication of neuroleptic medications often used in the management of individuals with dementia. Conducted in the 1980s, it predated establishment of cognition as an area of scholarly concentration in UMSN's doctoral program. Nonetheless, her work on early and correct identification of TD contributed to establishing a "pillar of excellence" within UMSN, according to then-dean Rhetaugh Dumas, and served as a foundation for the concentration as it emerged in the 1990s. Whall's paper also became a benchmark for the National Institute of Mental Health in its efforts to educate practitioners of the time (Whall, Engle,

Edwards, Bobel, & Haberland, 1983). Further, her extensive works in books and journal articles on nursing theory placed Whall in a foundational position within the curriculum of the doctoral program.

Following on in the area of dementia, in the late 1980s, Whall began early methodological work to examine another common care issue: aggressive behavior. Seeing the aggression of elders with dementia during care routines as a behavioral consequence of dementia placed her emerging work in this area squarely within UMSN's focus on cognition.

Algase joined UMSN in 1989 after completing an award-winning dissertation on the wandering behavior of people with dementia at Case Western Reserve University. Because studies of wandering were scarce and knowledge of it was limited, her independent program of research simultaneously advanced both method and theory. Foundational studies, completed with federal and foundation funding, and theoretical work were focused on measurement, description, and correlate identification, largely from the perspective of rhythm theory, explicating an association between wandering and the severity of cognitive impairment (e.g., Algase, Beattie, & Therrien, 2001). Through a series of peer-reviewed reference works and literature reviews (e.g., Algase, 1999), she developed the foundation for the establishment of wandering as a nursing diagnosis (North American Nursing Diagnosis Association, 2001).

Shortly thereafter, Algase was invited by Audrey Nelson, then director of the Patient Safety Center of Inquiry at the James A. Haley Veterans Hospital in Tampa, Florida, to help establish wandering as a field of inquiry at this veterans hospital. A productive collaboration was established that continued to refine definition, measurement, and correlate identification (e.g., Algase, Moore, Vandeweerd, & Gavin-Dreschnack, 2007), including an American Journal of Nursing award-winning book (Nelson & Algase, 2007). As of 2016, Algase continues to consult with the veterans hospital in their work on wandering.

The interactive work of Whall and Algase began in the mid-1990s, when Whall invited Algase and Dr. Cornelia Beck of the University of Arkansas for Medical Sciences to work jointly on developing a unified approach to the study of aggressive, vocal, and wandering behaviors of individuals with dementia. Aiming toward joint applications under NIH's Interactive Research Project Grant (IRPG) awards, they developed the need-driven, dementia-compromised behavior (NDB) model (Algase et al., 1996), which later served as the theoretical foundation for the only IRPG ever awarded by the National Institutes of Nursing and Aging. This work was widely cited and influential (for example, Donaldson, 2000); it posits that cognition, one of a group of background factors, directly influences wandering, aggression, and problematic vocalizations and that the relationship was mediated by dynamic personal and environmental factors (Algase et al., 1996). This relationship is supported for need-driven behaviors (e.g., Beck, Richards, Lambert, Doan, Landes, Whall, Algase, Kolanowski, & Feldman, 2011).

Much methodological (e.g., Algase, Yao, Son, et al., 2007), empirical (e.g., Algase, Antonakos, Beattie, Beel-Bates, & Yao, 2009), and theoretical work on need-driven behaviors (e.g., Algase, Yao, Beel-Bates, & Song, 2007) has been derived from the NDB model in the context of the IRPG studies. Secondary data analyses conducted by doctoral students have continued to expand knowledge derived from NDB studies (e.g., Jao, Algase, Specht, & Williams, 2015).

Postdoctoral fellows and doctoral students involved in IRPG projects of Algase and Whall at UMSN have had a national and an international impact. Of note nationally is Ann Kolanowski, whose work to mitigate NDB through interventions tailored to personality is exemplary. The leadership and collaborative efforts of Beattie, working within Australian infrastructures for dementia research and care across Australia, to advance quality of life initiatives in the care of affected elders is impressive (e.g., Beattie et al., 2015). Similarly, in Korea, Son Hong has adapted measurement of wandering and other concepts within the NDB model for use in Korea studies (e.g., Son, Song, & Lim, 2006) and, further, continues to examine culture and familiarity (a kind of cognitive structure) for its impact on wandering and agitation (Hong, 2011). Song has continued to examine wandering along with other dementia-related behaviors among Korean elders, including some intervention work based on the NDB model (e.g., Song, Lim, & Hong Son, 2008).

In addition to health problems dominantly cognitive in nature, such as the dementias, many other illnesses have implications for cognitive functioning. Faculty currently conducting work on cognition as it affects and is affected by illness include Drs. Susan Pressler and Cynthia Arslanian-Engoren, who are examining connections between congestive heart failure and cognitive impairment in elders without dementia. Their work is covered elsewhere in this book.

Conclusion

The study of cognitive function at UMSN has had a long and strong impact on its doctoral programs as well as on this field of study within the discipline of nursing and beyond. Involved scholars have developed impactful programs of research with national and international reach across an array of phenomena pertinent to cognition. While the body of work presented herein is extensive and impressive, it is not exhaustive of all research undertaken. Many doctoral students, scholars, and faculty members contributed to the development of these and other programs of prior and ongoing work that stretches well beyond the walls of UMSN.

References

Algase, D. L. (1999). Wandering in dementia. In J. J. Fitzpatrick (Ed.), *Annual Review of Nursing Research, 17* (pp. 185–217). New York, NY: Springer.

Algase, D. L., Antonakos, C., Beattie, E. R. A., Beel-Bates, C. A., & Yao, L. (2009). Empirical derivation and validation of a wandering typology. *Journal of the American Geriatrics Society, 57*(11), 2037–2045. PMID: 20121953

Algase, D. L., Beattie, E. R. A., & Therrien, B. (2001). Impact of cognitive impairment on wandering behavior. *Western Journal of Nursing Research, 23*, 283–295. PMID: 11291432

Algase, D. L., Beck, C., Kolanowski, A., Whall, A., Berent, S., Richards, K., & Beattie, E. (1996). Need-driven dementia-compromised behavior: An alternative view of disruptive behavior. *American Journal of Alzheimer's Disease, 11*, 10–19.

Algase, D. L., Moore, D. H., Vandeweerd, C., & Gavin-Dreschnack, D. J. (2007). Mapping the maze of terms and definitions in dementia-related wandering. *Aging & Mental Health, 11*, 686–698. PMID: 18074256

Algase, D., Yao, L., Beel-Bates, C. A., & Song, J. A. (2007). Theoretical models of wandering. In A. L. Nelson & D. L. Algase (Eds.), *Evidence-based protocols for managing wandering behaviors* (pp. 19–51). New York, NY: Springer.

Algase, D. L., Yao, L., Son, G. R., Beattie, E. R. A., Beck, C., & Whall, A. F. (2007). Initial psychometrics of the ambiance scale: A tool to study person-environment interaction in dementia. *Aging and Mental Health, 11*, 266–272. PMID: 17558577

Bay, E., Hagerty, B. K., Williams, R. A., Kirsch, N., & Gillespie, B. (2005). Chronic stress, salivary cortisol response, interpersonal relatedness, and depression among community dwelling survivors of traumatic brain injury. *Journal of Neuroscience in Nursing, 37*, 4–14.

Beattie, E., O'Reilly, M., Moyle, W., Chenoweth, L., Featherstonehaugh, D., Horner, B., . . . Fielding, E. (2015). Multiple perspectives on quality of life for residents with dementia in long-term care facilities: Protocol for a comprehensive Australian study. *International Psychogeriatrics, 27*(10), 1739–1747. doi:10.1017/S1041610215000435

Beck, C., Richards, K., Lambert, C., Doan, R., Landes, R., Whall, A., . . . Feldman, Z. (2011). Factors associated with problematic vocalizations in nursing home residents with dementia. *Gerontologist, 51*(3), 389–405. UI: 2129275210

Donaldson, S. K. (2000). Breakthroughs in scientific research: The discipline of nursing, 1960–1999. *Annual Review of Nursing Research, 18*, 247–311.

Hagerty, B. K., & Williams, R. A. (1999). The effects of sense of belonging, social support, conflict, and loneliness on depression. *Nursing Research, 48*(4), 215–219.

Hagerty, B. M., Lynch-Sauer, J., Patusky, K., Bouwsema, M., & Collier, P. (1992). Sense of belonging: A vital mental health concept. *Archives in Psychiatric Nursing, 6*, 172–177.

Hong, G. R. S. (2011). Effects of multisensory stimulation using familiarity: Persons with dementia in long-term care facility in Korea. *Journal of Korean Academy of Nursing, 41*(4), 528–538.

Jao, Y. L., Algase, D. L., Specht, J. K., & Williams, K. (2015). The association between characteristics of care environments and apathy in residents with dementia in long-term care facilities. *Gerontologist, 55*(Suppl. 1), S27–39.

Nelson, A. L., & Algase, D. L. (Eds.). (2007). *Evidence-based protocols for managing wandering behaviors.* New York, NY: Springer.

North American Nursing Diagnosis Association. (2001). *Nursing Diagnoses: Definitions and Classifications, 2001–2002.* Philadelphia, PA: Author.

Pierce, P. F. (1993). Deciding on breast cancer treatment: A description of decision behavior. *Nursing Research, 42*(1), 22–28.

Scisney-Matlock, M., Algase, D., Boehm, S., Coleman-Burns, P., Oakley, D., Rogers, A. E., . . . Yu, M. (2000). Measuring behavior: Electronic devices in nursing studies. *Applied Nursing Research, 13*(2), 97–102.

Scisney-Matlock, M., & Beard, M. (1999). Bootstrap methodology in validating accuracy of cognitive representations of hypertension scales. *Journal of Theory Construction & Testing, 3*(1), 20–24.

Scisney-Matlock, M., Brough, E., Daramola, O., Jones, M., Jones, L., & Holmes, S. (2015). A non-pharmacological approach to decrease unhealthy eating patterns and improve blood pressure in African Americans. In K. C. Ferdinand (Ed.), *Hypertension in high-risk African Americans: Current concepts, evidence-based therapeutics and future considerations* (pp. 35–58). New York, NY: Springer.

Scisney-Matlock, M., Kachorek, L., McClerking, C., & Glazewski, C. (2006). Development and evaluation of DASH diet tailored messages for hypertension treatment. *Applied Nursing Research, 19*, 78–87.

Scisney-Matlock, M., Makos, G., Saunders, T., Jackson, F., & Steigerwalt, S. (2004). Comparison of quality-of-hypertension-care indicators for groups treated by physician versus groups treated by physician-nurse team. *American Academy of Nurse Practitioners, 16*, 17–23.

Scisney-Matlock, M., & Watkins, K. (2003). Validity of the cognitive representations of hypertension scales. *Journal of Applied Social Psychology, 33*, 1–19.

Son, G.-R., Song, J., & Lim, Y. (2006). Translation and validation of the Revised-Algase Wandering Scale (community version) among Korean elders with dementia. *Aging & Mental Health, 10*(2), 143–150.

Song, J., Lim, Y. M., & Hong Son, G.-R. (2008). Wandering behavior in Korean elders with dementia residing in nursing homes. *Journal of Korean Academy of Nursing, 38*(1), 29–38.

Stein, K. F., Corte, C., Chen, D. G., Nuliyalu, U., & Wing, J. (2013). A randomized clinical trial of an identity intervention programme for women with eating disorders. *European Eating Disorders Review, 21*(2), 130–142.

Whall, A. L., Engle, V., Edwards, A., Bobel, L., & Haberland, C. (1983). Development of a screening program for tardive dyskinesia: Feasibility issues. *Nursing Research, 32*, 151–156.

Williams, R. A., Hagerty, B. M., Andrei, A.-C., Yousha, S. M., Hirth, R. A., & Hoyle, K. S. (2007). STARS: Strategies to assist Navy recruits' success. *Military Medicine, 72*, 942–949.

Williams, R. A., Hagerty, B., & Ketefian, S. (Eds.). (2005). *Depression research in nursing: Global perspectives.* New York, NY: Springer.

Williams, R. A., Hagerty, B. K., Yousha, S., Horrocks, J., Hoyle, K., & Liu, D. (2004). Psychosocial effects of the BOOT STRAP Intervention with Navy recruits. *Military Medicine, 169*, 814–820.

CHAPTER 4

Biobehavioral Research in Cancer Nursing

Laurel Northouse, PhD, RN, FAAN

Oncology nurse researchers in the biobehavioral concentration focused on cancer patients and their family caregivers. Their programs of research made important contributions to our understanding of problems experienced by cancer patients and their caregivers and ways to treat them. These programs in nursing research started in the mid-1980s at the University of Michigan School of Nursing (UMSN) when the cancer survivorship movement was just beginning. Nurse researchers focused on assessing survivors' cognitive function, addressing survivors' and caregivers quality of life (QOL), increasing their use of healthy behaviors, managing risk for cancers that run in families, and developing new alternative and complementary approaches to care. The sections below describe the research programs of six faculty members at UMSN in the biobehavioral concentration. The innovative interventions they developed, the new technologies they used, the areas they identified for future research, and the influence of their research on clinical practice have all made important contributions nationally and internationally.

Cancer Nursing

Cognitive Function and Attentional Fatigue

Dr. Bernadine Cimprich's scientific contributions since the early 1990s have focused on altered cognitive function associated with cancer diagnosis and treatment (Cimprich, 1992). In pioneering work, she contributed new knowledge about the intense mental demands in dealing with the diagnosis of breast cancer. These demands lead to early development of cognitive or attentional fatigue, with a measurable decrease in concentration, acquiring new information, or making decisions. She first demonstrated the efficacy of a theoretically based environmental intervention to counteract attentional fatigue and maintain and restore cognitive function in women with breast cancer. She extended her work using advanced technology with functional magnetic resonance imaging (fMRI) to better understand the development and sources of neurocognitive impairment as well as self-reported cognitive complaints in women treated with and without adjuvant chemotherapy for breast cancer. One of Cimprich's major contributions to the field is the development of the Attentional Fatigue Index. This was the first instrument developed to measure cancer patients' perceptions of attentional fatigue (Cimprich, Visovatti, & Ronis, 2011), and it has been used by many researchers in the United States and abroad to assess attentional fatigue in cancer and noncancer populations.

With funding from the National Institute of Nursing Research (NINR), Cimprich conducted a prospective randomized controlled trial (RCT) that tested the efficacy of a natural restorative environmental intervention that was designed to decrease attentional fatigue in women newly diagnosed with breast cancer. The intervention consisted of regular exposure to nature through activities such as gardening, sitting in a park, and bird watching. According to the Attention Restoration Theory, individuals who have limited attentional capacity can become fatigued under various conditions (such as dealing with the demands of breast cancer). Spending time in nature decreases demands on directed attention and can restore attentional capacity. Cimprich found that breast cancer patients who participated in the restorative environmental intervention for 120 minutes per week had significantly less attentional fatigue than women in the control condition. Those positive intervention effects persisted over the course of 1 year, regardless of the type of treatment women received (Cimprich & Ronis, 2003). Cimprich subsequently incorporated elements of this natural restorative intervention in another program for breast cancer survivors called Taking CHARGE (Cimprich et al., 2005).

Cimprich and her team were the first to use fMRI to assess attention and working memory in women treated for breast cancer (Cimprich et al., 2010; Reuter-Lorenz & Cimprich, 2013). In a prospective longitudinal study over the course of 1 year, her interdisciplinary team found that (a) pretreatment neural inefficiency in executive function was a better predictor of cognitive fatigue after treatment than exposure to chemotherapy (Askren et al., 2014) and that (b) worry is a significant contributor to neurocognitive dysfunction before any adjuvant treatment, and worry by itself may contribute to reports of "chemo brain" over the course of treatment (Berman et al., 2014).

Influence on clinical practice. Cimprich's program of research has influenced clinical practice in a number of ways. She has defined cognitive fatigue and cognitive decline in women with breast cancer, which was previously elusive or minimized by health professionals. Cimprich developed a measure that can assess attentional fatigue, and that measure is being used by others to assess cognitive problems with healthy and ill populations. She has extended patients' and professionals' understanding of "chemo brain," underscoring that factors prior to treatment can influence posttreatment cognitive function. She has also drawn attention to the important role of worry, not just adjuvant therapy, on cancer patients' cognitive function. She has provided an empirical foundation for others to study the benefits of restorative environments for improving cognitive function among various healthy and ill populations.

According to Cimprich, future research needs to delineate the sources of cognitive dysfunction in cancer. In particular, there is a need for research that develops pretreatment interventions that target deficits in cognitive performance, symptoms of worry and fatigue, and other sources of distress related to cognitive function in breast cancer survivors.

Quality of Life of Cancer Patients and Their Family Caregivers

Dr. Laurel Northouse's scientific contributions focus on describing and improving the quality of life of cancer patients and their family caregivers. Through a series of studies, Dr. Northouse was one of the first to report the high emotional distress reported by family caregivers of cancer patients and their need for information and support from nurses and other health professionals (Northouse & Swain, 1987). She documented the interdependence between patients' and their caregivers' emotional response to illness (Northouse, Templin, & Mood, 2001) and provided evidence across many studies that cancer patients and their family caregivers need to be treated together as the "unit of care" (Northouse, Williams, Given, & McCorkle, 2012).

Northouse was at the forefront of developing and testing programs of care for cancer patients and their family caregivers. She developed one of the first psychoeducational programs (FOCUS [which stands for the components of the program: family involvement, optimistic outlook, coping effectiveness, uncertainty reduction, and symptom management]) for women with recurrent breast cancer and their family caregivers, delivered to them jointly at home by a masters-prepared nurse. Findings from a large RCT indicated that patients and caregivers who received the FOCUS intervention had significantly better outcomes (e.g., less hopelessness, less negative appraisal of illness) than participants in the control condition (Northouse, Kershaw, Mood, & Schafenacker, 2005).

Subsequently, Northouse and colleagues adapted the FOCUS program for men with prostate cancer and their spouses/partners to determine the effects of the program on older adults who were managing a different type of cancer (Northouse et al., 2007), and they tested the modified program in a second large RCT. Significant intervention effects were found for prostate cancer patients and especially for their spouses, whose needs were seldom addressed by health professionals. Those who participated in the intervention reported less uncertainty, less hopelessness, more effective coping, higher self-efficacy, and better QOL.

In a third RCT, the effect of the FOCUS program was tested with patients with advanced lung, colorectal, prostate, or breast cancer and their caregivers. This study also examined (a) the effect of the intervention dose (i.e., three sessions versus six sessions) on outcomes and (b) whether the intervention outcomes differed for couples who were at high risk or low risk of distress (Northouse et al., 2013). Significant intervention effects were found for patients and their caregivers who participated in the FOCUS program, such as higher self-efficacy, more effective coping, and better QOL. Both doses of the intervention produced positive outcomes, and the intervention was effective for both high- and low-risk couples. Currently, the FOCUS program is being implemented in pilot effectiveness studies in Cancer Support Community agencies by social workers in three cities in the United States (Dockham et al., 2015)

Northouse collaborated with web designers at the University of Michigan to translate the nurse-delivered FOCUS program to a tailored, interactive web-based format that could reach more patients and their family caregivers, using fewer health care resources. This was one of the first psychoeducational, tailored, web-based dyadic interventions developed for cancer patients and their caregivers. Patients and caregivers who completed the program reported significant improvements in their benefits of illness (brought family closer together), self-efficacy, and QOL (Northouse et al., 2014). This innovative dyadic platform has become a model that is now being used by other researchers who are developing further web interventions for patients and caregivers.

Influence on clinical practice. Northouse's research has been used to develop professional guidelines for assessing and intervening with cancer patients and family caregivers. Her intervention programs and analysis of dyadic interventions (Northouse, Katapodi, Song, Zhang, & Mood, 2010) have been used by other researchers to guide intervention development with patients and caregivers. She has developed many educational materials for patients, caregivers, and professionals that are being distributed nationally and internationally by the National Cancer Institute's (NCI) Cancer Control P.L.A.N.E.T. and the Michigan Department of Community Health.

The FOCUS program and other psychoeducational programs need further testing with survivors and caregivers from more racially and socioeconomically diverse backgrounds. Future research also needs to examine the cost-effectiveness of these programs and determine if they can reduce health care costs (i.e., use of urgent care and hospitalizations).

Health Behavior Change in Cancer Patients

Since the 1990s, Dr. Sonia Duffy has developed a program of research on the science of health behavior change, primarily as it relates to the smoking behavior among cancer patients, veterans, inpatients, and healthy populations such as blue-collar workers. She was one of the first to report that health behaviors (i.e., smoking and sleep) affect cancer patients' biomarkers, such as IL-6, and have a significant effect on cancer recurrence and survival in cancer patients (Duffy et al., 2008)

One of Duffy's major contributions was the development of a nurse-administered intervention that focused on reducing smoking behavior, alcohol use, and depression in head and neck cancer patients (Veterans Affairs [VA] and funding from various foundations). This "bundled intervention" addressed multiple interrelated health behaviors in cancer patients (Duffy et al., 2006). Building on prior studies, Duffy became a leader in translational intervention research in smoking cessation. Although many studies documented the efficacy of smoking cessation programs, few programs were ever implemented in practice settings. Based on this work, she developed an innovative program called "Tobacco Tactics," which nurses delivered to VA inpatients to promote smoking cessation (Duffy, Karvonen-Gutierrez, Ewing, Smith, & Veterans Integrated Services Network 11 Tobacco Tactics, 2010). Following this study, she received a U01 grant to replicate this study in a larger number of hospitals outside of the VA (Duffy, Ronis, et al., 2012). In both studies, she found that the nurse-delivered Tobacco Tactics intervention significantly reduced smoking in the intervention hospitals, compared to no change in the control hospitals.

Even though Tobacco Tactics was successful in increasing smoking cessation rates and producing other positive health outcomes, Duffy realized that in order to extend the program's reach to other professionals and patients, this nurse-delivered program had to be translated to a web-based format. Using Blue Cross Blue Shield of Michigan Foundation and R21 grants, she developed a web-based version of Tobacco Tactics. The web program was supported by follow-up calls from nurses and chat rooms for outdoor workers and was tested among operating engineers (Duffy, Ronis, Waltje, & Choi, 2013). The intervention increased 30-day-quit rates in the experimental group, compared to the control group (Choi, Terrell, Pohl, Redman, & Duffy, 2013).

Noticing that these outdoor workers were at risk for melanoma due to sun exposure, Duffy developed the Sun Solutions intervention, which tested four interventions: education, education plus text message reminders, education plus mailed sunscreen, and education plus text reminders and mailed sunscreen. All four aims increased workers' sunscreen use, although those who received all four interventions improved the most (Lee et al., 2014).

Influence on clinical practice. Dr. Duffy's research has had a major influence on clinical practice. According to an editorial in *Cancer*, findings by Duffy et al. (2008) "help to validate inflammatory dysregulation as a contributor of head and neck cancer development and provide further support for biomarkers to enable clinicians to identify patients at high risk for recurrence of disease, or possibly even second primary tumors" (Leibowitz & Ferris, 2008). Duffy has published widely on the nurse-administered Tobacco Tactics intervention, which has been packaged into a toolkit to promote tobacco cessation among people with and without cancer. The Joint Commission has released new standards for treating inpatient smokers, and Duffy has exported the Tobacco Tactics intervention to many more hospitals outside of her studies. Her seminal research with bundling interventions documented their efficacy and cost-effectiveness, and her approach was recently supported by the 2009 NIH Conference on the Science of Behavior.

Since few comprehensive cancer centers provide smoking cessation to their patients, Duffy intends to do a multisite study to test different strategies to teach nurses in cancer centers to conduct tobacco cessation. Duffy is interested in moving the Tobacco Tactics intervention into the radiology setting. Since her work with operating engineers has shown that this population has many cancer-related risky behaviors (Duffy, Louzon, & Gritz,

2012), Duffy is continuing her work with smoking cessation and sun protection interventions with this population.

Hereditary Risk of Cancer in Families

Dr. Maria Katapodi's program of research focuses on cancer genetics and the management of hereditary cancer risk, including family communication and support, and their influence on decision making for genetic testing. Katapodi's research has broadened the management of hereditary cancer risk from focusing only on mutation carriers to include their high-risk relatives, who also need assistance to lower their cancer risk. She was one of the first researchers to explore the role of the family in the decision to use genetic testing for hereditary cancer. In a large community-based sample of cancer-free women, she found that 15% of the women had a family history indicative of increased risk for familial breast cancer. However, most of these high-risk women underestimated their breast cancer risk and did not follow recommended screening guidelines (Katapodi, Dodd, Lee, & Facione, 2009). An important contribution of Katapodi's research is determining the influence of the family environment on high-risk women and their relatives' decision to pursue genetic testing for hereditary breast and ovarian cancer (Katapodi, Munro, Pierce, & Williams, 2011; Katapodi, Northouse, Milliron, Liu, & Merajver, 2013; Katapodi, Northouse, et al., 2011).

With funding from the Robert Wood Johnson Foundation (RWJF), Katapodi developed one of the first communication-and-support interventions for families that carry a BRCA1 or BRCA2 mutation, predisposing them to the development of hereditary breast cancer. The intervention has four modules: knowledge of breast cancer genetics, managing the decisions about genetic testing, increasing adaptive coping, and increasing family communication about genetic test results. The intervention content was reviewed by focus groups of women at genetic risk of developing cancer and was extremely well received by those women because the intervention addresses a significant gap in current health care services (Katapodi, Northouse, Milliron, & Schafenacker, 2012).

Next, with funding from the Centers for Disease Control and Prevention, Katapodi conducted one of the largest state-wide cancer prevention and dissemination initiatives in Michigan. A large randomized controlled trial (RCT) was used to test the efficacy of two versions of a printed educational intervention (tailored vs. nontailored) designed to improve screening and genetic counseling among breast cancer survivors with a high suspicion of hereditary disease and their high-risk relatives. An innovative aspect of this RCT was that it used a public health approach to recruit a population-based random sample of 3,000 young women with breast cancer and their at-risk female relatives using Michigan's Cancer Registry (Katapodi, Northouse, Schafenacker, et al., 2013). Findings indicate that women and their family members at high risk for hereditary breast and ovarian cancer underuse cancer genetic services (genetic counseling and genetic testing) (Katapodi et al.,

2014). This is especially evident among African American breast cancer survivors (Jones, Katapodi, & Lockhart, 2015). Findings also have shown that women who are diagnosed with breast cancer at a young age do not necessarily perceive adequate family support, which in turn hinders family communication about hereditary cancer, risk factors, and cancer genetics (Katapodi et al., 2014).

To be able to provide the communication-and-support intervention originally developed as part of the RWJF funding to women carrying a BRCA1 or BRCA2 mutation and their high-risk relatives, Katapodi is testing the delivery of the Family Gene Toolkit. This is a web-based decision and family communication support intervention designed to be delivered by an advanced practice nurse with expertise in psycho-oncology and a genetic counselor.

Implications for clinical practice. Katapodi's pioneering research in cancer genetics has not only drawn attention to hereditary cancer in cancer patients but also extended the research to address the information and support needs of their high-risk relatives. Her research also supports a tailored approach to risk stratification and disease management, with an emphasis on the prevention of hereditary cancer syndromes among high-risk, cancer-free individuals.

There are a number of areas pertaining to women with hereditary cancer and their high-risk relatives that need further research. Katapodi is focusing on cascade screening in family members of known mutation carriers who have an increased risk for hereditary breast and colon cancer. Her goal is to advance public health genomics by integrating clinical and public health research methods for the benefit cancer patients and their family members.

Chemotherapy-Induced Peripheral Neuropathy

Dr. Ellen Lavoie Smith's scientific contributions focus on chemotherapy-induced peripheral neuropathy (CIPN), a common and painful condition associated with neurotoxic chemotherapy. Through a series of studies, Dr. Lavoie Smith discovered new ways to identify those at highest risk and to assess and treat this troubling chemotherapy-induced condition in adults and children. Smith has conducted extensive research to refine and develop new methods for assessing CIPN. She revised the Total Neuropathy Score (TNS) and developed two shorter versions (2- and 5-item) of the scale for use in busy oncology clinics (Lavoie Smith, Cohen, Pett, & Beck, 2011; Smith, Cohen, Pett, & Beck, 2010). She also made important contributions to pediatric clinical practice by establishing psychometrically strong approaches for assessing CIPN in children, which did not exist previously (Lavoie Smith, Li, et al., 2013), as well as documenting the psychometric properties of other instruments such as the EORTC-CIPN-20 (Lavoie Smith, Barton, et al., 2013).

Smith extended her research to determine which individuals are at higher risk than others for developing chronic CIPN-associated pain. She collaborated with an interdisciplinary team to explore if a physiologic and biobehavioral phenotype could predict who is more likely to develop CIPN following treatment for breast cancer. Smith's unique and important contribution in this area has been to discover ways to quantify the phenotype. Further, Smith collaborated with a second multidisciplinary team to identify pharmacogenetic predictors of vincristine-induced CIPN in children with leukemia. This is an extremely important line of research that will provide greater understanding of CIPN and chronic pain mechanisms.

Dr. Smith has devoted a significant amount of her research career to discovering new treatments for painful CIPN. She felt a sense of urgency to identify a treatment for this painful, life-altering condition, as none yet existed. She conducted landmark intervention studies that examined various pharmacologic interventions for CIPN. In the first study, she pilot-tested an evidence-based CIPN treatment algorithm and found preliminary evidence that the algorithm might be effective in reducing CIPN pain while improving patient function and satisfaction (Lavoie Smith et al., 2009; Smith et al., 2011). Subsequently, Smith conducted a national, multisite, placebo-controlled trial funded by the NCI that tested the effect of duloxetine as a treatment for CIPN. This study made an enormous contribution to the field because it provided evidence that duloxetine was effective in decreasing CIPN pain severity and improving functional capacity and quality of life in cancer patients (Smith et al., 2013).

In an attempt to translate research findings into practice, Smith obtained funding to pilot-test a web-based electronic platform for obtaining reliable and valid data about patients' CIPN and pain severity that can be integrated into the electronic medical record in the future. This cutting-edge research will determine whether the On Q platform can foster patient and provider engagement in the CIPN assessment as well as provider adherence to quality care standards—namely, CIPN symptom assessment and CIPN-associated pain management. Smith has also conducted pilot studies to determine if similar web-based platforms could engage patients and families in symptom assessment (Lavoie Smith et al., 2012; Skalla, Smith, Li, & Gates, 2013).

Influence on clinical practice. Smith's research has had an important impact on clinical practice in several ways. She has developed psychometrically sound assessment scales for CIPN that are brief and easy to use in clinical settings with adults and children. She has also discovered the first treatment for CIPN (duloxetine), which, according to NCI publications, is a "practice-changing" discovery. It is the only treatment for CIPN recommended for clinical practice by the *Journal of Clinical Oncology*, the official publication of the American Society of Clinical Oncology. This treatment is now available to treat painful, debilitating CIPN in cancer patients worldwide.

While duloxetine is the only drug with demonstrated efficacy for painful CIPN, it does not work for everyone. Further research is needed to test multimodality treatments that could result in more people experiencing a greater degree of relief from chronic and debilitating painful CIPN than is currently possible when using duloxetine alone. Additional research is needed to clarify the mechanisms associated with high-risk CIPN and to develop targeted interventions to prevent or ameliorate the devastating consequences experienced by children and adults.

Nonhormonal, Alternative, and Complementary Treatments for Managing Symptoms

Dr. Deborah Barton's contributions to science focus on symptoms resulting from cancer diagnosis and treatments and innovative ways to manage them. She has studied interventions for a number of symptoms including fatigue, hot flashes, peripheral neuropathy, sleep problems, cognitive changes, and sexual problems commonly experienced by cancer patients. A major contribution of Dr. Barton's research is the use of nonhormonal interventions and other alternative or complementary strategies to manage cancer patients' symptoms. Barton and colleagues have also spearheaded new methods to assess and reduce hot flashes, and those methods are now being used by many investigators in the United States and abroad (Barton & Loprinzi, 2004; Loprinzi et al., 2008). Her research also has made important contributions to our understanding of the underlying physiology of hot flashes (Loprinzi & Barton, 2009; Shanafelt, Barton, Adjei, & Loprinzi, 2002).

Barton began evaluating nonhormonal options, namely Vitamin E, to treat hot flashes and other menopausal symptoms because many breast cancer patients could not use estrogen, the standard treatment for hot flashes. In an early study, she found that breast cancer patients who received Vitamin E had a significant but marginal reduction in their hot flashes compared to a placebo-control group (Barton et al., 1998). This research led to numerous other studies with various nonhormonal agents; some suggested serotonin might be an important mechanism related to hot flash occurrence.

Barton continued to conduct randomized, double-blind trials to test the effect of nonhormonal treatments to manage hot flashes in women with breast cancer. In a large study, she evaluated the effects of citalopram (an antidepressant) versus a placebo to treat hot flashes in postmenopausal women, who had at least 14 bothersome hot flashes per week (Barton et al., 2010). Patients who received citalopram reported significantly less hot flashes. It documented that citalopram was an effective, well-tolerated intervention for managing hot flashes.

Barton extended her intervention research to several other symptoms (fatigue, cognition, sleep, chemotherapy-induced peripheral neuropathy, nausea and vomiting, and sexual health), examining a number of agents and, more recently, behavioral interventions. To date, she has completed 12 large multisite intervention trials and numerous phase II trials, which, collectively, have made important contributions to oncology symptom science; evaluated the effectiveness of dietary and herbal supplements to manage symptoms (Barton et al., 2011); and added credibility to this area of scientific inquiry (Barton & Bauer-Wu, 2009; Barton et al., 2006).

Barton's more recent intervention work has focused on three areas: (a) improving breast cancer patients' sexual health and their problems related to vaginal atrophy, libido, and self-image by developing a multicomponent intervention; (b) determining that American ginseng can have a positive effect on cancer-related fatigue (Barton et al., 2013); and (c) testing a topical treatment for chemotherapy-induced peripheral neuropathy without causing side effects.

Influence on clinical practice. Barton's research has had a major impact on clinical practice. She was part of the team that first demonstrated that nonhormonal treatments could effectively treat hot flashes in breast cancer patients who are not able to use standard estrogen treatments. This research has led to a better understanding of possible underlying mechanisms, such as serotonin depletion that affects hot flashes. She has also demonstrated that both pharmacological treatments (citalopram) and some herbal treatments (American ginseng) can be used effectively to treat cancer-related symptoms. Barton's studies have been mentioned in clinical practice guidelines for three distinct symptoms: chemotherapy-induced peripheral neuropathy, hot flashes, and fatigue.

In the future, Barton will continue to conduct innovative and cutting-edge research that will focus on finding new agents and alternative treatments to manage cancer-related symptoms. She plans to evaluate hypnosis as a mind-body intervention for improving sexual health and fatigue. She will also be examining the physiologic etiologies associated with various symptoms and then developing multicomponent interventions to address the complexities underlying symptom development and expression.

Synthesis

Faculty members in the biobehavioral concentration at UMSN have made significant contributions to cancer nursing research and to the well-being of cancer patients and their family caregivers. There are a number of characteristics that are evident within and across the six programs of research described that are summarized in this chapter.

Addressing Significant Clinical Problems

Researchers in the biobehavioral concentration addressed clinically important problems. Three of the researchers focused on symptom assessment and management in areas pertaining to cognitive function and attentional fatigue, peripheral neuropathy, and hot flashes. Cancer patients were now living longer due to new chemotherapy regimens, and they were reporting many troubling symptoms and side effects that were interfering with their quality of life. UMSN researchers examined the underlying mechanisms of these symptoms, developed new instruments for assessing them, and developed traditional and nontraditional interventions to help cancer patients manage them more effectively.

Researchers also focused on patients' social context and examined the effect that the illness had on their family members, especially those who assumed the role of primary caregiver. As chemotherapy administration moved from inpatient to outpatient settings, the demands of family caregivers grew exponentially as they were expected to help patients cope with the toxic effects of treatment, the physical changes associated with the disease, as well as the emotional turmoil that accompanied the illness. UMSN researchers assessed family members' needs, identified those at higher risk of having more problems over time, and developed interventions to address their patients' and caregivers' concerns and to help both groups maintain their quality of life. Furthermore, as the field of human genetics and hereditary cancers emerged, UMSN faculty conducted research that assessed those family members who were at a greater risk of developing hereditary cancer. They developed interventions that educated them about hereditary cancer and ways to cope with their increased risk.

UMSN scientists are at the forefront of examining health behaviors in cancer patients. They developed programs to promote smoking cessation, to increase sun protection, and to promote other cancer prevention programs that will increase survivors' well-being and length of survival.

Progress Through Systematic Research

A common characteristic of the programs of research is that they all developed in a systematic manner, often building on years of clinical experience, which leads to the identification of key clinical problems. For the most part, researchers' doctoral dissertation and studies helped launch the direction and content of their ongoing programs of research. Typically, researchers conducted descriptive studies to learn more about the clinical problem and then conducted exploratory studies to identify risk factors that helped or exacerbated the problem. Based on knowledge obtained from these preliminary studies, researchers developed interventions and tested the efficacy of the interventions to improved outcomes in randomized clinical trials. If the interventions were effective, they moved to research dissemination. From the programs described, it is clear that they were orderly, strategically planned, and carried out in a sound scientific manner.

It is also important to note that each researcher obtained sizeable external funding to conduct her program of research. Due to the scope of the problems that they were addressing, and the importance of the interventions they were developing, an essential element of their successful programs of research was seeking and successfully obtaining sufficient external funding. The large amount of research funding that they obtained further attests to the high quality of their research programs.

Developing Innovative Interventions

It is noteworthy that all the programs of research described in this chapter developed interventions to address the clinical problems they identified in prior research. The interventions were all innovative. For example, the theory on directed attention was used to develop an environmental intervention to restore cognitive function in breast cancer patients. A new pharmaceutical intervention was used to treat peripheral neuropathy in many patients. Web-based interventions were developed to increase quality of life in cancer patients and their family caregivers, as well as to promote smoking cessation for cancer patients. Finally, alternative treatments, such as hypnosis, were used to manage symptoms and side effects of cancer treatments. Each intervention was innovative and utilized new ways to address pressing clinical problems. Even more remarkable, all the programs described in the biobehavioral area have had significant practice-changing effects.

References

Askren, M. K., Jung, M., Berman, M. G., Zhang, M., Therrien, B., Peltier, S., . . . Cimprich, B. (2014). Neuromarkers of fatigue and cognitive complaints following chemotherapy for breast cancer: A prospective fMRI investigation. *Breast Cancer Research and Treatment, 147*(2), 445–455. doi:10.1007/s10549-014-3092-6

Barton, D. L., Atherton, P. J., Bauer, B. A., Moore, D. F., Jr., Mattar, B. I., Lavasseur, B. I., . . . Loprinzi, C. L. (2011). The use of Valeriana officinalis (Valerian) in improving sleep in patients who are undergoing treatment for cancer: A phase III randomized, placebo-controlled, double-blind study (NCCTG Trial, N01C5). *Journal of Supportive Oncology, 9*(1), 24–31. doi:10.1016/j.suponc.2010.12.008

Barton, D., & Bauer-Wu, S. (2009). The emerging discipline of integrative oncology. *Oncology (Williston Park), 23*(11 Suppl. Nurse Ed.), 46–49.

Barton, D. L., LaVasseur, B. I., Sloan, J. A., Stawis, A. N., Flynn, K. A., Dyar, M., . . . Loprinzi, C. L. (2010). Phase III, placebo-controlled trial of three doses of citalopram for the treatment of hot flashes: NCCTG trial N05C9. *Journal of Clinical Oncology, 28*(20), 3278–3283. doi:10.1200/JCO.2009.26.6379

Barton, D. L., Liu, H., Dakhil, S. R., Linquist, B., Sloan, J. A., Nichols, C. R., . . . Loprinzi, C. L. (2013). Wisconsin Ginseng (Panax quinquefolius) to improve cancer-related fatigue: A randomized, double-blind trial, N07C2. *Journal of the National Cancer Institute, 105*(16), 1230–1238. doi:10.1093/jnci/djt181

Barton, D., & Loprinzi, C. L. (2004). Making sense of the evidence regarding nonhormonal treatments for hot flashes. *Clinical Journal of Oncology Nursing, 8*(1), 39–42. doi:10.1188/04.CJON.39-42

Barton, D. L., Loprinzi, C., Jatoi, A., Vincent, A., Limburg, P., Bauer, B., . . . Sloan, J. (2006). Can complementary and alternative medicine clinical cancer research be successfully accomplished? The Mayo Clinic-North Central Cancer Treatment Group experience. *Journal of the Society of Integrative Oncology, 4*(4), 143–152.

Barton, D. L., Loprinzi, C. L., Quella, S. K., Sloan, J. A., Veeder, M. H., Egner, J. R., . . . Novotny, P. (1998). Prospective evaluation of vitamin E for hot flashes in breast cancer survivors. *Journal of Clinical Oncology, 16*(2), 495–500.

Berman, M. G., Askren, M. K., Jung, M., Therrien, B., Peltier, S., Noll, D. C., . . . Cimprich, B. (2014). Pretreatment worry and neurocognitive responses in women with breast cancer. *Health Psychology, 33*(3), 222–231. doi:10.1037/a0033425

Choi, S. H., Terrell, J. E., Pohl, J. M., Redman, R. W., & Duffy, S. A. (2013). Factors associated with sleep quality among operating engineers. *Journal of Community Health, 38*(3), 597–602. doi:10.1007/s10900-013-9656-2

Cimprich, B. (1992). Attentional fatigue following breast cancer surgery. *Research in Nursing and Health, 15*(3), 199–207.

Cimprich, B., Janz, N. K., Northouse, L., Wren, P. A., Given, B., & Given, C. W. (2005). Taking CHARGE: A self-management program for women following breast cancer treatment. *Psycho-Oncology, 14*(9), 704–717. doi:10.1002/pon.891

Cimprich, B., Reuter-Lorenz, P., Nelson, J., Clark, P. M., Therrien, B., Normolle, D., . . . Welsh, R. C. (2010). Prechemotherapy alterations in brain function in women with breast cancer. *Journal of Clinical and Experimental Neuropsychology, 32*(3), 324–331. doi:10.1080/13803390903032537

Cimprich, B., & Ronis, D. L. (2003). An environmental intervention to restore attention in women with newly diagnosed breast cancer. *Cancer Nursing, 26*(4), 284–292; quiz 293–284.

Cimprich, B., Visovatti, M., & Ronis, D. L. (2011). The Attentional Function Index—a self-report cognitive measure. *Psycho-Oncology, 20*(2), 194–202. doi:10.1002/pon.1729

Dockham, B., Schafenacker, A., Yoon, H., Ronis, D., Kershaw, T., Titler, M., & Northouse, L. (2015). Implementation of a psycho-educational program for cancer survivors and family caregivers at a Cancer Support Community Affiliate: A pilot effectiveness study. *Cancer Nursing.* doi:10.1097/NCC.0000000000000311

Duffy, S. A., Karvonen-Gutierrez, C. A., Ewing, L. A., Smith, P. M., & Veterans Integrated Services Network 11 Tobacco Tactics, Team. (2010). Implementation of the Tobacco Tactics program in the Department of Veterans Affairs. *Journal of General Internal Medicine, 25*(Suppl. 1), 3–10. doi:10.1007/s11606-009-1075-9

Duffy, S. A., Louzon, S. A., & Gritz, E. R. (2012). Why do cancer patients smoke and what can providers do about it? *Community Oncology, 9*(11), 344–352. doi:10.1016/j.cmonc.2012.10.003

Duffy, S. A., Ronis, D. L., Titler, M. G., Blow, F. C., Jordan, N., Thomas, P. L., . . . Waltje, A. H. (2012). Dissemination of the nurse-administered Tobacco Tactics intervention versus usual care in six Trinity community hospitals: Study protocol for a comparative effectiveness trial. *Trials, 13*, 125. doi:10.1186/1745-6215-13-125

Duffy, S. A., Ronis, D. L., Valenstein, M., Lambert, M. T., Fowler, K. E., Gregory, L., . . . Terrell, J. E. (2006). A tailored smoking, alcohol, and depression intervention for head and neck cancer patients. *Cancer Epidemiology, Biomarkers & Prevention, 15*(11), 2203–2208. doi:10.1158/1055-9965.EPI-05-0880

Duffy, S. A., Ronis, D. L., Waltje, A. H., & Choi, S. H. (2013). Protocol of a randomized controlled trial of sun protection interventions for operating engineers. *BMC Public Health, 13*, 273. doi:10.1186/1471-2458-13-273

Duffy, S. A., Taylor, J. M., Terrell, J. E., Islam, M., Li, Y., Fowler, K. E., . . . Teknos, T. N. (2008). Interleukin-6 predicts recurrence and survival among head and neck cancer patients. *Cancer, 113*(4), 750–757. doi:10.1002/cncr.23615

Jones, T. P., Katapodi, M. C., & Lockhart, J. S. (2015). Factors influencing breast cancer screening and risk assessment among young African American women: An integrative review of the literature. *Journal of the American Association of Nurse Practitioners, 27*(9), 521–529. doi:10.1002/2327-6924.12223

Katapodi, M. C., Dodd, M. J., Lee, K. A., & Facione, N. C. (2009). Underestimation of breast cancer risk: Influence on screening behavior. *Oncology Nursing Forum, 36*(3), 306–314. doi:10.1188/09.ONF.306-314

Katapodi, M. C., Munro, M. L., Pierce, P. F., & Williams, R. A. (2011). Psychometric testing of the decisional conflict scale: Genetic testing hereditary breast and ovarian cancer. *Nursing Research, 60*(6), 368–377. doi:10.1097/NNR.0b013e3182337dad

Katapodi, M. C., Northouse, L. L., Merajver, S., Duquette, D., Milliron, K. J., Mendelsohn-Victor, K. M., . . . Janz, N. K. (November 2014). *Family support and knowledge of breast cancer genetics in families at increased risk for breast cancer.* Paper presented at the International Society of Nurses in Genomics, Annual Congress, November 7–9, Scottsdale, Arizona.

Katapodi, M. C., Northouse, L. L., Milliron, K. J., Liu, G., & Merajver, S. D. (2013). Individual and family characteristics associated with BRCA1/2 genetic testing in high-risk families. *Psycho-Oncology, 22*(6), 1336–1343. doi:10.1002/pon.3139

Katapodi, M. C., Northouse, L. L., Milliron, K. J., & Schafenacker, A. M. (November 2012). *Development of a family-communication and decision-support intervention for women that carry a BRCA1 or BRCA2 mutation and their high-risk relatives.* Paper presented at the Oncology Nursing Society Connections: Advancing Care Through Science Conference, November 16–18, Phoenix, Arizona.

Katapodi, M. C., Northouse, L., Pierce, P., Milliron, K. J., Liu, G., & Merajver, S. D. (2011). Differences between women who pursued genetic testing for hereditary breast and ovarian cancer and their at-risk relatives who did not. *Oncology Nursing Forum, 38*(5), 572–581. doi:10.1188/11.ONF.572-581

Katapodi, M. C., Northouse, L. L., Schafenacker, A. M., Duquette, D., Duffy, S. A., Ronis, D. L., . . . Copeland, G. (2013). Using a state cancer registry to recruit young breast cancer survivors and high-risk relatives:

Protocol of a randomized trial testing the efficacy of a targeted versus a tailored intervention to increase breast cancer screening. *BMC Cancer, 13,* 97. doi:10.1186/1471-2407-13-97

Lavoie Smith, E. M., Bakitas, M. A., Homel, P., Fadul, C., Meyer, L., Skalla, K., & Bookbinder, M. (2009). Using quality improvement methodology to improve neuropathic pain screening and assessment in patients with cancer. *Journal of Cancer Education, 24*(2), 135–140. doi:10.1080/08858190902854715

Lavoie Smith, E. M., Barton, D. L., Qin, R., Steen, P. D., Aaronson, N. K., & Loprinzi, C. L. (2013). Assessing patient-reported peripheral neuropathy: The reliability and validity of the European Organization for Research and Treatment of Cancer QLQ-CIPN20 Questionnaire. *Quality of Life Research, 22*(10), 2787–2799. doi:10.1007/s11136-013-0379-8

Lavoie Smith, E. M., Cohen, J. A., Pett, M. A., & Beck, S. L. (2011). The validity of neuropathy and neuropathic pain measures in patients with cancer receiving taxanes and platinums. *Oncology Nursing Forum, 38*(2), 133–142. doi:10.1188/11.ONF.133-142

Lavoie Smith, E. M., Li, L., Hutchinson, R. J., Ho, R., Burnette, W. B., Wells, E., . . . Renbarger, J. (2013). Measuring vincristine-induced peripheral neuropathy in children with acute lymphoblastic leukemia. *Cancer Nursing, 36*(5), E49–60. doi:10.1097/NCC.0b013e318299ad23

Lavoie Smith, E. M., Skalla, K., Li, Z., Onega, T., Rhoda, J., Gates, C., . . . Scott, M. R. (2012). Assessing cancer survivors' needs using web-based technology: A pilot study. *Computers, Informatics, Nursing, 30*(2), 71–81. doi:10.1097/NCN.0b013e318246042e

Lee, C., Duffy, S. A., Louzon, S. A., Waltje, A. H., Ronis, D. L., Redman, R. W., & Kao, T. S. (2014). The impact of Sun Solutions educational interventions on select health belief model constructs. *Workplace Health and Safety, 62*(2), 70–79.

Leibowitz, M. S., & Ferris, R. L. (2008). Recurrence in head and neck squamous cell carcinoma [Editorial]. *Cancer, 113*(4), 671–673. doi:10.1002/cncr.23616

Loprinzi, C. L., & Barton, D. L. (2009). On hot flash mechanism, measurement, and treatment. *Menopause, 16*(4), 621–623. doi:10.1097/gme.0b013e3181a85107

Loprinzi, C. L., Barton, D. L., Sloan, J. A., Novotny, P. J., Dakhil, S. R., Verdirame, J. D., . . . Christensen, B. (2008). Mayo Clinic and North Central Cancer Treatment Group hot flash studies: A 20-year experience. *Menopause, 15*(4 Pt 1), 655–660. doi:10.1097/gme.0b013e3181679150

Northouse, L. L., Katapodi, M. C., Song, L., Zhang, L., & Mood, D. W. (2010). Interventions with family caregivers of cancer patients: Meta-analysis of randomized trials. *CA: A Cancer Journal for Clinicians, 60*(5), 317–339. doi:10.3322/caac.20081

Northouse, L., Kershaw, T., Mood, D., & Schafenacker, A. (2005). Effects of a family intervention on the quality of life of women with recurrent breast cancer and their family caregivers. *Psycho-Oncology, 14*(6), 478–491. doi:10.1002/pon.871

Northouse, L. L., Mood, D. W., Schafenacker, A., Kalemkerian, G., Zalupski, M., LoRusso, P., . . . Kershaw, T. (2013). Randomized clinical trial of a brief and extensive dyadic intervention for advanced cancer patients and their family caregivers. *Psycho-Oncology, 22*(3), 555–563. doi:10.1002/pon.3036

Northouse, L. L., Mood, D. W., Schafenacker, A., Montie, J. E., Sandler, H. M., Forman, J. D., . . . Kershaw, T. (2007). Randomized clinical trial of a family intervention for prostate cancer patients and their spouses. *Cancer, 110*(12), 2809–2818. doi:10.1002/cncr.23114

Northouse, L., Schafenacker, A., Barr, K. L., Katapodi, M., Yoon, H., Brittain, K., . . . An, L. (2014). A tailored web-based psychoeducational intervention for cancer patients and their family caregivers. *Cancer Nursing, 37*(5), 321–330. doi:10.1097/NCC.0000000000000159

Northouse, L. L., & Swain, M. A. (1987). Adjustment of patients and husbands to the initial impact of breast cancer. *Nursing Research, 36*(4), 221–225.

Northouse, L., Templin, T., & Mood, D. (2001). Couples' adjustment to breast disease during the first year following diagnosis. *Journal of Behavioral Medicine, 24*(2), 115–136.

Northouse, L., Williams, A. L., Given, B., & McCorkle, R. (2012). Psychosocial care for family caregivers of patients with cancer. *Journal of Clinical Oncology, 30*(11), 1227–1234. doi:10.1200/JCO.2011.39.5798

Reuter-Lorenz, P. A., & Cimprich, B. (2013). Cognitive function and breast cancer: Promise and potential insights from functional brain imaging. *Breast Cancer Research and Treatment, 137*(1), 33–43. doi:10.1007/s10549-012-2266-3

Shanafelt, T. D., Barton, D. L., Adjei, A. A., & Loprinzi, C. L. (2002). Pathophysiology and treatment of hot flashes. *Mayo Clinic Proceedings, 77*(11), 1207–1218. doi:10.4065/77.11.1207

Skalla, K. A., Smith, E. M., Li, Z., & Gates, C. (2013). Multidimensional needs of caregivers for patients with cancer. *Clinical Journal of Oncology Nursing, 17*(5), 500–506. doi:10.1188/13.CJON.17-05AP

Smith, E. M., Bakitas, M. A., Homel, P., Piehl, M., Kingman, L., Fadul, C. E., & Bookbinder, M. (2011). Preliminary assessment of a neuropathic pain treatment and referral algorithm for patients with cancer. *Journal of Pain and Symptom Management, 42*(6), 822–838. doi:10.1016/j.jpainsymman.2011.03.017

Smith, E. M., Cohen, J. A., Pett, M. A., & Beck, S. L. (2010). The reliability and validity of a modified total neuropathy score-reduced and neuropathic pain severity items when used to measure chemotherapy-induced peripheral neuropathy in patients receiving taxanes and platinums. *Cancer Nursing, 33*(3), 173–183. doi:10.1097/NCC.0b013e3181c989a3

Smith, E. M., Pang, H., Cirrincione, C., Fleishman, S., Paskett, E. D., Ahles, T., . . . Alliance for Clinical Trials in Oncology. (2013). Effect of duloxetine on pain, function, and quality of life among patients with chemotherapy-induced painful peripheral neuropathy: A randomized clinical trial. *JAMA, 309*(13), 1359–1367. doi:10.1001/jama.2013.2813.

Building a Healthy Nation Through Nursing Science

Advancing the Science of Health Promotion for Children, Adolescents, and Their Families

Carol Loveland-Cherry, PhD, RN, FAAN
Nola J. Pender, PhD, RN, FAAN

Advancing the science of health promotion and translating science to clinical practice is essential to address health disparities and create a culture of health in the United States and globally. Scientists at the University of Michigan School of Nursing (UMSN) have made important contributions to emerging knowledge about promoting the health of children, adolescents, and families. In this chapter, we describe the organizational structures undergirding these scientific contributions and the investigative work of specific UMSN faculty, doctoral graduates, and postdoctoral fellows.

Organizing Structures for Advancing the Science of Health Promotion

Educational Initiatives

Evolution of academic structural changes. Historically, the administrative academic units within UMSN were organized into traditional clinical areas, whereby acute and chronic care of individuals were central considerations in the programs. Development of research foci in the PhD program preceded and guided a restructuring of the academic units that resulted in three subunits within the newly created Division of Health Promotion and Risk Reduction (HPRR): (a) Parent/Child Nursing/Pediatric Nurse Practitioner; (b) Community Health Nursing/Occupational Health, Adult Nurse Practitioner, Family Nurse Practitioner; (c) and Women's Health/Nurse Midwifery. Dr. Jean Goeppinger was the first director of HPRR. She was succeeded by Dr. Carol Loveland-Cherry as division director, followed by Dr. Kristy Martyn. The creation of the Child/Adolescent Health Behavior Research Center in 1991 was a catalyst for bringing together a group of faculty, doctoral students, and postdoctoral fellows with similar research interests and supporting their growing body of work. As the focus in health care shifted to a greater emphasis on health promotion and risk reduction, a parallel shift was evident in research at the UMSN, especially in community health, pediatrics, women's health, and obstetrical nursing.

Doctoral and postdoctoral education. The growing cadre of faculty conducting HPRR research externally funded by the National Institutes of Health (NIH) and other agencies and organizations provided the basis for the development of a T32 research training grant. Dr. Shaké Ketefian was the principal investigator (PI) on the first T32 and several competing renewals for support of doctoral and postdoctoral training. Loveland-Cherry, in collaboration with Dr. Caroline Sampselle and other HPRR faculty, was responsible for conceptualizing the T32 competing renewals within an HPRR framework; Loveland-Cherry subsequently assumed the PI role on the grant, and with each renewal, the T32's focus continued to be on HPRR but was updated to include new knowledge and new faculty. Funding continued for a period of 21 years and supported four predoctoral students and four postdoctoral fellows for each of those years. The HPRR nursing concentration enabled students to develop an in-depth understanding of health promotion and risk reduction interventions. Courses examined conceptual and methodological issues in health behavior; empirical research, and theory related to the study of families in health and illness; behavioral analysis in health and illness; interventions directed to health promotion with regard to individuals, families, and aggregates; community-level health, stress, and coping processes; physical activity across the life-span; and parenting across the life-span, including interrelationships among parenting, environment, health, family demographics, and sociocultural/technological developments that influence parenting roles. The nurse scientists who were supported in part by the HPRR T32 have continued to conduct cutting-edge research and function in faculty and leadership roles. The works of several of the nurse scientists who were supported by the HPRR T32 are presented in this chapter (Youngblut, Villarruel, Kinter, Robbins), along with descriptions of the works of former faculty members Drs. Loveland-Cherry, Pender, and Martyn.

Research Initiatives

Health promotion as a major research emphasis. For centuries, community health nurses have been at the forefront of encouraging proper sanitation, good nutrition, prenatal care, well-child care, and prevention of epidemics. However, only in the 1980s and onward has attention been given to developing the behavioral sciences undergirding health counseling, behavior change, and adoption of healthy lifestyles. As people lived longer, the incidence of chronic illness and related disabilities increased, thus compromising quality of life and work productivity. The need to keep people healthy throughout the life-span became a major public health issue. Further, the cost of health care grew exponentially, bringing attention to gaps in science that needed to be addressed to decrease health disparities, create a healthier society, and lower health care costs. The Division of HPRR took leadership in organizing a cadre of scientists with a commitment to building nursing knowledge about health across the life-span and the science for effective health promotion interventions.

Child/Adolescent Health Behavior Research Center (CAHBRC). The faculty in HPRR was committed to not only developing the science of health promotion and prevention of illness but also providing doctoral students and postdoctoral fellows with an ongoing mentoring and support structure for research training. Faculty collaborated to submit a proposal to NIH for an exploratory center grant. An exploratory center grant provides the infrastructure for faculty and students alike to collaborate in a focused area of research. In 1991, UMSN was funded for 3 years (P20 NR02962-01) by the National Institute of Nursing Research (NINR) for the Child/Adolescent Health Behavior Research Center (CAHBRC) to conduct research and develop knowledge about promoting the health of children, adolescents, and their families. Dr. Nola Pender served as principal investigator/center director and Loveland-Cherry served as codirector. The center incorporated the research efforts of multiple faculty to achieve synergy and optimize the impact of their respective scientific investigations. Research studies in the center focused on sexual health, preventing substance abuse, promoting physical activity, and understanding the mechanisms of eating disorders in adolescents.

Center activities included regular meetings to develop research ideas, discuss issues in the design and conduct of research, assist with proposal development, provide statistical assistance, review manuscripts prior to submission, and arrange press coverage of ongoing research. The center integrated doctoral students and postdoctoral fellows into ongoing activities, providing valuable mentoring and research training. Pilot work at CAHBRC resulted in a number of intervention studies that were subsequently funded by NIH.

Contributions to the Science of Health Promotion

School- and Family-Based Interventions for Alcohol/Drug Abuse Prevention, Dr. Carol Loveland-Cherry

As a community health nurse, Loveland-Cherry worked in community settings, including family homes; well-child, prenatal, and immunization clinics; and schools to promote the health and well-being of infants, children, adolescents, and their families. Her practice emphasized the importance of health promotion, and she became acutely aware of the limited empirical knowledge base for health promotion and risk reduction with these populations. Her master's in public health expanded her practice perspective within a community context, but it did not fill the need for a stronger theoretical and empirical base. Consequently, she decided to pursue a PhD at Wayne State University College of Nursing to begin her research career. Her dissertation, *Health Promotion in Single-Parent and Two-Parent Families with School-Age Children*, was supported by a grant from Sigma Theta Tau International.

Early in her career, Loveland-Cherry recognized the importance and value of building strong, collaborative working relationships. This lesson was reinforced in her research career and fostered the development of important relationships with colleagues. While in the PhD program, she was fortunate to meet and work with Mary Horan. As they were both completing their PhD programs, they discovered a shared interest in health promotion in childbearing and child-rearing families. They were funded by an R01 from NINR and NIH for a study of preterm infants and their families. After completing her PhD, Loveland-Cherry assumed a faculty position at Wayne State University College of Nursing and then moved to a faculty position at UMSN. Dr. Joanne Youngblut, at the time a doctoral student at UMSN, joined the project as a research assistant. Her strong neonatal intensive care unit (NICU) clinical experience added to the expertise of the research team. Her dissertation research was a secondary analysis of data from this R01 and served as the foundation for her highly productive research career.

Loveland-Cherry's research focus shifted back to her original interest of health promotion and risk reduction in families with school-age children. Based on her research with children and their families in the community, Dr. Ted Dielman, a faculty member in postgraduate medicine at the University of Michigan, invited her to work with him as he expanded his program of research on school-based interventions to reduce alcohol risk and use in adolescents to include a family component. They worked together until his retirement, after which Loveland-Cherry served as the PI for the ongoing research. The research included two randomized controlled trials (RCTs) supported by R01 grants from the National Institute on Drug Abuse and the National Institute on Alcohol Abuse and Alcoholism.

When Dr. Antonia Villarruel joined the UMSN faculty, she was well into her program of research focused on health promotion and risk reduction in the area of sexual health in Mexican American adolescents and wanted to include a family intervention component. Loveland-Cherry joined her research team and worked with Villarruel to expand her program of research with a family intervention that brought together components from her research and components and experience from Loveland-Cherry's family-focused research. The work was funded by NINR and resulted in a second grant that moved the family component to a computer-based format. Villarruel's work is presented later in this section.

Contributions to science. Loveland-Cherry's research and scholarship in health promotion and risk reduction included some of the early RCTs in nursing that focused on families in communities as a locus for intervention. The findings demonstrated the viability of changing individual behaviors through changing family beliefs and capabilities (Loveland-Cherry, Kaufman, & Ross, 1999). The instrumentation and theory-based intervention strategies developed in her work with families have served as models for work by other researchers, both nationally and internationally.

Loveland-Cherry's research and scholarship in health promotion and risk reduction had major implications for academic programs in HPRR, for doctoral and postdoctoral studies, and for the research training of students and fellows. Ketefian was the PI for several of the initial T32s funded by NINR, as part of her role as director of doctoral and post-doctoral studies. The role of PI then devolved to Loveland-Cherry, who transformed the training grant to focus on health promotion and risk reduction. She chaired or cochaired 30 dissertations focused on health promotion and prevention.

Promoting the Health of Families With Critically Ill Children, Dr. Joanne M. Youngblut

Youngblut's program of research is focused on critically ill children and their families after the child's hospital discharge or death to identify family members at risk for adverse physical and mental/emotional health and dysfunction of the parent dyad and the family system. These data provided the foundation for tailored interventions to promote health and decrease risk for adverse parent, child, and family outcomes. She has been the PI of four NINR-funded R01s (two with multiple principal investigator Brooten) and a research subproject funded by the National Institute of General Medical Sciences through a program for minority-serving institutions. Most studies of parents experiencing a child's death have focused on cancer. Youngblut extended research to ICU deaths and included grandparents (NR R01 009120).

Impact of a child's ICU death on family members. Research findings identified the effects on parents and grandparents of a child's death in a neonatal or pediatric intensive care unit (NICU/PICU) (Youngblut & Brooten, 2013; Youngblut, Brooten, Blais, Kilgore, & Yoo, 2015; Youngblut, Brooten, Cantwell, del Moral, & Totapally, 2013). Youngblut's and Brooten's current study (NR R01 012675) focuses on children's responses to the death of a sibling in the NICU/PICU, the emergency department, or at the scene. Hispanic, Black non-Hispanic, and White non-Hispanic school-age children and adolescents throughout Florida are being recruited. Data on grief, depression, anxiety, and relationships with parents, siblings, and friends will be collected from all eligible children in a family.

Effects of children's critical illness and PICU hospitalization on parents. Youngblut and Jay (1991) found that parents were most concerned about the child's survival and potential future disabilities. Fathers' concerns about the child and parenting increased as the illness severity increased (Youngblut & Shiao, 1992). After discharge, the longer the child's hospital stay, the more satisfied fathers were with their families. The longer the child was intubated, the less satisfied mothers were with their families and the less cohesive they perceived their families to be (Youngblut & Shiao, 1993). Compared to parents after a child's general care unit (GCU) hospitalization, PICU parents rated family relationships as less satisfying and less cohesive (Youngblut & Lauzon, 1995). In a study of preschool children hospitalized for head trauma and their families (NR R01 04430), mothers had more stress if their child was in the PICU versus the GCU. Mother-father couples rated their child's injury severity similarly, but mothers had more stress than fathers (Youngblut,

Brooten, & Kuluz, 2005). Parents' perceptions of their child's injury severity were negatively related to quality of family functioning at 2 weeks postdischarge (Youngblut & Brooten, 2006) and to mothers' mental health at 3 months after discharge (Youngblut & Brooten, 2008). Mothers with greater stress and poorer mental health during their child's hospitalization might be at risk for negative mother-child and family outcomes.

Effects of maternal employment on child outcomes pre-welfare reform. Youngblut conducted one of the first studies of maternal employment effects for preterm infants (F31 NR 06152) in two-parent families (as part of a larger study [Youngblut, Loveland-Cherry, & Horan, R01 NR 01390, 1986–1989]) and later studied preschoolers born preterm in female-headed, single-parent families (R01 NR 02707). In the study of preterm infants in two-parent families, child development outcomes were the same for preterm infants with employed mothers and those with nonemployed mothers (Youngblut, Loveland-Cherry, & Horan, 1993). In a study of preschoolers in female-headed, single-parent families (66% African American, 75% nonemployed), the preschoolers' outcomes were better if their single mothers were employed (Youngblut, Brooten, Singer, Standing, Lee, & Rodgers, 2001). Employed single mothers provided a more enriching home environment and had more positive attitudes about their preschoolers than nonemployed single mothers (Youngblut, Singer, Madigan, Swegart, & Rodgers, 1998).

Contributions to science. Youngblut's highly productive program of research has created new knowledge about the impact of the NICU and PICU experience on the parents, siblings, and extended family of children who are critically ill. She has investigated how parents and other family members respond to the death of a child in these care settings. Her research findings have resulted in more effective support systems for stressed and bereaved families. Further, her research on the effects of maternal employment on child outcomes was highlighted in television and print media. Her work influenced legislation by addressing concerns about the impact that welfare reform provisions would have on children and about the availability of sufficient alternate child care arrangements.

Physical Activity Among Children and Adolescents, Dr. Nola Pender

Since the 1970s, Pender's scholarly work has focused on developing and testing the health promotion model (HPM) as a theoretical framework for understanding motivation for healthy behaviors. Empirical evidence indicates that positive health practices increase quality of life, prevent illness, and minimize health care costs. Her early research in health promotion was funded by the American Association of Fitness in Business (AAFB) and Signature Corporation, a subsidiary of Montgomery Ward. At four major companies in Chicago, she evaluated the effects of a corporate fitness program on state-trait anxiety, job-related strain, absenteeism, and work productivity. The results indicated that absenteeism was significantly lower and productivity significantly higher with the fitness center members compared to nonmembers, who reported no differences in anxiety or job-related strain (Pender, Smith, & Vernof, 1987).

In 1985, Pender was funded by the newly founded National Center for Nursing Research (P01NR01121) for a research program grant (Pender, Sechrist, Stromborg, & Walker, 1987) that included four large-scale studies to test the power of the HPM to explain motivation for health-promoting behaviors among young working adults (N. Pender), community-dwelling older adults (S. Walker), cardiac rehabilitation patients (K. Sechrist), and cancer patients in remission from their disease (M. Stromborg). Five years of funding resulted in extensive testing of the original HPM and revisions of the model to further increase its explanatory power. Valid and reliable instruments in English and Spanish to measure model variables were designed. Multiple research publications resulted (Pender, Walker, Stomborg, & Sechrist, 1990).

At the University of Michigan, Pender and her colleagues were funded by NINR for 3 years (1 P20 NR02962-01) to establish the CAHBRC, which focused on the development of knowledge about promoting the health of children, adolescents, and their families. With center funding for her individual project, Pender developed HPM-based instruments to measure physical activity in preadolescents and adolescents as a basis for application of the model to these populations. Her research team conducted qualitative research in multiple schools with multiethnic students, using the HPM as a framework to understand perspectives on physical activity among adolescent girls. Based on these data, HPM-based instruments were developed and used to explore beliefs about physical activity and how the transition from elementary school to junior high school changed physical activity beliefs and behaviors of adolescent girls (Garcia, Pender, Antonakos, & Ronis, 1998). International colleagues at the University of Michigan tested the HPM in Korean and Thai populations (Shin, Yun, Pender, & Jang, 2005; Wu & Pender, 2001). The HPM had adequate explanatory and predictive power for levels of physical activity among adolescent girls to suggest its usefulness in developing physical activity interventions.

Pender was funded by the Robert Wood Johnson Foundation to develop and test a computer-based physical activity counseling intervention for adolescent girls called "Girls on the Move." This was a collaborative effort with the University of Michigan Center for Health Communications Research directed by Dr. Victor Strecher. The latest computer technology was used to individualize the health behavior counseling program. A large data bank of tailored messages was used to provide individualized assessments and interventions for adolescent girls. This computerized program was designed for use by school nurse practitioners and nurse practitioners in primary care as part of an overall counseling program to increase physical activity among adolescent girls. The feasibility study indicated that the program was attractive to the girls, but parental involvement had to be increased to address parents' perception of physical activity as a waste of time and their discouragement of physical activity. Based on these findings, the program was modified to increase its impact.

Dr. Lorraine Robbins is testing the modified intervention in a large-scale project that is being funded from 2011 until 2017.

Contributions to science. The HPM as a framework for behavioral counseling to promote healthy lifestyles among adolescents and adults has been tested nationally and internationally in descriptive and intervention research. Hundreds of articles cite the HPM as the framework for their research. HPM-based research and clinical instruments have been translated into multiple languages. Clinicians have used the HPM to structure health promotion counseling in multiple settings. The University of Michigan maintains an active HPM website to disseminate information and instruments related to the model. Pender's contributions to theory development are recognized nationally and internationally by her inclusion in the Fuld Institute for Technology in Nursing Education video series, "Nursing Theorists: Portraits of Excellence."

Interventions to Promote Physical Activity Among Children and Adolescents in Diverse Populations, Dr. Lorraine Robbins

Lorraine Robbins began her productive research career with a 2-year predoctoral award (T32 NR07073) and a postdoctoral award (F32 NR007509) from NINR to explore cognitive and affective responses of adolescent boys and girls to physical activity as well as their physical activity behaviors. Her research clarified definitions of physical activity variables, illuminated gender differences in perceptions of physical activity, underscored the low level of physical activity among adolescents and its link to obesity while also demonstrating the importance of personalized approaches to addressing the problem (Robbins, Pender, & Kazanis, 2003; Robbins, Pender, Ronis, & Kazanis, 2004).

Subsequently, she was coinvestigator with Pender on a study funded by the Robert Wood Johnson Foundation to develop and test a computer-based physical activity counseling program for adolescent girls. This intervention was based on the HPM and was one of the early studies of computerized interventions for health promotion. Robbins collaborated in designing the intervention with the University of Michigan Center for Health Communications Research. Recognizing her early research contributions and her potential to emerge as a leading nurse scientist in physical activity research, Robbins received the UMSN Award for New Investigators.

Upon completion of her postdoctoral work, Robbins joined the College of Nursing faculty at Michigan State University. Continuing her research momentum, she was funded by NIH for an ongoing program of research to test the feasibility (R21HL090705) and the efficacy (R01HL109101) of "Girls on the Move," a multicomponent, school-based physical activity counseling and behavior change intervention. She integrated the HPM with motivational interviewing to create a roadmap for counselors to follow in personally encouraging adolescents to increase their physical activity. She trained numerous health professionals in nursing, public health, education, and other disciplines across Michigan to use the intervention. This ongoing research program includes 1,500 underserved urban girls in grades five through eight and provides them with an opportunity to engage in various physical activity programs to promote their health and well-being. This research has resulted in many collaborative publications (Robbins, Sikorskii, Hamel, Wu, & Wilbur, 2009; Robbins, Talley, Wu, & Wilbur, 2010).

Robbins's research has contributed to the science of process evaluation in physical activity counseling programs and knowledge about strategies for maintaining the fidelity of physical activity counseling interventions in school and community settings (Wu, Robbins, & Hsieh, 2011). Through her research, Robbins is committed to reducing health disparities and promoting child, adolescent, and family health and positive behavior change. Her ultimate goal is to significantly impact public health policy and decrease the problem of childhood and adolescent obesity, a precursor to many of the chronic health problems that children and adults experience (Vanden Bosch, Robbins, Pfieffer, Kazanis, & Maier, 2014).

Robbins collaborates with the Healthy Schools Initiative Committee for the Lansing School District to work on transforming school policies to promote child and adolescent health. She brings the accumulating knowledge gained from her research directly to the public to improve the quality of the lives of children and families.

She coauthored one of the first reviews of the state of the science of physical activity interventions and reports her research on health promotion nationally and internationally. She keynoted the first International Conference on Research in Health Promotion and Disease Prevention in Barranquilla, Colombia, and presented health promotion workshops for faculty and students at Simón Bolívar University.

Contributions to science. Robbins's research has changed approaches to promoting physical activity among adolescents in Michigan, and her work has influenced school-based programs in other states. She has contributed to decreasing health disparities across ethnic and racial groups by decreasing obesity among adolescents. The theory-based counseling road map and tools she provides to multiple professionals working with adolescents greatly enhance their effectiveness as health promotion counselors. Her use of adolescent-friendly technologies as part of her interventions augments her impact on the health of the nation's youth. The frequent invitations Robbins receives to present her work at national and international conferences attest to the broad impact of her research.

Interventions to Reduce Sexual Risk Among Adolescents From Diverse Populations, Dr. Kristy Kiel Martyn

As a faculty member at UMSN from 1999 to 2013, Martyn developed and evaluated the first clinical intervention event history calendar (EHC). This EHC was designed to reduce adolescent sexual risk and improve person-centered assessment of sexual risk and subsequent communication by health care providers (Martyn & Hutchinson, 2001; Martyn

& Belli, 2002). EHC methods were originally developed at UM by researchers at the Institute for Social Research (ISR). Dr. Deborah Oakley introduced Martyn to scientists at ISR when she came to UMSN as a new PhD graduate in 1999. This collaboration with ISR scientists resulted in the development of a clinical EHC intervention for adolescents (Martyn, Reifsnider, & Murray, 2006).

Martyn's adolescent EHC intervention research was funded by NIH/NIMH (R34 MH082644) and NIH/NINR (P30 NR009000), the latter as part of a center grant headed by Sampselle. With this funding at the University of Michigan, she evaluated further the adolescent sexual risk EHC and conducted an RCT. This RCT showed improved adolescent-provider assessment and communication (Martyn et al., 2013) and increased adolescent awareness of sexual risk behaviors and intentions to use condoms in the intervention group. This investigative work was conducted with a collaborative team of researchers at the University of Michigan including Drs. Cindy Darling-Fisher, Antonia Villarruel, David Ronis, Michelle Pardee, and Michelle Munro.

Further funding provided the opportunity for Martyn to apply the EHC internationally within the Sexual Risk Assessment Project and the Mexico Adolescent HIV Risk Intervention Project, both headed by Villarruel. Application of the EHC methodology to an internationally diverse group of adolescents expanded the cross-cultural dimension of her work. This research resulted in an important international publication on patient-centered communication and health assessment with youth (Martyn et al., 2013). The EHC uses a retrospective approach and relies on personal cues to enhance recall of specific life events. In research with Black, Latina, and White females aged 15–19, the participants reported that the EHC accurately reflected their health history information and could be highly useful in personalized interventions to decrease sexual risk and promote adolescent sexual and reproductive health. The EHC helps provider and patients work together to recognize repetitive patterns of nonproductive and risky behavior (Martyn & Faleer, 2013). The 2013 SAGE Research Methods Case publication (Martyn & Faleer, 2013) provided a description of her adolescent event history calendar and expanded application of this important research methodology beyond traditional uses with populations for demographic studies and mental health research.

Contributions to science. Martyn's EHC research has influenced the research of colleagues at the University of Michigan, including PhD students (e.g., Saftner, Gultekin), postdoctoral fellows (e.g., Danford), faculty (e.g., Darling-Fisher, Pardee, Kao, Brush), and interdisciplinary colleagues in the United States and globally. Clinical researchers at the University of Groningen in the Netherlands have adapted the EHC to explore the mental health of adolescents. Further, the EHC has been applied in Canada and Korea to explore other health-promoting behaviors of diverse populations.

Martyn has improved the health of adolescents and their families through fostering thoughtful decisions regarding sexual health and sexual behavior. Reflection on past memories of sexual behavior and resulting outcomes can help adolescents make better decisions that support sexual health in adolescence and adulthood. In 2014, her work with adolescents was recognized by appointment to the Independence Chair in Nursing at Emory School of Nursing.

Reducing Sexual Risk Among Mexican and Latino Adolescents, Dr. Antonia Villarruel

Villarruel's program of research focuses on the development, testing, dissemination, and scale-up of interventions designed to reduce sexual risk behavior among Latino and Mexican youth. Studies include RCTs to test *¡Cuídate!* (Take Care of Yourself), an adolescent behavioral intervention in the United States and Mexico, and the efficacy of *¡Cuídalos!* (Take Care of Them), a parent-adolescent communication intervention in the United States, Mexico, and Puerto Rico, using a small-group format and web-based/computer-based formats. Ecodevelopmental theory, theory of reasoned action/planned behavior, and cognitive social theory served as the basis for the interventions. Scale-up and dissemination of efficacious interventions have incorporated the use of technology, specifically virtual environments and web-based applications.

Adolescent studies. These studies examine the efficacy of a behavioral intervention to reduce sexual risk behavior among Latino adolescents (Villarruel, Jemmott, & Jemmott, 2006). *¡Cuídate!* is a cultural- and theory-based HIV sexual risk reduction program designed for Latino youth. It incorporates cultural beliefs that are common among Mexican, Puerto Rican, and Latino subgroups that abstinence and condom use are culturally accepted and effective ways to prevent unwanted pregnancy and sexually transmitted diseases, including HIV/AIDS. In an RCT in Philadelphia, Pennsylvania, adolescents recruited from community and school settings were randomly assigned to a 6-hour sexual risk reduction intervention or a health promotion control intervention. Data were collected preintervention; postintervention; and at 3-, 6-, and 12-month follow-ups. Adolescents in the intervention group were less likely to report sexual intercourse, multiple partners, or days of unprotected intercourse and more likely to report consistent use of condoms. Attitudes, norms, and control beliefs mediated the intervention effects on sexual behavior and condom use intentions. In an RCT in Monterrey, Mexico (Gallegos, Villarruel, Loveland-Cherry, Ronis, & Zhou, 2008), adolescents (n = 829) 14 to 17 years of age and one of their parents (n = 791) were recruited from schools and communities and randomly assigned to a sexual risk reduction intervention or a general health promotion control condition. Data were collected preintervention; postintervention; and at 3- (adolescents only), 6-, and 12-month follow-ups with 83%–97% retention rates. Adolescents in the sexual risk reduction intervention group were more likely to be older at first sex, use contraception at first sex, and use condoms at first sex than those in the general health promotion control group.

Parent studies. In the study in Monterrey, parents in ¡*Cuídalos!* received an intervention focused on sexual risk communication with their adolescents. Results indicated more general communication, sexual risk communication, and comfort with communication than those in the control group. Prevention beliefs, reaction beliefs, and communication efficacy mediated the effect of the intervention on general communication, sexual communication, and comfort with sexual communication. Familialism mediated intervention effects on all communication outcomes. Parent reports of parent-child sexual risk communication were shown to mediate the effect of the intervention on adolescents' intentions to use condoms (Villarruel, Loveland-Cherry, Gallegos Cabriales, Ronis, & Zhou, 2008).

The small-group intervention was converted to a computer-based format for parents with limited education and low literacy. Spanish-speaking parents and adolescents were recruited from community-based organizations and schools in Detroit, Michigan, and randomly assigned to the intervention group or a 3-month wait list control group. For parents in the computer-based intervention group, general communication and sexual risk communication were increased at the 3-month follow-up and were higher as compared to the wait list control group at the 3-month follow-up. Attitudes, perceived behavioral control, and intentions to communicate with adolescents about sex and contraceptives and condoms were higher in the intervention group. Results from these studies formed the basis of a current RCT to test a web-based version of ¡*Cuídalos!* with Puerto Rican parents.

Contributions to science. ¡*Cuídate!* is recognized as an effective evidence-based program by the Centers for Disease Control and Prevention and the Office of Adolescent Health (a division of the Department of Health and Human Services). It is part of a group of interventions that must be used in conjunction with federal funding. More than 30 States and Puerto Rico are implementing the program, providing evidence of the value of Villarruel's intervention research. Her work was part of the body of evidence that changed federal policy from an abstinence-only approach to a safer sex approach. This program of research is one of the few that has focused on Latino families, providing evidence-based programs to families and communities to reduce sexual risk behavior and promote adolescent health and well-being.

Promoting Competent Self-Care and Health in Children With Asthma, Dr. Eileen Kintner

Asthma is the most common chronic, life-threatening childhood condition affecting more than 9 million children in the United States. Half of these children have experienced acute exacerbation of asthma symptoms in the last year. Using an ecological approach and lifespan development perspective, Kintner has conducted qualitative and quantitative studies to explore and address the multiple factors that impact asthma control, quality of life, and use of health care services.

Her early work was funded at UMSN by an institutional postdoctoral fellowship from the NINR (T32). She explored student reasoning about asthma, worked on refining her theoretical thinking, and further developed and refined instrumentation to measure asthma-related variables. Her research activities are focused on improving the health and self-care of diverse populations of intercity youth with asthma who are of lower socio-economic status and medically underserved. For more than two decades, Kintner and her colleagues have evaluated and refined the acceptance of asthma model (AAM) for school-age children and early adolescents. Qualitative investigations enriched the science undergirding the model, and subsequent quantitative studies have tested the psychometric properties of eight instruments to measure model variables (Kintner & Sikorskii, 2008).

Kintner led an interdisciplinary research team of health care professionals, school personnel, and community partners in the development, implementation, and evaluation of school-based asthma education programs based on the AAM. These efforts culminated in development of the theory-guided, evidence-based asthma health education and counseling program for older school-age students with asthma and members of their social networks titled Staying Health-Asthma Responsible and Prepared (SHARP). The program is integrated into existing school curricula focused on healthy lungs for life. SHARP has a school-based component and a community component, including a sibling program. Kintner was funded by NIH (in collaboration with NINR and three other institutes) to conduct an intervention study of the feasibility of SHARP as a school- and community-based intervention. Her findings established the feasibility of SHARP with students, caregivers, siblings, school personnel, and community partners demonstrating willingness, readiness, and the ability to fully implement the program. Further, improvements occurred in student knowledge of asthma, reasoning abilities for management of acute episodes, episode management behaviors, use of effective risk reduction, and acceptance and taking control of asthma compared to a usual care control group. These effects were stable over a 12-month period (Kintner & Sikorskii, 2009).

The successful feasibility study was followed by NIH funding for a 6-year, large-scale randomized, longitudinal clinical trial titled, Comparison of Asthma Programs for Schools (CAPS). When CAPS students were compared to a control group that received a well-established nonacademic asthma education program, Open Airways for Schools (OAS), students in the SHARP program demonstrated statistically significant increased levels of knowledge and reasoning about symptom management, increased openness to sharing and learning about their condition, and increased vigilance and taking control. In addition, there were statistically significant decreases in the severity of asthma and increased levels of undisturbed sleep and participation in life activities (Kintner, Cook, & Lewis, 2012; Kintner et al., 2015). The SHARP program can be disseminated widely to diverse school settings to decrease health disparities among vulnerable groups.

Contributions to science. Kintner's research funding has supported doctoral and master students' work and contributed to the development of a strong health promotion and risk reduction training program at all levels of the curriculum at her university. She led the way in developing academics-based programs for the control of asthma in young school-age children. By mainstreaming information about asthma, children become more knowledgeable about asthma, and those with asthma become more assertive in taking control of their asthma and its effect on their sleep and activities. Additionally, peers are able to provide more support during acute episodes.

National and International Impact of Scientific and Theoretical Work

UMSN faculty, doctoral program graduates, and postdoctoral fellows have made major contributions to the science of health promotion for children, adolescents, and their families. Not only have they clarified the nature of health promotion behaviors, but they have contributed to the development of important theoretical perspectives and methods in health promotion research. Theories of health behavior such as the HPM and new methods for exploring health behaviors such as the EHC are the results of their empirical work. Further, UMSN scientists have developed evidence-based interventions to address pressing adolescent health problems. For example, Loveland-Cherry developed school- and family-based interventions to prevent substance use and abuse among children and adolescents; Youngblut developed interventions to promote the health of families with a critically ill child or following a child's death; Pender and Robbins developed computerized counseling interventions to increase physical activity and combat adolescent obesity; Villarruel, Martyn, and Loveland-Cherry developed widely disseminated interventions to reduce risky sexual behaviors in adolescents from diverse populations; and Kintner developed interventions to promote optimal self-care among children with asthma from low socioeconomic populations. Major federal investment in UMSN-driven research and both national and global dissemination of the theories, methods, instruments, and interventions of UMSN nurse scientists attests to the major impact that their work has had in promoting the health of underserved and low socioeconomic populations.

Future Research to Promote the Health of Children, Adolescents, and Their Families

The impact of UMSN-based health promotion research to date is impressive, but there is much left to be done. The studies reported in this chapter examined health promotion in ethnically, racially, and economic diverse groups of children and adolescents and offered culturally appropriate, evidence-based interventions. A next step is wide dissemination of these interventions in family-, school-, and community-based programs and evaluation of their sustainability and impact on health policies; health disparities; community environments; and family, child, and adolescent behaviors. There is also a need for descriptive research and intervention studies for displaced families, families experiencing major life changes, refugee families, and LGBT families. Establishing the efficacy and effectiveness of interventions for these groups will continue to advance the science of health promotion for children, adolescents, and their families both in the United States and globally.

References

Gallegos, E. C., Villarruel, A. M., Loveland-Cherry, C., Ronis, D. L., & Zhou, Y. (2008). Intervention to reduce sexual risk behavior in adolescents. Results of a randomized control trial. *Salud Publica de Mexico, 50*, 1–10.

Garcia, A. W., Pender, N. J., Antonakos, C. L., & Ronis, D. L. (1998). Changes in physical activity beliefs and behaviors of boys and girls across the transition to junior high school. *Journal of Adolescent Health, 22*(5), 394–402.

Kintner, E. K., Cook, G. D., & Lewis, K. (2012). Feasibility and benefits of a school-based academic and counseling program for older school-age students with asthma. *Research in Nursing and Allied Health, 35*(5), 507–517. Advance online publication. doi:10.1002/nur.21490

Kintner, E. K., Cook, G., Marti, C. N., Allen, A., Stoddard, D., Harmon, P., . . . Van Egeren, L. A. (2015). Effectiveness of a school- and community-based academic asthma health education program on use of effective asthma self-care behaviors in older school age students. *Journal for Specialists in Pediatric Nursing, 20*(1), 62–75, doi:10.1111/jspn.12099

Kintner, E. K., & Sikorskii, A. (2008). Reliability and construct validity of the Participation in Life Activities Scale for children and adolescents with asthma: An instrument evaluation study. *Health and Quality of Life Outcomes, 6*(43), 1–10. doi:10.1186/1477-7525-6-4

Kintner, E. K., & Sikorskii, A. (2009). Randomized clinical trial of a school-based academic and counseling program for older school-age students with asthma. *Nursing Research, 58*(5), 321–331. doi:10.1097/NNR.0b013e3181b4b60e

Loveland-Cherry, C. J., Kaufman, S. R., & Ross, L. T. (1999). Effects of a family intervention to decrease adolescent alcohol use and misuse. *Journal of Studies in Alcoholism* (Suppl. 13), 94–102.

Martyn, K. K., & Belli, R. F. (2002). Retrospective data collection using event history calendars. *Nursing Research, 51*, 270–274.

Martyn, K. K., & Faleer, H. E. (2013). Event History Calendar: Adolescent sexual risk research and clinical use. In *Sage research cases*. London: SAGE Publications.

Martyn, K. K., & Hutchinson, S. A. (2001). Low-income African American adolescents who avoid pregnancy: Tough girls who rewrite negative scripts. *Qualitative Health Research, 11*, 238–256.

Martyn, K. K., Munro, M. L., Darling-Fisher, C. S., Ronis, D. L., Villarruel, A. M., Pardee, M., . . . Fava, N. M. (2013). Patient-centered communication and health assessment with youth. *Nursing Research, 62*, 383–393.

Martyn, K. K., Reifsnider, E., & Murray, A. (2006). Improving adolescent sexual risk assessment with event history calendars: A feasibility study. *Journal of Pediatric Health Care, 20*(1), 19–26.

Pender, N. J. (n.d.). Listing of articles by N. J. Pender in University of Michigan Library database. Retrieved from http://deepblue.lib.umich.edu/browse?value=Pender%2C+Nola+J.&type=author

Pender, N. J., Sechrist, K. R., Stromborg, M., & Walker, S. N. (1987). Collaboration in developing research program grant. *Image, 19*(2), 75–77.

Pender, N. J., Smith, L. C., & Vernof, J. A. (1987). The effects of a corporate fitness program on absenteeism, productivity, anxiety, and job-related strain. *AAOHN Journal, 35*(9), 386–390.

Pender, N. J., Walker, S. N., Stromborg, M. F., & Sechrist, K. R. (1990). Predicting health promoting lifestyles in the workplace. *Nursing Research, 39*(6), 326–332.

Robbins, L. B., Pender, N. J., & Kazanis, A. S. (2003). Barriers to physical activity perceived by adolescent girls. *Journal of Midwifery and Women's Health, 48*(3), 206–212.

Robbins, L. B., Pender, N. J., Ronis, D. L., & Kazanis, A. S. (2004). Physical activity self-efficacy and perceived exertion among adolescents. *Research in Nursing and Health, 27*(6), 435–446.

Robbins, L. B., Sikorskii, A., Hamel, L. Wu, T. Y., & Wilbur, J. (2009). A comparison of benefits of and barriers to physical activity perceived by middle school boys and girls. *Research in Nursing and Health, 32*(2), 163–176.

Robbins, L. B., Talley, H. C., Wu, T. Y., & Wilbur, J. (2010). Sixth-grade boys perceived benefits of and barriers to physical activity and suggestions for increasing physical activity. *Journal of School Nursing, 26*(1), 65–77.

Shin, Y. H., Yun, S. K., Pender, N. J., & Jang, H. J. (2005). Test of the health promotion model as a causal model of commitment to a plan of exercise among Korean adults with chronic disease. *Research in Nursing and Health, 28*(2), 117–125.

Vanden Bosch, M. L., Robbins, L. B., Pfeiffer, K. A., Kazanis, A. S., & Maier, K. S. (2014). Demographic, cognitive, affective, and behavioral variables associated with overweight and obesity in low-active girls, *Journal of Pediatric Nursing, 29*(6), 576–585. PMCID: 4252398

Villarruel, A. M., Jemmott, J. B., III, & Jemmott, L. S. (2006). A randomized controlled trial testing an HIV prevention intervention for Latino youth. *Archives of Pediatrics & Adolescent Medicine, 160*(8), 772–777.

Villarruel, A. M., Loveland-Cherry, C., Gallegos Cabriales, E. C., Ronis, D., & Zhou, Y. (2008). A parent-adolescent intervention to increase sexual risk communication: Results of a randomized controlled trial. *AIDS Education and Prevention, 20*(5), 371–383.

Wu, T. Y., & Pender, N. J. (2001). Determinants of physical activity among Taiwanese adolescents: An application of the health promotion model. *Research in Nursing and Health, 25*, 25–26.

Wu, T. Y., Robbins, L. B., & Hsieh, H. F. (2011). Instrument development and validation of perceived physical activity self-efficacy scale for adolescents. *Research & Theory for Nursing Practice: An International Journal, 25*(1), 39–54.

Youngblut, J. M., & Brooten, D. (2006). Pediatric head trauma: Parent, parent-child and family functioning 2 weeks after hospital discharge. *Journal of Pediatric Psychology, 31*, 608–618. doi:10.1093/jpepsy/jsj066. PMCID: 2424404

Youngblut, J. M., & Brooten, D. (2008). Mother's mental health, mother-child relationship, and family functioning 3 months after a preschooler's head injury. *Journal of Head Trauma Rehabilitation, 23*, 92–102. doi:10.1097/01. HTR.0000314528.85758.30. PMCID: 2442865

Youngblut, J. M., & Brooten, D. (2013). Parent report of child response to sibling death in a neonatal or pediatric ICU. *American Journal of Critical Care, 13*, 474–481. doi:10.4037/ajcc2013790. PMCID: 3881261

Youngblut, J. M., Brooten, D., Blais, K., Kilgore, C., & Yoo, C. (2015). Health and functioning in grandparents after a young grandchild's death. *Journal of Community Health, 40*(5), 956–966. doi:10.1007/s10900-015-0018-0. PMCID: 4556735

Youngblut, J. M., Brooten, D., Cantwell, G. P., del Moral, T., & Totapally, B. (2013). Parent health and functioning 13 months after infant or child NICU/PICU death. *Pediatrics, 132*(5), e1295–1301 [Epub]. doi:10.1542/peds.2013-1194. PMCID: 3813397

Youngblut, J. M., Brooten, D., & Kuluz, J. (2005). Parent reactions at 24–48 hrs after a preschool child's head injury. *Pediatric Critical Care Medicine, 6*, 550–556. PMCID: 2614927

Youngblut, J. M., Brooten, D., Singer, L. T., Standing, T., Lee, H., & Rodgers, W. L. (2001). Effects of maternal employment and prematurity on child outcomes in single parent families. *Nursing Research, 50*, 346–355. PMCID: 2792577

Youngblut, J. M., & Jay, S. S. (1991). Emergency admission to the pediatric ICU: Parental concerns. *AACN Clinical Issues in Critical Care Nursing, 2*, 329–337.

Youngblut, J. M., & Lauzon, S. (1995). Family functioning following pediatric intensive care unit hospitalization. *Issues in Comprehensive Pediatric Nursing, 18*, 11–25.

Youngblut, J. M., Loveland-Cherry, C. J., & Horan, M. (1993). Maternal employment, family functioning, and preterm infant development at 9 and 12 months. *Research in Nursing & Health, 16*, 33–43. PMCID: 3601196

Youngblut, J. M., & Shiao, S.-Y. P. (1992). Characteristics of a child's critical illness and parents' reactions: Preliminary report of a pilot study. *American Journal of Critical Care, 1*(3), 80–85 [Corrected Table 2 printed in *2*(1), 101 (1993)].

Youngblut, J. M., & Shiao, S.-Y. P. (1993). Child and family reactions during and after pediatric ICU hospitalization: A pilot study. *Heart & Lung, 22*, 46–54.

Youngblut, J. M., Singer, L. T., Madigan, E. A., Swegart, L. A., & Rodgers, W. L. (1998). Maternal employment and parent-child relationships in single-parent families of LBW preschoolers. *Nursing Research, 47*, 114–121. PMCID: 2792580

CHAPTER 6

Promoting Worker Health and Safety

Sally L. Lusk, PhD, RN, FAAN, FAAOHN

Community health nursing, with its focus on community/public health, had always included worker health in its purview, but had not offered a defined major directed to this target population. In 1982, Professors Don Chaffin, College of Engineering, and Larry Fine, School of Public Health met with Dr. Violet Barkauskas, chair of Community Health Nursing (CHN) and Dr. Sally Lusk, associate professor of CHN to explore the possibility of the School of Nursing offering a master's degree program in Occupational Health Nursing (OHN). Master's degree programs in the College of Engineering and the School of Public Health were already part of the University of Michigan Center for Occupational Health and Safety (COHSE), an education and research center funded by the National Institute of Occupational Safety and Health (NIOSH). There was a desire to comprehensively include all the major professional specialties in occupational health and safety in COHSE. The proposed expansion would increase the interdisciplinary focus of COHSE, consistent with evolving NIOSH goals for centers to offer four or more academic master's programs. This proposal would require the School of Nursing to develop an occupational health nursing master's degree (MS) program and to partner with the Schools of Engineering and Public Health to submit a request for funding to support the program. Dr. Barkauskas asked Dr. Lusk to take leadership in developing this program and assisted her in doing so.

During the 1983–1984 and 1984–1985 academic years, the School of Nursing successfully applied to NIOSH for program planning funds. These funds were used to collect data regarding the need for and the interest in an OHN program. Joanne Disch, a PhD student in the School of Nursing, was employed to assist Dr. Lusk with two studies: (a) a survey of a random sample of Forbes 500 companies regarding their interest in employing occupational health nurses with advanced preparation and the responsibilities these companies wanted them to assume (Lusk, Disch, & Barkauskas, 1988b) and (b) a survey of a random sample of licensed registered nurses in Michigan regarding their interest in an OHN MS program and their availability and preferences for class schedules (Lusk, Disch, & Barkauskas, 1988a). Using the results from these studies, a proposal was submitted to NIOSH, and the occupational health nursing program was funded beginning January 1987.

Concomitant with the establishment of the OHN MS degree program as part of the NIOSH-funded Education and Research Center, a research focus on worker health and safety was initiated. This focus then was narrowed to workers' use of personal protective equipment (PPE) and ultimately, more specifically, use of hearing protection devices (HPDs) to prevent noise-induced hearing loss (NIHL).

Problem of Noise-Induced Hearing Loss

Studies have demonstrated the many negative effects of noise exposure: increases in hearing loss, tinnitus, cardiovascular diseases, stress, anxiety, depression, somatic complaints, accidents, and sickness absences and decreases in cognitive performance, social behavior, and job satisfaction (Melemed, Harari, & Green, 1993; Melamed, Luz, & Green, 1992; WHO, 2011). When engineering controls do not sufficiently mitigate noise, the use of HPDs, federally mandated in worksites by the Occupational Health and Safety Administration (OSHA), is critical to reduce exposure to noise and to prevent NIHL, the most common work-related injury (NIOSH, 1988). However, workers do not consistently use HPDs, even though they are mandated by law and by employers' policies. Prior to the studies conducted by Dr. Lusk and her teams at the University of Michigan, research related to HPDs conducted by NIOSH, or by manufacturers of HPDs, had tested only their efficacy, with no attention to the user. The two studies found (Ewigman, Kivlahan, Hosokawa, & Horman, 1990; Zohar, Cohen, & Azar, 1980) that tested an intervention to increase use were not based on conceptual models or empirically identified factors associated with workers' decisions to use HPDs.

NIHL has many deleterious effects on quality of life, negatively impacting communication, relationships, employability, and safety. NIHL is not reversible, and hearing aids never fully restore hearing. Most importantly, NIHL is entirely preventable by avoiding high noise exposure (Lusk & Kelemen, 1993).

Research Programs

This section describes the projects and outcomes of research conducted by former and current scientists at the University of Michigan School of Nursing to develop and test interventions to increase the use of HPDs to prevent NIHL. Included in this volume are the research briefs describing the research conducted by the PhD alumni (see Section 6). Although the focus of the projects was on worksite noise, environmental noise is also a threat to hearing and health, and information regarding these hazards was also incorporated into the interventions delivered to the workers.

The Beginnings: The Formation of a Research Team

As I was entrusted to provide leadership for the OHN master's program, I saw it was necessary to simultaneously launch a research program in order to not only grow the specialty, as it was very new within nursing, while engaging and educating graduate students in research methods but also contribute to the practice field. This section describes my journey and formation of the research team.

With support from NIOSH funds, the health promotion model (Pender, 1987) (Figure 6-a) provided the basis for small preliminary studies conducted to develop and test instruments to measure workers' health behaviors, attitudes and beliefs regarding noise, hearing loss, and use of HPDs. Students participated in these studies to enhance their research experience. Data were obtained through questionnaires, focus groups, and interviews (Lusk & Kelemen, 1993).

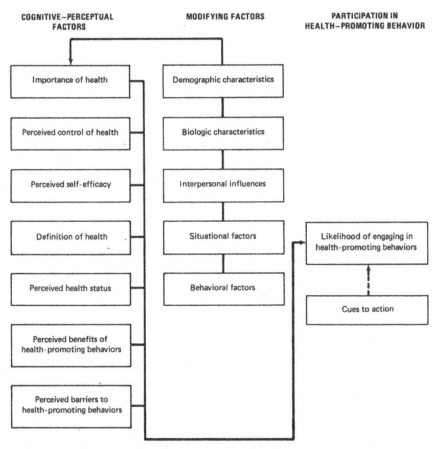

Figure 6-a. Health promotion model.
Pender, N. J. (1987). *Health promotion in nursing practice* (2nd ed.). Norwalk, CT: Appleton and Lange, 58.

Results from these studies were used to apply for funding from the National Center for Nursing Research (NCNR). In 1989, the proposal to test a model to explain workers' use of HPDs was funded, Preventing Noise-Induced Hearing Loss (R01NR02050 NCNR, NIDCD, NIH).

Adapting the health promotion model (Pender, 1987) to address the behaviors specific to attitudes and beliefs about hearing and protection, this project identified the most important predictors of workers' use of HPDs. These factors accounted for 49.2% of the variance in use in male and female blue-collar and skilled-trade workers in the factory setting, with three of the cognitive-perceptual factors in the model having significant direct paths to use of HPDs (Lusk, Ronis, Kerr, & Atwood, 1994). This result, with the unusually large amount of variance accounted for by the model, justified its use as a basis for designing interventions (Lusk, Ronis, & Kerr, 1995). Other significant components of this project were the comparison of observations and self-reporting of the behavior. Because it is often difficult or not feasible to observe behavior outside the laboratory, self-reporting must be considered; however, there is always concern about its reliability. This study documented that self-reporting was a reliable measure: self-reported use of HPDs correlated at .89 with the observed behavior of the individual workers (Lusk, Ronis, & Baer, 1995). This is particularly significant in light of the fact that workers were secure in reporting nonuse of a federally mandated and employer-required behavior (i.e., use of HPDs). These findings have aided researchers in justifying the use of self-reporting over observations, which had been considered the "gold standard" despite their many limitations. A supplement to this enabled the addition of more female workers to analyze for gender differences. Overall use of HPDs did not differ by gender, but the relative importance of significant factors in the model predicting use did differ between men and women (Lusk, Ronis, & Baer, 1997)

This project and its supplement made significant contributions to science, provided a foundation for developing interventions, and resulted in a total of nine publications in peer-reviewed journals. In addition to Dr. Lusk (principal investigator [PI]), Dr. David Ronis (statistician), and Ms. Madeleine Kerr (doctoral student), more than 25 persons participated in the project as consultants, data collectors, and students. Significant findings from this project were also presented at national and international meetings.

Because NIHL is insidious, frequently taking years to develop, workers often are not motivated to prevent it. For example, they are much more compliant in using protective eyewear to avoid foreign bodies because they are felt immediately, impacting vision and causing pain. An opportunity became available to seek funding to document the hazardous effects of noise exposure beyond hearing loss when the United Auto Workers-General Motors called for proposals to assess other effects of worksite noise. This study, Noise Effects on Cardiovascular and Stress-Related Diseases (funded by UAW-GM National Joint Committee on Health and Safety [NJCHS] and its Occupational Health Advisory Board), was conducted in an automotive plant in two phases. The first phase of the study examined the chronic effects of noise on blood pressure and heart rate in 374 workers at the plant. Resting blood pressure, heart rate, and body mass index were obtained. Noise exposure levels were extracted retrospectively from company records for each participant for the past 5 years. After controlling for demographic and a wide array of potentially confounding variables, the use of hearing protection in high-noise areas was a significant predictor of lower systolic (SBP) and diastolic blood pressures (DBP). The results suggested that the reduction of noise exposure by means of engineering controls or by consistent use of hearing protection by workers may positively affect health outcomes (Lusk, Hagerty, Gillespie, & Caruso, 2002).

In the second phase of the study, the acute effects of exposure to noise on SBP and DBP and heart rate were measured in 46 workers in a Midwestern automobile assembly plant while they wore ambulatory blood pressure monitors and personal noise dosimeters during one work shift. After adjustment for the covariates of cardiovascular function, SBP and DBP, along with heart rate, were shown to be significantly positively associated with noise exposure. For example, for each increase of 10 decibels of noise, or of 5 decibels between the average and the maximum decibels, SBP was increased by 2 mmHg. Further, SBP was reduced by 5.5 mmHg. for those observed to be wearing HPDs (Lusk, Hagerty, Gillespie, & Ziemba, 2004). The results of this and other studies suggested that reducing acute noise exposure reduces cardiovascular stress.

The investigative team for this study included Drs. Lusk, PI; Bonnie Hagerty, then assistant professor of nursing; a statistician from the Center for Statistical Consultation and Research; Ms. Ziemba, a doctoral student in nursing who served as project manager; and Ms. Caruso, a doctoral student in nursing who assisted with data analyses and collected data for her dissertation. In addition to the project team, a large number of data collectors and students contributed to the study and gained a great deal of knowledge and experience in conducting research in a manufacturing plant. Significant findings were reported in two publications in interdisciplinary peer-reviewed journals and in Dr. Caruso's dissertation and subsequent publication, as well as in presentations at national and international conferences.

The next large-scale project promoting use of HPDs, Preventing Noise-Induced Hearing Loss in Construction Workers (R01 OHO3136, NIOSH), designed and tested the effectiveness of a theory-based, multifaceted intervention program. The effectiveness of the intervention to increase the use of HPDs was tested with a regional sample of three groups of construction workers (operating engineers, carpenters, and plumber-pipefitters; n = 798) and with a national sample of plumber-pipefitters attending a trainer certification program (n = 234).

The project was conducted in three phases. In Phase 1, a sample of 356 workers from the three trade groups completed questionnaires measuring the factors associated with their use of HPDs. The predictors of use of hearing protection model (PUHPM) (based on the health promotion model; Pender, 1987) served as the basis for the questionnaires to determine important predictors. Variables in the model—benefits, barriers, and self-efficacy—related to use of HPDs, Noise Exposure, and Interpersonal Influences accounted for more than 50% of the variance in the use of HPDs and were used to design the intervention (Lusk, Hogan, & Ronis, 1997). Demographic characteristics of the trade group samples varied among the trades, but all were predominately White males with perceived hearing losses and low reported use of HPDs.

In Phase 2, the intervention package (a video on hearing health and conservation presented by actors portraying construction workers and a nurse, a practice session guided by trainers, and a brochure) based on the identified predictors of use was tested with a sample of 33 construction workers. These workers completed feedback forms and participated in focus groups to provide further evaluation of the training program. Project staff and consultants used these data to revise the intervention program.

In Phase 3, the effectiveness of the intervention package delivered to groups was assessed using a Solomon four-group design and random assignment to the groups. Postintervention measures occurred 10 to 12 months following the intervention. Self-reported posttest use of HPDs was the same in the carpenter group and higher in the operating engineers and plumber-pipefitters groups than the pretest use, but a significant effect of the intervention was found only in the plumber-pipefitter trade group (Lusk, Hong, Ronis, Kerr, Eakin, & Early, 1999; Lusk, Kerr, & Kauffman, 1998).

In order to make the training program available for use with construction workers, a trainers manual was developed and a contract was signed with the American Industrial Hygiene Association to market the package as part of their portfolio of continuing education programs for workers. Further, Drs. Kerr and Hong also used material from the intervention package to develop and test interventions in their studies with laborers and operating engineers.

In addition to Drs. Lusk, Ronis, and Madeleine Kerr, Drs. Mary Hogan, assistant professor of nursing, and OiSaeng Hong, a postdoctoral fellow, joined the research team, along with more than 22 other persons who served as consultants, staff, or data collectors for this project. One of the staff served as project manager and media development coordinator. Significant findings from this study were published in five articles in peer-reviewed journals and presented at multiple national and international conferences.

Although model variables accounted for a high level of variance in use of HPDs by construction workers, the intervention significantly affected behavior in only one trade group. Because the intervention package was delivered to groups and the technology to tailor messages to individuals was just then becoming available, it was decided the next project would develop and test a computer-based individually tailored intervention.

This large randomized controlled trial, Interventions to Prevent Workers' Hearing Loss (2R01NR0250, National Institute of Nursing Research), compared the effectiveness of three computer-based programs delivered in soundproof booths in an automobile plant and tested the effect of booster interventions. The PUHPM (Figure 6-b) derived from previous studies provided the basis for the design of the intervention. Workers were randomly assigned to receive one of three interventions: (a) an individually tailored, predictor-based intervention based on their responses; (b) a predictor-based intervention not tailored to their responses; and (c) a commercially developed control intervention. The first two of these were developed and tested by the project team (Eakin, Brady, & Lusk, 2001), and the latter was integrated into the computer delivery with the permission of the vendor (Barkauskas, Lusk, & Eakin, 2005). Following their annual audiometric test to assess hearing, workers were invited to enter the project's booth. Regardless of the type of intervention they would receive, workers first completed questionnaires via the computer to provide data regarding their use and type of HPDs, their perceived hearing ability, and their beliefs and attitudes regarding use of HPDs (based on the predictors in the model). Following this data collection, workers were randomly assigned to receive one of the three interventions.

Posttest data collected at the time of the workers' (n = 1325) next annual audiometric test showed that only the tailored intervention significantly increased workers' use of HPDs (Lusk, Ronis, Kazanis, Eakin, Hong, & Raymond, 2003). The PUHPM as a causal model of use of HPDs fit well and accounted for 35% of the variance in use at the pretest and 69% at posttest, with the pretest use included in the model where it was the strongest predictor. At pretest, the strongest predictors were benefits and social norms of use of HPDs. At posttest, the strongest predictors were prior use and social norms, indicating more stability than change in the behavior and that changes in the perceived norm for use of HPDs are associated with changes in use. Findings were consistent with the PUHPM's emphasis on behavior-specific factors as determinants of use of HPDs. Several of the strongest predictors in the model were the behavior-specific factors: benefits, barriers, social norms, and social models (Ronis, Hong, & Lusk, 2006). While no individual factors in the model proved to be a significant predictor, the relationships found were all in the expected directions.

Colorful printed booster interventions were mailed to workers' homes (n = 5,393). Workers were randomly assigned to one of four groups to receive postintervention boosters: (a) at 30 days, (b) at 90 days, (c) at 30 and 90 days, and (d) no booster at all. Although there was a significant main effect for boosters at 30 days to the tailored intervention group, post hoc comparisons found no significant differences in changes in mean use of HPDs by different booster groups (Lusk, Eakin, Kazanis, & McCullagh, 2004). Effects of the interventions and booster interventions on use of HPDs did not differ by gender and race subgroups of workers (African American, White, Hispanic, and non-Hispanic), and no significant interactions in the effects of the interventions or the boosters were found on use of HPDs by gender or racial status or by hearing ability (Hong, Lusk, & Ronis, 2005; Raymond, Hong, Lusk, & Ronis, 2006).

In addition to the scientific team comprising Drs. Lusk (PI), Kerr (coinvestigator), Ronis (statistician), Barkauskas (associate professor), and Hong (research scientist), more than 17 other persons served as consultants, project staff, or student assistants. Ms. Brenda

Eakin served as the project manager and media development coordinator. Significant findings from this study were published in six articles in peer-reviewed journals and presented at multiple national and international conferences. A CD containing the tailored intervention program was produced and made available for download on the web for use by others.

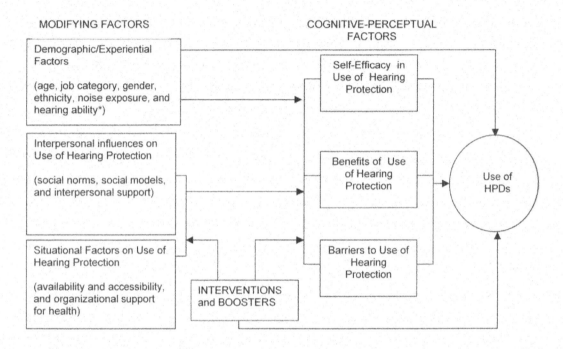

*Perceived hearing ability and by audiometric test

Figure 6-b. Predictors of use of hearing protection model.

Studies Conducted by Alumnae From the UMSN

It is believed that the University of Michigan School of Nursing was the first, or one of the first, schools of nursing to receive funding from NIOSH to support PhD students specializing in occupational health nursing and conducting research in occupational health and safety. Three alumnae, two from the doctoral program and one from a postdoctoral experience went on to develop their own programs of research to prevent NIHL in various populations. Brief summaries of their many contributions to preventing NIHL follow, with more detailed descriptions of their work in Section 6.

In her dissertation study, Dr. Kerr collected original data to identify the most important predictors for use of HPDs by Mexican American garment factory workers (Kerr, 1994; Kerr, Lusk, & Ronis, 2002). Factors from the health promotion model (Pender, 1987) that directly influenced the use of HPDs by Mexican American garment workers (n = 119) were benefits and barriers to HPD use, clinical conception of health, self-efficacy in the use of HPDs, and perceived health status, accounting for 25% of the variance in use. With the addition of two environmental factors that were directly related to the use of HPDs—required use of HPDs and plant site—55% of the variance in use was accounted for. These results suggested that Mexican American workers' use of hearing protection could be supported by interventions based on the PUHPM's cognitive-perceptual factors and the implementation of appropriate administrative policies.

In subsequent studies, Dr. Kerr designed and tested tailored and nontailored interventions based on the PUHPM. These were delivered to general construction workers and laborers via computer tablets (Kerr, Savik, Monsen, & Lusk, 2007). Both interventions were in an innovative animated "Mission Impossible" game format with actor Peter Graves providing the narration. The PUHPM accounted for 58% of the variance in workers' use of HPDs. Both interventions significantly increased posttest use of HPDs, with the tailored intervention resulting in greater use. She also tested booster interventions, which increased use in participants who received a booster over those who did not. The combination of the tailored intervention and booster resulted in a 30% increase in use over baseline, providing support for both tailoring and boosters.

Dr. Marjorie McCullagh came to the university with a history of collaboration with farm worker groups to improve and protect their health. She continued serving that population by conducting dissertation research to determine the self-reported prevalence of hearing loss and use of HPDs and to develop and validate instruments to measure the factors predicting their use of HPDs (McCullagh, 2000; McCullagh, Lusk, & Ronis, 2002). She continued to carefully establish a research trajectory by developing and testing a conceptual model of farm workers' use of HPDs using a random sample of workers. Her farmers' use of hearing protection model correctly predicted the use of HPDs in 74% of the cases (McCullagh, Ronis, & Lusk, 2010). A qualitative study that included videos of farmers describing their experiences with using HPDs provided valuable insights for refining data collection instruments and also provided resources that could be incorporated in interventions as persuasive testimonials (McCullagh & Robinson, 2009).

Dr. McCullagh's recently completed project tested the effectiveness of a web-based intervention delivered to a sample of 491 farmers in 13 states. A comparison of the effectiveness of information-based materials singly or in combination with a mailed sample of assorted HPDs found that although a web-based intervention was effective in increasing HPD use among farm operations, the mailed samples were more effective in changing behavior (McCullagh, Banerjee, Cohen, & Yang, 2016).

Currently under way is a randomized controlled trial of a community-based intervention designed to compare the effectiveness and the sustainability of approaches to increase farm youths' use of hearing conservation strategies (i.e., turn it down, walk away, use protection). Farm youth are exposed to high noise from an early age, but most have not been served by hearing health programs. This study is being carried out with funding from the National Institutes of Health for the 2015–2018 period.

In addition to the intervention programs described, Drs. Kerr and McCullagh collaborated to better describe the problem of occupational hearing loss and workers' awareness of their hearing ability. A cross-sectional survey compared a functional ability questionnaire to audiometric screening and demonstrated the need for development of improved self-reported measures of hearing ability (Kerr, McCullagh, Savik, & Dvorak, 2003). A subsequent comparison of the perceived and measured hearing ability of factory workers (McCullagh, Kerr, Raymond, & Lusk, 2011) showed hearing loss was highly prevalent, and self-reported hearing ability was poorly related to audiometric results, suggesting that using workers' perceptions of their hearing ability is an insufficient measure to classify hearing ability in studies of NIHL.

Upon her arrival, Dr. Hong, a postdoctoral fellow, joined the NIHL research projects in progress. After gaining experience with the team, she built upon Dr. Lusk's study with construction workers by developing a project focused solely on operating engineers. She added a self-administered hearing screening test to the computer-based tailored intervention originally designed for factory workers but modified it to be relevant for operating engineers by incorporating some assets (video clips, computer programming, and tailoring algorithms) from the previous interventions tested with construction workers and factory workers. Results from this self-administered hearing test provided the first published estimate of the prevalence of hearing loss in this worker group (Hong, 2005).

Workers receiving the tailored intervention, as opposed to the control, reported a significantly greater intention to use HPDs immediately following the intervention, but at 1 year posttest, the two groups' reports of use of HPDs did not significantly differ. The interpretation of the hearing test included in the tailored intervention may have played a role in increasing their immediate intention to use HPDs (Hong, Ronis, Lusk, & Kee, 2006). Three of psychosocial factors in the PUHPM (benefits, barriers, and social norms), two demographic variables (hearing ability and noise exposure), and supervisor climate were significant predictors of intention to use, but they accounted for only 22% of the variance (Hong, Ronis, Lusk, & Kee, 2006.)

Dr. Hong's subsequent projects have addressed NIHL in firefighters, an occupational group that heretofore received inadequate attention regarding this hazard. A self-directed, self-study web-based intervention to specifically address the unique needs of firefighters and their profession was tested with 35 fire departments in several states through a project titled SIREN (Safety Instruction to Reduce Exposure to Noise and Hearing Loss). This innovative project was the first nursing intervention study to be funded by the Department of Homeland Security (Hong, Eakin, Chin, Feld, & Vogel, 2013).

Recognizing that hearing loss can also be caused by exposure to ototoxic (i.e., having a harmful effect on the organs or nerves concerned with hearing and balance) chemicals, Dr. Hong utilized the data from a large NIH-funded longitudinal study of Latinos above age 60, Sacramento Area Latino Study of Aging (SALSA). She found that exposures to noise and ototoxic chemicals, after controlling for the effect of aging, were significantly associated with hearing loss among older populations of Latino Americans (Hong, Chin, & Kerr, 2015).

Outcomes and Impacts From These Programs of Research

All of the studies described in this chapter have made significant contributions to the field of occupational health nursing, the health and safety of workers, and the science of developing and testing behavioral interventions. This research has significantly impacted practice, research, and policy nationally and internationally. The following are examples of these specific outcomes and their impact:

1. Attention to the behavioral factors influencing workers' use of HPDs and other types of PPE.

   Prior to Dr. Lusk's first project, the only research conducted regarding use of HPDs was testing their efficacy, with no studies of the workers' perspectives or the factors that would influence their use. NIOSH had never funded studies of the behavioral aspects of workers' use of PPEs. Now NIOSH does fund such extramural projects and, in fact, has established an internal division to conduct such studies. Thus Dr. Lusk's work has influenced the program objectives of a national agency, thereby influencing national policy.

2. Attention to underserved worker groups and the distribution of effective interventions.

   Three of the OHN program alumni have gone on to develop their own significant programs of research to prevent hearing loss with attention to underserved worker groups: Dr. Kerr, focusing on laborers and Latinos; Dr. McCullagh, focusing on agricultural workers; and Dr. Hong, continuing work with the construction worker population and firefighters.

   Interventions developed and tested through these projects were effective in increasing workers' use of HPDs to prevent NIHL. The training programs developed through these projects have been made available for widespread use in training workers.

3. Increased use of HPDs and reduction of noise exposure, leading to improved health.

   Increasing the use of HPDs for those in high noise settings decreases the incidence of NIHL, reduces the negative effects of noise exposure (tinnitus, cardiovascular diseases, stress, anxiety, depression, somatic complaints, accidents, and sickness absences), and improves learning, social behavior, and job satisfaction. A recent study (Swinburn, Hammer, & Neitzel, 2015) documented the effect of noise exposure on costs associated with cardiovascular disease and estimated that a reduction of 5 decibels of exposure would save $3.9 billion each year in health care costs. A World Health Organization report (2011) estimates a total of more than 1.6 disability-adjusted-life-years lost in Europe that are attributable to effects of noise on ischemic heart disease, sleep, annoyance, tinnitus, and the cognitive impairment of children. Thus these and many other sources offer evidence that reductions in noise exposures will have significant effects on the health of our nation and the cost of health care.

4. Documentation of the reliability of self-reporting.

    The finding that observations and self-reporting were very highly correlated has aided many researchers designing studies, allowing them to justify use of self-reporting to measure behavior and behavior changes.

5. Development and testing of conceptual models.

    A model specific to predicting workers' use of HPDs was developed. Beginning with the health promotion model, the most significant factors from that model, along with a few additional factors important to the use of HPDs, evolved into PUHPM (Figure 6-b). This model served as the basis for the development of the farmers' use of hearing protection model and other models guiding the studies conducted by Kerr (Kerr, 1994: Kerr, Lusk, & Ronis, 2002; Kerr, Savik, Monson, & Lusk, 2007) and Hong (Hong, Lusk, & Ronis, 2005; Hong, Ronis, Lusk, & Kee, 2006). Further, the development of models specific to different worker groups will facilitate future research on worker health and safety. These models are being used in other studies and are modified based on new findings and the unique characteristics of the target populations.

    In addition, these studies provided additional support for the value of the components of the health promotion model in predicting a protective behavior (use of HPDs), thereby not limiting its application to health-promoting behaviors. The results of these studies validated the assumption that model factors must be specific to the behavior of interest and to the target population.

6. Availability of data collection instruments.

    The instruments developed to collect data to measure the factors in the health promotion model and PUHPM have been placed in the Health and Psychosocial Instruments (HaPI) repository at Behavioral Measurement Database Services (http://www.bmdshapi.com/contact.html), which makes them available to other researchers around the world at no cost. A significant number of researchers and students here and abroad have made use of the instruments to conduct their own studies.

7. Provision of research experiences.

    Many faculty and students of all levels and representing a variety of nursing specialties have gained valuable research experience through participation in these projects. A large number of students in nursing and other disciplines were employed on these projects as research assistants. Further, six participating doctoral students, two of whom were not specializing in occupational health nursing, used data collected through these projects for their dissertation research. Data from the first research project were used for a master's degree thesis, and subsequent research projects provided data for master's degree projects and classroom exercises. Further, a significant number of researchers and students, nationally and internationally, have used the model described in Figure 6-b and the instruments developed through these projects to conduct their own studies.

8. Increased awareness of workers' health issues.

These studies and their reports in nursing and occupational health literature have heightened the awareness of workers as a target population for nursing research and the importance considering behavioral factors in occupational health and safety.

Summary

In summary, the research initiated by the University of Michigan School of Nursing faculty, and continued by its alumni and faculty, has significantly impacted worker health and safety, aspects of health of the nation, and federal policy. For the future, efforts must be directed toward continuing to design and test effective interventions to prevent NIHL and the deleterious effects of noise. This mission is not complete until all workers always wear HPDs 100% of the time when needed.

While most of the work to date has focused on noise associated with work, interventions delivered to workers always informed them of the hazards of environmental and recreational noise exposure. The next critical frontier is to reduce environmental noise exposure for everyone. With the known deleterious effects of noise exposure already described, reductions will result in enhanced health and reduced health care costs. In addition to focused research projects, reducing noise exposure will require education of the public to change individual behavior, changes in federal policies, and drafting new local, state, and national laws. This is the mission for the future!

It is well recognized that occupational health nursing must work to increase its evidence base for practice (Robert Wood Johnson Foundation, 2015). The research conducted at the University of Michigan School of Nursing and by alumni of the program has served as a model for the development and conduct of research in occupational health nursing and has demonstrated the importance of addressing the workers' perspectives in regard to any behavior change. In the United States, and other countries, it is clear that unsafe and unhealthy conditions exist for workers. No one should have to sacrifice health for employment. The research described here has contributed to one aspect of promoting worker health, but much additional research is needed to ensure healthy workplaces for workers everywhere.

References

Barkauskas, V. H., Lusk, S. L., & Eakin, B. L. (2005). Selecting control interventions for clinical outcome studies. *Western Journal of Nursing Research, 27*(3), 346–363.

Eakin, B. L., Brady, J., & Lusk, S. L. (2001). Creating a tailored, multimedia computer-based intervention. *Computers in Nursing Journal 19*(4), 152–163.

Ewigman, B. G., Kivlahan, C. H., Hosokawa, M. C., & Horman, D. (1990). Efficacy of an intervention to promote use of hearing protection devices by firefighters. *Public Health Reports, 105,* 53–59.

Hong, O. (2005). Hearing loss among operating engineers in American construction industry. *International Archives of Occupational and Environmental Health, 78*(7), 565–574.

Hong, O., Chin, D., & Kerr, M. (2015). Lifelong occupational exposures and hearing loss among Latino American elderly. *International Journal of Audiology, 54*(Suppl. 1), S57–64.

Hong, O., Eakin, B., Chin, D., Feld, J., & Vogel, S. (2013). An Internet-based tailored hearing protection intervention for firefighters: Development process and users' feedback. *Health Promotion Practice, 14*(4), 572–579. doi:10.1177/1524839912462031. PMID: 23149759

Hong, O., Lusk, S. L., & Ronis, D. L. (2005). Ethnicity differences in predictors for hearing protection behavior in Black and White workers. *Research & Theory for Nursing Practice: An International Journal, 19*(1), 63–76.

Hong, O., Ronis, D. L., Lusk, S. L., & Kee, G. S. (2006). Efficacy of a computer-based hearing test and tailored hearing protection intervention. *International Journal of Behavioral Medicine, 13*(4), 304–314.

Kerr, M. J. (1994). Factors related to Mexican-American workers' use of hearing protection. *UMI Dissertations,* 9501083.

Kerr, M. J., Lusk, S. L., & Ronis, D. L. (2002). Explaining Mexican American workers' hearing protection use with the health promotion model. *Nursing Research, 51*(2), 100–109.

Kerr, M. J., McCullagh, M., Savik, K., & Dvorak, L. A. (2003). Perceived and measured hearing ability in construction laborers and farmers. *American Journal of Industrial Medicine, 44*(4), 431–437.

Kerr, M. J., Savik, K., Monsen, K. A., & Lusk, S. L. (2007). Effectiveness of computer-based tailoring versus targeting to promote use of hearing protection. *Canadian Journal of Nursing Research, 39*(1), 80–97.

Lusk, S. L., Disch, J. M., & Barkauskas, V. H. (1988a). Barriers to advanced education for OHNs. *AAOHN Journal, 36*(11), 457–463.

Lusk, S. L., Disch, J. M., & Barkauskas, V. H. (1988b). Interest of major corporations in expanded practice of occupational health nurses. *Research in Nursing and Health, 11,* 141–151.

Lusk, S. L., Eakin, B. L., Kazanis, A. S., & McCullagh, M. C. (2004). Effects of booster interventions on factory workers' use of hearing protection. *Nursing Research, 53*(1), 53.

Lusk, S. L., Hagerty, B. M., Gillespie, B., & Caruso, C. C. (2002). Chronic effects of workplace noise on blood pressure and heart rate. *Archives of Environmental Health: An International Journal, 57*(4), 273–281.

Lusk, S. L., Hagerty, B. M., Gillespie, B., & Ziemba, R. (2004). Acute effects of workplace noise on blood pressure and heart rate. *Archives of Environmental Health: An International Journal, 59*(8), 392–399.

Lusk, S. L., Hogan, M. M., & Ronis, D. L. (1997). Test of the health promotion model as a causal model of construction workers' use of hearing protection. *Research in Nursing & Health, 20*(3), 183–194.

Lusk, S. L., Hong, O. S., Ronis, D. L., Kerr, M. J., Eakin, B. L., & Early, M. R. (1999). Effectiveness of an intervention to increase construction workers' use of hearing protection. *Human Factors, 41*(3), 487–494.

Lusk, S. L., & Kelemen, M. J. (1993). Predicting use of hearing protection: A preliminary study. *Nursing Research, 10*(3), 189–196.

Lusk, S. L., Kerr, M. J., & Kauffman, S. A. (1998). Use of hearing protection and perceptions of noise exposure and hearing loss in construction workers. *American Industrial Hygiene Association Journal, 59,* 466–470.

Lusk, S. L., Ronis, D. L., & Baer, L. M. (1995). A comparison of multiple indicators: Observations, supervisors' report, and self-report as measures of workers' hearing protection use. *Evaluation and the Health Professions, 18*(1), 51–63.

Lusk, S. L., Ronis, D. L., & Baer, L. M. (1997). Gender differences in use of hearing protection. *Women & Health, 25*(4), 69–89.

Lusk, S. L., Ronis, D. L., Kazanis, A. S., Eakin, B. L., Hong, O. S., & Raymond, D. M. (2003). Effectiveness of a tailored intervention to increase factory workers' use of hearing protection. *Nursing Research, 52*(5), 289–295.

Lusk, S. L., Ronis, D. L., & Kerr, M. J. (1995). Predictors of workers' use of hearing protection: Implications for training programs. *Human Factors, 37*(3), 635–640.

Lusk, S. L., Ronis, D. L., Kerr, M. J., & Atwood, J. R. (1994). Test of the health promotion model as a causal model of workers' use of hearing protection. *Nursing Research, 43*(3), 151–157.

McCullagh, M. (2000). Factors affecting use of hearing protectors among farmers. *UMI Dissertations, 61*(2), AAT 9959819.

McCullagh, M. C., Banerjee, T., Cohen, M. A., & Yang, J. J. (2016). Effects of interventions on use of hearing protectors among farm operators: A randomized controlled trial. *International Journal of Audiology, 55*(Suppl 1): S3–S12. doi:10.3109/14992027.2015. 1122239. PMID: 26766172.

McCullagh, M. C., Kerr, M. J., Raymond, D. M., & Lusk, S. L. (2011). Prevalence of hearing loss and accuracy of self-report among factory workers. *Noise & Health, 13*(54), 340–347. doi:10.4103/1463-1741.85504

McCullagh, M. C., Lusk, S. L., & Ronis, D. L. (2002). Factors influencing use of hearing protection among farmers: A test of the Pender health promotion model. *Nursing Research, 51*(1), 33–39.

McCullagh, M. C., & Robinson, C. (2009). Too late smart: Farmers' adoption of self-protective behavior in response to exposure to hazardous noise. *AAOHN Journal, 57*(3), 99–105.

McCullagh, M. C., Ronis, D. L., & Lusk, S. L. (2010). Predictors of use of hearing protection among a representative sample of farmers. *Research in Nursing and Health, 33*(6), 528–538.

Melamed, S., Harari, G., & Green, M. (1993). Type A behavior, tension and ambulatory cardiovascular reactivity in workers exposed to noise stress. *Psychosomatic Medicine, 5,* 185–192.

Melamed, S., Luz, J., & Green, M. S. (1992). Noise exposure, noise annoyance, and their relation to psychological distress, accident, and sickness absence among blue-collar workers—the Cordis Study. *Israel Journal of Medical Science, 28*(8–9), 629–635.

National Institute of Occupational Safety and Health. (1988). *A proposed national strategy for the prevention of work-related noise-induced hearing loss* (Department of Health and Human Services Publication No. 89-135). Washington, DC: U.S. Government Printing Office.

Pender, N. J. (1987). *Health Promotion in Nursing Practice* (2nd ed.). Norwalk, CT: Appleton and Lange, 58.

Raymond, D. M., Hong, O., Lusk, S. L., & Ronis, D. (2006). Comparison of predictors of hearing protection use for Hispanic and non-Hispanic White factory workers. *Research and Theory for Nursing Practice: An International Journal, 20*(2), 127–140.

Robert Wood Johnson Foundation. (2015). The value of nursing in building a culture of health (part 2): Helping employers create safe and productive workplaces. *Charting Nursing's Future: Reports that Can Inform Policy and Practice, 26.*

Ronis, D. L., Hong, O., & Lusk, S. L. (2006). Comparison of the original and revised structure of the health promotion models in predicting construction workers' hearing protection. *Research in Nursing and Health, 29*(1), 3–17.

Swinburn, T. K., Hammer, J. D., & Neitzel, R. L. (2015). Valuing quiet: An economic assessment of U.S. Environmental Noise as a cardiovascular health hazard. *American Journal of Preventive Medicine, 49*(3), 345–353.

World Health Organization. (2011). *Burden of disease from environmental noise: Quantification of healthy life years lost in Europe.* Bonn, Germany: WHO European Centre for Environment and Health, World Health Organization.

Zohar, D., Cohen, A., & Azar, N. (1980). Promoting increased use of ear protectors in noise through information feedback. *Human Factors, 22,* 69–79.

Note: Instruments developed by Dr. Lusk's team are available on the Behavioral Measurement Database Services website: http://www.bmdshapi.com/contact.html.

Behavioral Measurement Database Services
PO Box 110287
Pittsburgh, PA 15232–0787
Phone: 412–687–6850; Fax: 412–687–5213

CHAPTER 7

Primary Care and Nurse-Managed Health Centers

Research Team 1998–2013

Joanne M. Pohl, PhD, APRN-BC, FAAN, FAANP
Violet H. Barkauskas, PhD, MPH, RN, FAAN

SHORT PAPERS SUBMITTED FOR THIS CHAPTER

Debra J. Barksdale
Ramona A. Benkert
Deborah Vincent

Increased attention is being given to the development of primary care services, specifically since the Patient Protection and Affordable Care Act (PPACA) was passed in 2010 and enrollment in insurance plans began in 2013. Research related to the role of advanced practice registered nurses (APRNs) in primary care as well as nurse-led care in nurse-managed health centers (NMHCs) was limited in the 1990s when Dr. Joanne Pohl first joined the faculty of the University of Michigan School of Nursing (UMSN). Much of the data were based on small practices and not generalizable. As a primary care nurse practitioner, Pohl's interest in contributing to the body of literature on the impact of APRNs in primary care and community health drove her research focus for more than two decades. As studies were developed, faculty and students with similar interests joined the research initiatives.

This chapter focuses on the development and growth of the work related to primary care in NMHCs, first regionally and then nationally. Three major grants and one bridge funding, on which Pohl was the primary investigator, moved this work forward. The emphasis in all the grants addressed the Triple Aim (Institute for Health Improvement, http://www.ihi.org/engage/initiatives/tripleaim/Pages/default.aspx)—improving the patient experience (including quality and satisfaction), addressing cost of care, and improving the health of populations, which for NMHCs means focusing on some of the most vulnerable and often uninsured groups. As with many such funded projects, the work was based on a large team and for all cases a consortium across universities and NMHCs—first in Michigan and then nationally.

Three UMSN PhD students had an important role in this work at various stages and then went on to pursue academic careers and research related to primary care and vulnerable populations. A summary of their work is presented in their self-authored brief reports. Dr. Deborah Vincent completed her dissertation using the NMHCs at the University of Michigan and other NMHCs across the country to study the financial aspects of managing NMHCs. Her work was important in guiding some of the financial models in our first W. K. Kellogg Foundation (WKKF) funding. She continued this focus of developing and testing cost-effective interventions and models of health care delivery, specifically focusing on Mexican Americans and diabetes management. Dr. Debra Barksdale participated in the first WKKF grant, managing one of the NMHCs and its data collection at an African American church in Detroit, Michigan. She continued her doctoral focus on hypertension to explore the relationship of stress and biobehavioral biomarkers related to hypertension in Black Americans. In 2010, Barksdale was invited to serve as the only nurse on the board of the Patient Centered Outcomes Research Institute (PCORI), formed under the PPACA. Dr. Ramona Benkert participated in all three of the funded projects described in this chapter as she joined the Wayne State University (WSU) faculty as associate professor after completing her PhD. She coauthored many of the manuscripts on the three funded projects discussed. Her research trajectory addressed the effect that the primary health care dyad has on racial and ethnic minorities' utilization of and satisfaction with health care services and the resultant influence on health outcomes. UMSN faculty member Dr. Violet Barkauskas had a major leadership role in the broad evaluation process for the first two WKKF grants. As a postdoctoral fellow, Dr. Susan Vonderheid contributed substantially to the first funded WKKF project, moving the financial sustainability issues forward. She authored and coauthored multiple papers.

References identified within the text of this chapter are all fully referenced in the list of publications following each section.

1998–2003: Michigan Academic Consortium: Nurse-Managed Primary Care Project Funded by the W. K. Kellogg Foundation

The focus of this work was to study the nine NMHCs across four public Michigan universities: the University of Michigan, Grand Valley State University, Michigan State University, and Wayne State University. The Michigan Public Health Institute (MPHI) was an important fifth "neutral" partner and functioned as the fiduciary in addition to providing oversight of the evaluation process. This grant was funded at a time when the state was looking for data on primary care sites that were addressing vulnerable populations, including the Medicaid population. The WKKF contributed significant funding ($4.2 million) to understand nursing's role in primary care in Michigan a 5-year period. A robust consortium (Michigan Academic Consortium [MAC]) was developed to educate nurse practitioners (NPs) to deliver more cost-effective and community-responsive primary care to unserved, underserved, and Medicaid patients. Additional goals included increasing access to quality, cost-effective care delivered by NPs in interdisciplinary, collaborative practices. The development of strong business models and the delivery of community-responsive care were emphasized.

Findings. The breadth of impact of this work was consistent with the overall goals. A uniquely broad and comprehensive evaluation component was implemented and completed including a pilot of quality outcome measures using national standards (the first of this type of analysis across NMHCs) and comprehensive financial data (also the first of its kind in NMHCs). Students, faculty, patients, communities, and consortium members were all included in this very extensive evaluation process, with Barkauskas providing leadership.

Quality of care was studied across all the sites, and graduate students gained experience with quality assessment processes as they used project-developed measures for their required scholarly papers across universities. The outcomes were then used by practices to better understand areas that needed improvement as well as those in which they exceeded the national Healthcare Effectiveness Data and Information Set (HEDIS) benchmarks. NMHCs outcome data often exceeded national benchmarks, especially in the area of chronic disease (Barkauskas, Pohl, Benkert, & Wells, 2005).

Access to care for very high-need populations at all universities increased, with patient volume tripling over the course of this first grant. Working with the Michigan Primary Care Association, we addressed the commonalities between federally qualified health centers (FQHCs) and NMHCs (Pohl, Vonderheid, Barkauskas, & Nagelkerk, 2004). These findings of similarity, but different financial support, were the first to be published and eventually contributed to policy changes.

Data supported that NMHCs provided a unique clinical experience for undergraduate and graduate students that they did not receive in more traditional health care practices, and this experience included a strong community focus (Tanner, Pohl, Ward, & Dontje, 2003). In the final year of the study, 69 graduate students and 187 undergraduate students from the four universities had some clinical experience across all nine participating NMHCs, reflecting a substantial increase in student participation from the first year. Findings also emphasized the importance of strong business plans and reimbursement for the successful management and sustainability of NMHCs.

Impact. NMHC data were shared regularly with state legislators and key stakeholders through policy briefs, in the form of postcards. Data helped inform language for the U.S. Senate and House subcommittees working on the Health Care Safety Net Amendments of 2001 that would allow nurse-managed centers a 2-year waiver to become community health centers/FQHCs. Numerous (55) presentations and 18 publications resulted from WKKF funding.

Selected publications. All members of the consortium, including students, were encouraged to participate in publications, which modeled the partnership and teamwork central to this work. Those marked with an asterisk (*) are data based, and those with a caret (^) are postdoctoral fellow first-authored. They are listed chronologically to give a sense of the progression of the work. Of the 18 publications, three were student first-authored and two were first authored by a postdoctoral scholar.

Pohl, J. M., Bostrom, A., Talaarczak, G., & Cavanagh, S. (2001). Development of an academic consortium: Nurse managed primary care. *Nursing and Health Care Perspectives, 22*(6), 308–313.

*Breer, L. B., Pohl, J. M., Stommel, M., Barkauskas, V., Schillo, B., & Oakley, D. (2002). Attitudes toward managed care: A comparison of nurse practitioner students and medical residents. *Journal of Professional Nursing, 18*, 263–270.

*Benkert, R., Barkauskas, V., Pohl, J. M., Tanner, C., & Nagelkerk, J. (2002). Patient satisfaction outcomes in nurse managed centers. *Outcomes Management for Nursing Practice, 6*(4), 174–181.

*^Vonderheid, S., Pohl, J. M., Barkauskas, V., Gift, D., & Hughes-Cromwick, P. (2003). Financial performance of academic nurse-managed primary care centers. *Nursing Economics, 21*(4), 167–175.

*Tanner, C., Pohl, J. M., Ward, S., & Dontje, K. (2003). Education of nurse practitioners in academic nurse managed centers: Student perspectives. *Journal of Professional Nursing, 19*(6), 354–363.

*^Vonderheid, S., Pohl, J. M., Schafer, P., Forrest, K., Poole, M., Barkauskas, V., & Mackey, T. (2004). Using FTE and RVU performance measures to assess the financial viability of academic nurse-managed primary care centers. *Nursing Economics, 22*(3), 124–134.

*Pohl, J. M., Vonderheid, S., Barkauskas, V., & Nagelkerk, J. (2004). The safety net: Academic nurse-managed centers' role. *Policy, Politics, and Nursing Practice, 5*(2), 84–94.

*Barkauskas, V., Pohl, J. M., Breer, L., Tanner, C., Bostrom, A., Benkert, R., & Vonderheid, S. (2004). Academic nurse-managed centers (ANMCs): Approaches to evaluation. *Outcomes Management, 8*(1), 57–66.

*Benkert, R., Tanner, C., Oakley, D., Guthrie, B., & Pohl, J. M. (2005). Cultural competence in nurse practitioner students: A Consortium's experience. *Journal of Nursing Education, 44*(5), 1–10.

*Barkauskas, V. H., Pohl, J. M., Benkert, R., & Wells, M. (2005). Measuring quality in nurse-managed centers using HEDIS measures. *Journal for Healthcare Quality, 27*(1), 4–14.

Bostrom, A. C., Scshafer, P., Dontje, K., Pohl, J. M., Nagelkerk, J., & Cavanagh, S. J. (2006). Electronic health record: Implementation across the Michigan Academic Consortium. *CIN: Computers, Informatics, Nursing, 24*(1), 44–52.

*Benkert, R., George, N., Tanner, C., Barkauskas, V. H., Pohl, J. M., & Marszalek, A. (2007). Satisfaction with a school based teen health center: A report card on care. *Pediatric Nursing, 33*(2), 103–109.

*Pohl, J. M., Sebastian, J. G., Barkauskas, V. H., Breer, L., Williams, C., Stanhope, M., . . . Rogers, M. K. (2007). Characteristics of nursing schools operating academic nurse-managed centers. *Nursing Outlook, 55*(6), 289–295.

2003–2004: Bridge Funding From W. K. Kellogg Foundation

Based on the success of the first grant, the WKKF offered the consortium additional funding to do a national survey of NMHCs and hold a national data consensus conference on the key clinical and financial data elements needed to sustain NMHCs.

Findings. The first record of NMHCs connected to academic programs was developed based on a survey of all American Association of Colleges of Nursing (AACN) members. The first national standardized data tool to report clinical and financial data from NMHCs was also developed. This positioned the consortium well for its next large funding from the WKKF and for moving the data warehouse concept forward.

Publications

*Barkauskas, V. H., Schafer, P., Sebastian, J. G., Pohl, J. M., Benkert, R., Nagelkerk, J., . . . Tanner, C. L. (2006). Clients served and services provided by academic nurse-managed centers. *Journal of Professional Nursing, 22*(6), 331–338.

Pohl, J. M., Breer, L., Tanner, C., Barkauskas, V., Bleich, M., Bomar, M., . . . Werner, K. (2006). National consensus on data elements for nurse managed health centers. *Nursing Outlook, 54*(2), 81–84.

Pohl, J. M., Vonderheid, S., Barkauskas, V., & Nagelkerk, J. (2006). Critical elements for tracking financial data in academic nurse managed centers. *American Journal for Nurse Practitioners, 10*(4), 10–16.

2003–2008: Institute for Nursing Centers

Funding from the WKKF enabled the consortium to advance the focus of previous work to a national level. A national network, called the Institute for Nursing Centers (INC), was created, and we developed and managed the first and only standardized national clinical and financial database and warehouse for NMHCs (including the infrastructure for data warehousing at MPHI). The goal was to inform policy and identify benchmarks for best practices for NMHCs. This work promoted NMHCs as a viable health care option while also generating and marketing educational and business products and services. For 4 years, NMHCs across the country submitted standardized data to our data warehouse at MPHI. These data were summarized for each center and provided to them along with feedback for improvement. The data were also used to develop aggregate reports of NMHCs that were shared publicly with stakeholders through high-quality reports.

Our survey was based on the earlier consensus work, with specific support and advice from Medical Group Management Association and the U.S. Health Resources and Services Administration (via their Uniform Data System). In addition, we piloted quality outcome measures from the largest NMHCs using national benchmarks (HEDIS measures) for four quality indices: breast cancer screening, cervical cancer screening, diabetes, and hypertension. This work represented another first for national NMHC data reporting. As our work became nationally known, investigators were often invited to speak at national multidisciplinary conferences such as the Patient Centered Primary Care Consortium and the Annual Summit in Washington, DC. In addition to the publications listed, we disseminated findings at more than 30 regional, national, and international meetings. Many of the presentations were invited and included predominantly multidisciplinary groups. In addition to publications, four annual reports summarizing the national NMHC aggregate data were disseminated broadly.

Findings. The first and only set of national standardized data on NMHCs over a 4-year period was obtained and published (Pohl, Tanner, Barkauskas, Gans, Nagelkerk, & Fiandt, 2010). National standardized quality outcomes on NMHCs were measured and published

(Barkauskas, Pohl, Tanner, Onifade, & Pilon, 2011). National outcomes again often matched or exceeded national indicators. We again updated the data on NMHCs when compared to FQHCs (Pohl, Tanner, Pilon, & Benkert, 2011) and found that NMHCs' cost of care was slightly lower than FQHCs, while outcomes of care were comparable.

Impact. The findings from this work informed policy at the national level. The *Clinical and Financial Data Survey and Codebook* remain the first and only standardized tools for comprehensively assessing and evaluating NMHCs. The survey and codebook are in the public domain and now housed at the National Nursing Center Consortium in Philadelphia, Pennsylvania. The data warehouse remains at MPHI. By linking NMHC data to FQHCs, we were able to report on the similarities of our patient population, clinical services, costs, and quality of care when compared to FQHCs. The data were used by national policy groups to obtain funding for NMHCs in the initial years of the PPACA.

Selected Data-Based Publications

Vonderheid, S., Pohl, J. M., Tanner, C., Newland, J., & Gans, D. (2009). CPT coding patterns at nurse managed centers: Data from a national survey. *Nursing Economics, 27*(4), 211–220.

Pohl, J. M., Tanner, C., Barkauskas, V. H., Gans, D., Nagelkerk, J., & Fiandt, K. (2010). Toward a national nurse managed health center dataset: Findings and lessons learned over three years. *Nursing Outlook, 58*(2), 97–103.

Barkauskas, V. H., Pohl, J. M., Tanner, C., Onifade, T. J., & Pilon, B. (2011). Quality of care in nurse managed health centers. *Nursing Administration Quarterly, 25*(1), 35–41 doi:10.1097/NAQ.0b013e3182032165

Pohl, J. M., Tanner, C., Pilon, B., & Benkert, R. (2011). Comparison of nurse managed health centers with community health centers as safety net providers. *Policy, Politics, & Nursing Practice, 12*(2), 90–99.

2007–2011: R18 Agency for Health Care Research Grant— A Partnership for Clinician Electronic Health Record Use and Quality of Care

Electronic health record (EHR) work had started as part of our NMHC work in the first WKKF grant (Bostrom, Schafer, Dontje, Pohl, Nagelkerk, & Cavanagh, 2006). For the Agency for Health Care Research (AHRQ) grant, we partnered with a network of FQHCs in Chicago, the Alliance of Chicago, that was very interested in collaborating with NMHCs. As a result, INC—in partnership with the Alliance of Chicago—was awarded a R18 AHRQ grant, A Partnership for Clinician EHR Use and Quality of Care. We implemented the same EHR product across four NMHCs nationally and three FQHCs in Chicago. The goals of the project were to study the effectiveness of a partnership that shares resources and uses a data-driven approach to promote full use of an EHR by clinicians in settings that serve vulnerable populations in order to improve the quality and safety of care in the areas of preventive care, chronic disease management, and medication management.

Findings. The complexities of implementing an EHR in smaller NMHCs was profound. The NMHCs were all affiliated with universities, and university systems did not consistently appreciate the challenges involved. The small (by comparison to the FQHCs) NMHCs also experienced challenges in terms of their financial practices and business plans. Overall, however, the EHR heightened emphasis on patient safety (see published articles for this section), especially for medication safety and drug-to-drug interactions, which were exceptionally low (Pohl, Tanner, Hamilton, Kaleba, Rachman, White, & Zeng, 2013). When measuring quality outcomes using the same EHR product across multiple sites across the country, we found the quality of chronic disease care in safety net centers improved over time.

Publications

*Data-Based Papers; Listed Chronologically

*Dennehy, P., White, M., Hamilton, A., Pohl, J. M., Tanner, C., Onifade, T. J., & Zheng, K. (2011). A partnership model for implementing electronic health records in resource-limited primary care settings: Experiences from two nurse managed health centers. *Journal of the American Informatics Association, 18*(6), 820–826. doi:10.1136/amiajnl-2011-000117. PMID: 21828225

Pohl, J. M., Nath, R. Zheng, K., Rachman, F., Gans, D., & Tanner, C. (2013). Use of a comprehensive patient safety tool in primary care practices. *Journal of the American Association of Nurse Practitioners, 25*(8), 415–418. doi:10.1111/1745-7599.12021

*Pohl, J. M., Tanner, C., Hamilton, A., Kaleba, E. O., Rachman, F. D., White, J., & Zeng, K. (2013). Medication safety after implementation of a commercial electronic health record system in five safety-net practices: A mixed methods approach. *Journal of the American Association of Nurse Practitioners, 26*(8), 438–444. doi:10.1002/2327-6924.12089

*Benkert, R., Dennehy, P., White, J., Hamilton, A., Tanner, C., & Pohl, J. M. (2014). Diabetes and hypertension quality measurement among four safety-net clinics in the U.S. *Applied Clinical Informatics, 5*(3), 757–772.

Future Directions for Primary Care Research

The contributions of the research described here impacted knowledge and policy in the area of nurse-led primary care—specifically, the care of vulnerable populations and the sustainability of NMHCs. That work continues with ongoing efforts related to access to care in the context of the PPACA. As of September, 2015, the Health and Human Services Administration reported a total of 17.6 million persons insured due to the PPACA through the Insurance Marketplace, Medicaid expansion, young adults staying on their parents' plan, and other coverage provisions. The primary care workforce is considerably challenged, with the number of new primary care physicians staying flat. Although 1,965 U.S. medical student graduates matched to primary care specialties in 2015, that represented no appreciable increase from the previous year. At the same time, there were 800 *more* primary care NPs graduated than the previous year, with a total of 14,400 primary care NP

graduates in 2014 (http://healthaffairs.org/blog/2015/07/01/primary-care-workforce-the
-need-to-lower-barriers-for-nurse-practitioners-and-physicians). Although some NMHCs
had closed nationally (largely due to financial sustainability issues) before the PPACA,
they are now needed more than ever to provide access to care as the number of people with
insurance has increased significantly.

There is also a trend for NMHCs becoming FQHCs, developing strong business plans
with financial models that lead to sustainability, or partnering with larger health care organizations. Data from all these models need to be examined. Interprofessional models of
care need to be analyzed with new research to better understand the impact of each provider in primary care. The Institute of Medicine report *The Future of Nursing* calls for all
nurses to work to their fullest educational preparation (IOM. *The Future of Nursing: Leading change, advancing health*. 2010. Washington, DC. The National Academies Press). For
primary care, that has weighty impacts. Removing barriers to full practice authority for
APRNs remains a challenging policy issue for the 27 states lacking such measures. There
is strong evidence on workforce, quality and safety of care, and financial impact when
APRNs practice to their fullest preparation. Although that evidence needs to be monitored
in the future, the positive research findings are overly abundant.

Primary care and a strong public health system are the foundation of a robust health
care system. With the PPACA covering many more Americans, nursing at all levels has
much to offer this foundation in terms of access, quality outcomes, and reasonable cost of
care. The next generation of nurse researchers will need to study the impact of interprofessional teams and the effectiveness of strategies that are unique to NPs and also examine the
best-practice models and value added when NPs are actively involved in and leading our
evolving health care system.

Reference

Pohl, J., Barksdale, D., & Werner, K. (2015, July 1). Primary care workforce: The need to lower barriers for
nurse practitioners and physicians. *Health Affairs Blog*. Retrieved from http://healthaffairs.org/blog/2015/07/01/
primary-care-workforce-the-need-to-lower-barriers-for-nurse-practitioners-and-physicians

The Many Facets of Cardiovascular Health Disparities in Black Americans

Debra J. Barksdale, PhD, FNP-BC, ANP-BC, CNE, FAANP, FAAN

Early in my career as a family nurse practitioner, I became interested in stress and its effects on the health of Black Americans. My program of research was inspired by my clinical practice in the DC metro area, where I saw a large number of young Black males who had high blood pressure but who did not exhibit many of the other risk factors that are often associated with hypertension (HTN). Nevertheless, they often told me how stressed they were. This was foundational to my program of research, which began during my PhD studies at the University of Michigan School of Nursing.

Great disparities in health exist for Black Americans. As a group, they have a higher incidence of chronic diseases and greater morbidity and mortality, which result in fewer healthy life years. Stress has been implicated as one factor in the adverse outcomes of Black Americans. In my dissertation research, *Everyday Life for Black American Adults; Stress, Emotions and Blood pressure* (Brown, 2004), in a sample of 211 adults between the ages of 25 and 79, socioeconomic status had a significant effect on chronic stress and chronic stress contributed to negative affect. From my dissertation data, I was able to do several other studies based on secondary data analysis. For example, we were able to show that based on the criteria of the *Seventh Report of the Joint National Committee on Prevention, Detection, Evaluation, and Treatment of High Blood Pressure* (U.S. Department of Health and Human Services, 2004), only 28.9% of the participants who had no history of HTN and who were not taking antihypertensive medications were actually normotensive. Thus more than 70% of the participants had elevated blood pressure (Brown & Metiko, 2005).

My program of research expanded to include a biobehavioral focus that led to the inclusion of multiple noninvasive physiological biomarkers such as cortisol, ambulatory blood pressure, heart rate variability, arterial stiffness, and other indicators of allostatic load. The study, titled *Stress, Cortisol, and Nighttime Blood Pressure Dipping in Nonhypertensive Black American Women*, showed that nearly one third of the subjects did not have an adequate blood pressure dipping of 10%–20% when they were asleep. These women also tended to report greater stress, more negative affect (emotions), and a greater likelihood of a positive family history of hypertension than women who displayed normal blood pressure dipping. This study highlights the need for providers to look at the entire risk profile of women who may appear normotensive while awake in the clinical setting (Barksdale, Woods-Giscombe, & Logan, 2013).

This work and others provided the foundation for my recent NIH K23 grant on hypertension in Black Americans. The purpose of this study was to examine the underlying hemodynamic determinants of HTN, particularly sleep blood pressure and sleep total peripheral resistance, as well as the cortisol awakening response. The study also explored whether individual differences in trait emotions and chronic active coping (John Henryism) moderated the influence of chronic psychosocial stressors on physiological systems. Chronic active coping is based on the legend of John Henry. In a competition against a steam-powered drill, John Henry won the contest but then died from mental and physical exhaustion. *John Henryism* is defined as a strong personality and behavioral predisposition to directly confront chronic psychosocial stressors through hard work and determination (James, Keenan, Strogatz, Browning, & Garrett, 1992). The sample consisted of 24 men and 56 women between the ages of 25 and 56. There were no differences in daily stress, perceived racial discrimination, or financial strain between those with and without HTN; however, those with HTN had a significantly greater body mass index. The relation of blood pressure dipping to daily hassles did not differ between HTN groups. HTN classification did affect the relation of dipping to racial discrimination. The HTN positive group differed significantly from the normal and the pre-HTN groups. The correlation of dipping and racial discrimination was .56 in the normal group, –.06 in the pre-HTN group and –.75 in the HTN group. The HTN positive group differed significantly from the pre-HTN group. The correlation of dipping and racial discrimination was –.33 in the normal group, .29 in the pre-HTN group, and –.33 in the HTN group (findings not yet published).

I have been fortunate to work with talented doctoral and postdoctoral students who have extended my work. In addition to research publications, we have published aspects of our work in clinical journals for nurse practitioners and other providers. Drs. Jeongok Logan and Minhee Suh extended my work to Korean Americans and have gone on to have successful careers of their own as junior faculty (e.g., Logan, Barksdale, Carlson, Carlson, & Rowsey, 2012; Suh, Barksdale, & Logan, 2013, 2014). Dr. Carolyn Lekavich has expanded aspects to include the mechanism of heart failure (Lekavich & Barksdale, 2016).

My education at the University of Michigan and my research career at the University of North Carolina at Chapel Hill have collectively contributed to my appointment to the Patient Centered Outcomes Research Institute (PCORI). I am currently the only nurse serving on the Board of Governors, and I chair the Engagement, Dissemination, and Implementation Committee, one of the three major strategy committees. The committee's charge is to provide recommendations to the board regarding the development of (a) the Institute's communications and branding work, (b) strategies to engage all stakeholders in the work of PCORI, and (c) methodologically sound approaches to disseminating and implementing the research results and ensuring their utility to patients and clinicians.

PCORI was created by the Patient Protection and Affordable Care Act of 2010 to address the challenges of closing the gap between research and real-life questions that patients, their families, and clinicians face daily. PCORI aims to close the gap between evidence to improve health, health care, and patient outcomes by focusing on research needed to inform health using a patient-centered perspective (Barksdale, Newhouse, & Miller, 2014; Newhouse, Barksdale, & Miller, 2015). An integral part of my work with PCORI has also focused on engaging more nurses in clinical comparative effectiveness research and patient-centered research.

References

Barksdale, D. J., Newhouse, R., & Miller, J. (2014). The Patient-Centered Outcomes Research Institute: Opportunities for academic nursing. *Nursing Outlook, 62*(3), 192–200. doi:10.1016/j.outlook.2014.03.001

Barksdale, D. J., Woods-Giscombe, C., & Logan, J. (2013). Stress, cortisol, and nighttime blood pressure dipping in nonhypertensive Black American women. *Biological Research for Nursing, 15*(3), 329–336. doi:10.1177/1099800411433291

*Brown, D. J. (2004). Everyday life for Black American adults: Stress, emotions and blood pressure. *Western Journal of Nursing Research, 26*(5), 499–514. doi:10.1177/0193945904265667

*Brown, D. J., & Metiko, E. B. (2005). Prevalence of hypertension in a sample of Black adults using JNC 7 classifications. *Journal of the National Black Nurses Association, 16*(2), 1–5.

James, S. A., Keenan, N. L., Strogatz, D. S., Browning, S. R., & Garrett, J. M. (1992). Socioeconomic status, John Henryism and blood pressure in Black Adults, The Pitt County Study. *American Journal of Epidemiology, 135*, 69–67.

Lekavich, C., & Barksdale, D. J. (2016). A critical evaluation of the representation of Black patients with heart failure preserved ejection fraction in clinical trials: A Literature Review. *Journal of Cardiovascular Nursing, 31*(3), 202–208. doi:10.1097/JCN.0000000000000237.

Logan, J., Barksdale, D. J., Carlson, J., Carlson, B., & Rowsey, P. (2012). Psychological stress and arterial stiffness in Korean Americans. *Journal of Psychosomatic Research, 73*(1), 53–58. doi:10.1016/j.jpsychores.2012.04.008

Newhouse, R., Barksdale, D. J., & Miller, J. (2015). Research done differently: The patient centered outcomes research institute, *Nursing Research, 64*(1), 72–77. doi:10.1097/NNR.0000000000000070

Suh, M., Barksdale, D. J., & Logan, J. (2014). Morning blood pressure surge and nighttime blood pressure in relation to nocturnal sleep pattern and arterial stiffness. *Journal of Cardiovascular Nursing, 29*(2), 439. doi:10.1097/JCN.0b013e318291ee43

Suh, M., Barksdale, D. J., & Logan. (2013). An exploratory study on relationships among stress, sleep and blood pressure dipping in Korean American. *Clinical Nursing Research, 22*(1), 112–129. doi:10.1177/1054773812455054

U.S. Department of Health and Human Services, National Heart, Lung, and Blood Institute. (2004). *Seventh report of the Joint National Committee on prevention, detection, evaluation, and treatment of high blood pressure.* Washington, DC: Author.

*Name changed to Barksdale.

The Effect of Cross-Cultural Provider-Patient Dyadic Relationships on Health Outcomes

Ramona A. Benkert, PhD, RN

My program of research focuses on identifying interactions among cultural and socioeconomic processes that influence health outcomes among racial and ethnic minority populations. My primary program has studied the effect that the primary health care dyad has on racial and ethnic minorities' utilization of and satisfaction with health care services and the resultant influence on health outcomes. I have studied provider cultural competence, racial and ethnic concordance, the patients' perceptions of racism and ethnic discrimination, and coping with racism. My research is relevant to an interdisciplinary audience of both researchers and clinicians.

Major Findings

The major findings from my research are summarized in four areas: (a) cross-racial provider-patient dyadic relationships, (b) patient perspectives of the provider and health system, (c) provider cultural competence, and (d) health services outcomes. Each of these areas is described below.

Cross-cultural provider-patient dyadic relationships. My primary area of research interest has been on the cross-cultural provider-patient relationship, particularly the influence that perceived racism and discrimination and the provider's interaction style have on health outcomes. My research has focused on non-Hispanic White American providers (nurse practitioners and physicians) and African American patients in primary care dyads. My dissertation research used qualitative methods to study the growing but little understood dyads of nurse practitioners and patients in primary health care (Benkert, Pohl, & Coleman-Burns, 2004). I found that African American female patients and non-Hispanic White nurse practitioners (NPs) had distinct perceptions of the relationship. Both members of the dyad were shaped by life experiences, their interpersonal interactions, and the phase of the relationship. These cross-racial relationships proceeded through three distinct phases. In a secondary analysis of the dissertation data, I also discovered that African American women developed distinct ways of coping with the prejudice and racism they experienced in health care. African American women reported using the coping strategies of "anger," "learning to unlearn," "being assertive," and finally "walking away" when exposed to prejudice, strategies that had not been previously reported in the health care literature (Benkert & Peters, 2005). Overall, I found that patients described a mistrust of the non-Hispanic White NPs (and other non-Hispanic White providers) based on their White skin color, which the NPs were unaware existed. Although these findings were not new to multicultural counseling and clinical psychology research, no studies utilizing these concepts could be found in the nursing or medicine research at that time. These findings led me to explore the concepts of cultural mistrust, race concordance, racial/ethnic identity, and privilege awareness in the primary health care arena.

Patients' perspectives of the provider and the health system. Although it is well known that African American patients rate their primary care physician lower than non-Hispanic White patients, little or no research had been conducted to examine African American patients' trust in and satisfaction with health care delivered by an NP. This gap in knowledge provided the basis for a study that examined the NP provider-patient dyad, as well as the quality of care provided to urban African Americans with hypertension. The study found interactions between the length of the provider-patient relationship, race concordance, perceived racism, cultural mistrust, type of setting (nurse practitioner managed versus jointly managed), trust in the provider, and satisfaction with the provider (Benkert, Peters, Clark, & Keves-Foster, 2006). The study provided the first published framework (using path analysis) of the interactions between exposure to lifetime racism, cultural mistrust, and diminished trust and satisfaction with primary care providers. Further findings suggested that trust in and satisfaction with primary care differed between NPs and physicians and between nurse-managed clinics and joint-managed clinics, even when care was provided by NPs in the joint-managed clinic. The results of these findings were new and added significantly to our understanding of African American patients' perspectives of primary care NPs (Benkert, Peters, Tate, & Dinardo, 2008). In another study, I examined the impact of racial identity, medical mistrust, and cultural mistrust as predictors of satisfaction with NP-delivered primary care from three distinct clinic types and a more socioeconomically heterogeneous African American patient population. The findings confirmed that cultural mistrust is negatively associated with patient trust and satisfaction with NP-delivered care, and patients with a flexible racial identity were more satisfied with NP care. The data also suggested that trust and satisfaction ratings by patients in a joint-managed clinic servicing older populations of African Americans were similar to those of the nurse-managed clinic (Benkert, Hollie, Nordstrom, Wickson, & Binns-Emerick, 2009). In addition, race concordance was correlated with satisfaction. Having explored the underlying cultural and socioeconomic processes among African American patients and the interactions of these processes with trust and satisfaction, I sought to understand NP processes that may impact provider-patient dyads. I had theorized that both providers and patients come to the dyadic interaction as complex humans. This led me to study provider cultural competence and diversity experiences among NPs.

Provider cultural competence. The primary avenue recommended for diminishing the health disparities of African Americans (and other racial and ethnic minorities) at the provider-patient encounter level is cultural competence training of the provider. Few studies have focused on primary care or practicing physicians, and still fewer have focused on practicing NPs. To fill this gap in knowledge, my research, both collaboratively and independently, has focused on the measurement of cultural competence and understanding the predictors of cultural competence among nurses, and more specifically NPs. In order to better understand cultural competence among NPs, I conducted a study using a stratified random national sample of underrepresented and rarely studied nurse practitioners (NPs of color and male NPs). My review of the literature suggested that one of the limitations of cultural competence research is its narrow assessment of the provider, and research is often conducted as a "one size fits all" philosophy. My study of NP cultural competence used multigroup structural equation modeling techniques to explore the multitude of predictors of NPs of color and male NPs. The findings suggested that life experience along with diversity, social justice beliefs, cultural competence awareness, sexual orientation, and diversity training predicted 27% of the variance in cultural competence behaviors (Benkert, Templin, Schim, Doorenbos, & Bell, 2011). Moreover, the data suggested that the predictors varied by the race and ethnicity of the NP.

Health outcomes. My research program is ultimately designed to improve the primary health care and health outcomes of ethnic minority populations. My early research findings (in teams and independently) led me to examine the influence of the psychosocial aspects of care on hypertension and patient satisfaction outcomes among low-income African Americans. To evaluate the provider-patient dyad and health service outcomes, I have used the Donabedian Quality Assessment framework. Several studies with my colleague Dr. Rosalind Peters using the Donabedian framework found that previous experiences of racism lead to a lack of trust in health care providers and lower satisfaction with care, but there is no direct link to hypertension outcomes. More recently, I have begun to assess the interactions between the trust of obstetric providers (including nurse midwives) and pregnancy outcomes (Peters, Benkert, & Templin, & Cassidy-Bushrow, 2014). The most recent study (Peters et al., 2014) found high trust of providers had limited associations with common pregnancy outcomes (e.g., use of prenatal vitamins, appointment follow-up, and low birth weight). We argued that the long-standing relationships between the obstetric providers and the high percentage of multiparous women influenced our results.

References

Benkert, R., Hollie, B., Nordstrom, C. K., Wickson, B., & Binns-Emerick, L. (2009). Trust, mistrust, racial identity and patient satisfaction in Urban African American primary care patients of nurse practitioners. *Journal of Nursing Scholarship, 41,* 211–219.

Benkert, R., & Peters, R. (2005). African American women's coping with healthcare prejudice. *Western Journal of Nursing Research, 27,* 863–889.

Benkert, R., Peters, R., Clark, R., & Keves-Foster, K. (2006). Effects of perceived racism, cultural mistrust, and trust in providers on satisfaction with care. *Journal of the National Medical Association, 98,* 1532–1540.

Benkert, R., Peters, R., Tate, N., & Dinardo, E. (2008). Low-income African Americans trust of nurse practitioners and physicians. *Journal of the American Academy of Nurse Practitioners, 20,* 273–280.

Benkert, R., Pohl, J., & Coleman-Burns, P. (2004). Creating cross-racial nurse practitioner-patient relationships in a nurse-managed center. *Journal of Cultural Diversity, 11,* 88–99.

Benkert, R., Templin, T., Schim, S., Doorenbos, A., & Bell, S. E. (2011). Testing a multi-group model of cultural competence behaviors among underrepresented nurse practitioners. *Research in Nursing and Health, 34,* 327–341.

Peters, R., Benkert, R., Templin, T., & Cassidy-Bushrow, A. (2014). Measuring African American's trust in provider during pregnancy. *Research in Nursing and Health, 37,* 144–154.

Culturally Tailored, Community-Based Diabetes Prevention and Management Interventions

Deborah Vincent, PhD, RN

My primary research has focused on developing and testing cost-effective interventions and models of health care delivery. Specifically, I have concentrated on designing and implementing culturally tailored diabetes prevention programs as a means of improving costs and health outcomes. Diabetes is a serious and deadly disease for all, but it is especially problematic in the Mexican American population of the United States-Mexico border region. This area has a high population of people of Mexican descent, and many are predominantly Spanish speakers. In addition, prevalence of diabetes is higher in Latinos than it is in the non-Hispanic population, and Latinos also have higher rates of diabetes complications and prediabetes (Vincent, Pasvogel, & Barrera, 2007). These combined factors result in a population at high risk for developing diabetes and complications of diabetes and lead to significant personal and societal costs.

My initial research focused on improving diabetes self-management behaviors in Latinos with type 2 diabetes. To enhance the understanding of barriers and facilitators of diabetes self-management, we conducted focus groups with patients and family caregivers

(Vincent, Clark, Marquez-Zimmer, & Sanchez, 2006) and used these results to inform a feasibility study of a culturally tailored diabetes self-management intervention for Spanish-speaking Latinos. First, we translated a widely used diabetes self-management assessment tool into Spanish, assessed its psychometric properties, and found it to be both reliable and valid (Vincent, McEwen, & Pasvogel, 2008). This instrument has been used by other researchers in many countries and has been cited more than 30 times.

Next, we conducted a small feasibility study of a culturally tailored diabetes intervention in which participants were randomly assigned to an intervention or control group condition. Feasibility was assessed by examining ease of recruitment and retention rates, and changes in diabetes knowledge, self-management behaviors, weight, and blood glucose were examined. The most effective recruitment strategy was personal referral—retention rates were 100% for the intervention group and 80% for the control. Findings from this study suggest that the intervention had a positive clinical and statistical effect on diabetes knowledge, weight, and body mass index. Improvements were noted in blood glucose, HbA1C levels, and self-efficacy scores, although they did not reach statistical significance (Vincent, Pasvogel, & Barrera, 2007); the results of this study influenced our next steps in research.

As I continued my research in culturally tailored interventions, I became increasingly convinced that diabetes prevention was a public health imperative. While the Diabetes Prevention Program (DPP) had clearly demonstrated that progression to diabetes could be delayed or prevented, it was resource intensive and was not easily replicated. Community-based programs offered in convenient and familiar locations were needed to reach underserved populations, such as Spanish-speaking Latinos, and decrease barriers to participation.

Our next study, therefore, was to determine the feasibility of translating and culturally tailoring the DPP into a community-based program for overweight Mexican American adults and to estimate the effect size of this intervention on weight loss. The randomized controlled trial, funded by the National Institute of Health (NIDDK, 1R34DK085195-01), compared the effects of a 5-month educational intervention with an attention control group. The intervention was called *Un Estilo De Vida Saludable* (EVS), which means "healthy lifestyle" in Spanish. EVS adopted the DPP goals of weight loss and increased physical activity but culturally tailored the implementation format into a community-based program for the target population. The primary study outcome was weight loss. Other outcomes included a change in waist circumference and diet and exercise self-efficacy.

EVS used a multimodal delivery format that incorporated culturally familiar methods such as small groups (*charlas*) and stories (*fotonovela*) to relay important lifestyle modification information for achieving weight loss and, therefore, preventing diabetes. Additionally, a bilingual community health worker (*promotora*) delivered the intervention.

Community advisory boards (CABs) have long been used in community-based research, and our study was no exception. A CAB was established over several years that built on collaborative relationships with a local community health center, their *promotora*, and a Latina public health student at the clinic. These individuals served as culture brokers and introduced me to other key members of the community and organizations who became critical to conducting research in the community. An outcome of this collaboration was two small studies that included the *promotora* and student as grant team members (Vincent, McEwen, Hepworth, & Stump, 2013; Vincent, McEwen, Hepworth, & Stump, 2014), both of whom continued to serve on the CAB during the EVS study.

Building on my community connections, I partnered with the faith-based and non-faith-based community leaders to recruit participants and deliver the intervention. To determine the effectiveness of various recruitment strategies, we assessed multiple passive and active recruitment tactics and found that presentations on healthy living strategies given at local churches were the most effective. Passive recruitment tactics such as flyers and radio announcements were ineffective as they do not rely on personal relationships, which are important when working with people of Mexican descent.

Findings support the conclusion that a community-based, culturally tailored intervention is effective in reducing diabetes risk factors. There were significant intervention effects for weight, waist circumference, body mass index, and diet self-efficacy, with the intervention group doing better than the control group.

Seven peer reviewed publications (*Diabetes Educator, Biological Research for Nursing, Journal of Transcultural Nursing*, and *Journal of the American Academy of Nurse Practitioners*) and national conference presentations resulted from this pilot work in diabetes. The *Biological Research for Nursing* article was ranked number 15 in their 50 most-read articles and was in the top 20 of their most-frequently-cited articles. Other accomplishments include our culturally tailored program being designated by the Canadian Diabetes Association as one of the "best and promising practices" in diabetes education in their Catalog of Best Practices and being listed in the Aging Texas Well Evidence-Based Clearinghouse as an evidence-based practice.

Based on my research and community partnerships, I was asked to participate in a project funded by the Centers for Disease Control and Prevention that brought together government, religious, and community leaders to develop local policies that promote healthy lifestyles and decrease the prevalence of obesity and diabetes in our community. Some of the results from this project were changes in health policies that established year-round farmers markets throughout Pima County, promoted physical activity awareness, and assisted faith-based organizations in developing or expanding health ministries to address obesity and diabetes in community-based settings. I was privileged to serve on the Health and Faith-Based Team, which worked with more than 183 faith-based organizations to develop health and wellness programs or health ministries.

References

Vincent, D., Clark, L., Marquez-Zimmer, L., & Sanchez, J. (2006). Using focus groups to design a culturally sensitive diabetes self-management program for Mexican-Americans. *Diabetes Educator, 32*(1), 89–97.

Vincent, D., Pasvogel, A., & Barrera, A. (2007). A feasibility study of a culturally tailored diabetes intervention for Mexican-Americans. *Biological Research for Nursing, 9*(2), 130–141.

Vincent, D., McEwen, M., Hepworth, J., & Stump, C. (2013). Challenges and success of recruiting and retention for a culturally tailored diabetes prevention program for adults of Mexican descent. *Diabetes Educator, 39*(2), 222–230. doi:10.1177/0145721713475842

Vincent, D., McEwen, M., Hepworth, J., & Stump, C. (2014). The effects of a community-based, culturally tailored diabetes prevention intervention for high risk adults of Mexican descent. *Diabetes Educator, 40*(2), 202–213.

Vincent, D., McEwen, M., & Pasvogel, A. (2008). The validity and reliability of a Spanish version of the summary of Diabetes Self-Care Activities Questionnaire. *Nursing Research, 57*(2), 101–106.

SECTION III

Advancing the Health
of Women Globally

CHAPTER 8

Three Decades of Research to Improve Women's Health

Carolyn Sampselle, PhD, RN, FAAN

SHORT PAPERS SUBMITTED FOR THIS CHAPTER

Carol J. Boyd
Jody Lori
Lisa Kane Low
Zxy-Yann Jane Lu
Janis Miller
Carolyn Sampselle
Julia S. Seng

Nursing is rooted in a history of strong women whose courageous actions have served to better human health. In the process of establishing professional nursing, Florence Nightingale left a comfortable life in England to challenge health and hygiene practices in battle-torn Crimea. The resulting declines in mortality and morbidity justified major changes in policy as well as increases in resources. Clara Barton forged a substantial role for nurses in the American Civil War and founded the Red Cross to promote healing efforts following natural disasters. Margaret Sanger risked personal danger to ensure women's access to the life-expanding option of fertility control. Mary Breckenridge demonstrated the public health impact that could be accomplished with evidence-based maternal child care and established the Frontier Nursing Service, an agency that continues to benefit the health of women and their families, especially in low-resource settings. Although these pioneers of modern nursing did not overtly acknowledge being motivated by a feminist rationale, it is not difficult to link the outcomes generated by their work to feminist precepts. They exemplified the value of a feminist voice raising worthy concerns and speaking truth to power. And they clearly based their reform efforts on the unrestricted agency of women that stemmed from an unequivocal respect for the innate strength that women needed in order to navigate a gender-biased world. The vision and commitment our forbearers modeled can be found in contemporary programs of research led by women's health nurse scientists at the University of Michigan School of Nursing (UMSN) and in the wider world of women's health scholarship.

This chapter highlights the research impact of UMSN Women's Health faculty as it fits within the broader literature of women's health scholarship. It is organized into three sections:

- the evolution of women's health scholarship
- the fit and contribution of UMSN women's health faculty to women's health scholarship
- future projections for women's health scholarship at UMSN

The Evolution of Women's Health Scholarship

Three decades ago, the operative scientific paradigm underlying clinical research was in sharp contrast to that of the present day because the majority of clinical research was conducted on men. This practice was based on the assumption that any results could simply be extrapolated to women. This was rooted in the belief that with the exception of reproductive system differences, males could be considered appropriate stand-ins for females. The rationale supporting this view was that it was too complicated and expensive to design research that would take women's hormonal cycles into account. An additional looming concern was raised, given the unintended consequences of prenatal drugs on fetal development; the justification was that an inadvertent or undisclosed pregnancy while participating in a clinical trial might lead to serious birth defects. Women of childbearing age were barred from clinical research participation by the Food and Drug Administration, implying that women were either unaware of or could not be trusted to disclose their exposure to pregnancy. Given the draconian restrictions on women's acceptability as clinical research participants, it is not surprising that in 1985, the U.S. Public Health Service reported that there existed insufficient "biomedical and behavioral research on conditions and diseases unique to, or more prevalent, in women in all age groups," a deficiency that compromised the evidence base that was available upon which to base women's health care (U.S. Department of Health and Human Services, 1985).

It is surprising that the documented dearth of research available to address women's health issues did not raise a public outcry when it was disclosed. In fact, 8 years elapsed before congressional action was taken in the form of the National Institutes of Health (NIH) Revitalization Act. Passed in 1993, this legislation required that women and minorities be included in all NIH-sponsored research. One wonders if a "protective" attitude might have underlain the lack of public opposition to the restriction of women from clinical research; such an attitude might have stemmed from an antiquated view of women as property rather than as independent individuals with agency in their own right.

Historically, the legal status of women was as the property of the man who headed their particular household, whether father or husband. This circumstance gave women limited sovereignty not only over their personal property but also over their own bodies. In fact, in many states, a wife had no legal recourse should marital rape occur. Evidence of the persistence of this narrow perspective was seen well into the 21st century in, for example, a societal view of violence against women guided by a belief that such violence was a "family matter" and not appropriate for external intervention. Using a similar line of reasoning, decisions to ban women from clinical research for their own good can be understood as a positive, humane practice on the part of well-intentioned individuals. But regardless of the good intentions that may have fueled it, this restrictive practice gave rise to scientifically insufficient data upon which to base women's health care.

The substantial changes that have occurred in these attitudes can be credited in large measure to women's health scholarship and the activism that insights of feminist scholars generated within the public at large. What follows are the most influential shifts that have occurred over the past three decades.

Women's Biological Differences Require Their Inclusion in All Phases of Clinical Trials

The concerns about sex bias in the nation's research portfolio were initially raised by women's health scholars. The Society for Women's Health Research, founded in 1990, sponsored a number of professional forums, public meetings, and congressional briefings to raise awareness about insufficient attention to women's health as a field of inquiry. Lay groups such as the Boston Women's Health Book Collective provided a powerful and influential voice with the widely disseminated publication *Our Bodies, Ourselves* (1973), which spoke resoundingly to the value of women's agency.

Concern about the inadequacy of women's health research to address the multiplicity of conditions affecting the health of women grew among the general public and among elected representatives, including Patricia Schroeder, Olympia Snowe, and Henry Waxman. The Office of Research on Women's Health was established in 1990. In 1993, the National Institutes of Health Revitalization Act was passed, requiring the inclusion of women and minorities in all NIH-funded clinical trials. These are tangible results that were taken to address sex bias concerns raised by advocacy, congressional, professional, and scientific groups. It is noteworthy that accomplishing the goal of research equity for women provided an incontrovertible imperative to address racial/ethnic equity as well.

Women's Health Is More Than Reproductive Health

Feminist critique highlighted the limitation of the predominant view of women's health as simply the pathology of the reproductive system. The NIH Office of Research on

Women's Health (ORWH) provides the following explanation on their website: "The field has expanded far beyond its roots in reproductive health and includes the study of health throughout the lifespan and across the spectrum of scientific investigations: from basic research and laboratory studies to molecular research, genetics, and clinical trials. Researchers are investigating healthy lifestyles and behavior, risk reduction and disease prevention as well as searching for best ways to diagnose and treat chronic conditions" (ORWH, n.d.). Nancy Woods (1994), a member of the ORWH-appointed Task Force on Opportunities for Research on Women's Health, described the process to develop recommendations for the NIH Research Agenda on Women's Health. In addition to recommended research on conditions such as toxemia, habitual abortion, and menopause that are specific to the reproductive system, recommendations extended well beyond anatomical and physiological differences to include such topics as the development of self-esteem, health promotion across the life-span, and caretaker burden. These topics entail behavioral and ecological studies in addition to physiological parameters. Despite this more holistic approach, Woods offered an insightful critique: she pointed out that simply assuring sex equity by way of balanced sex representation among clinical research participants and increasing the number of women researchers would not solve the problem; rather Woods advised the necessity of a change in the very nature of the science conducted in order to fully illuminate the ecology of women's experiences and to serve emancipatory goals (Woods, 1994).

To advance the mandate of this critique, scientific rigor requires that a full understanding of health for women be based on awareness of their location in society and interface within their physical and social environment. Daly (1978) lifted up the inadequacy of gynecology defined as the study of disease and routine care of women's reproductive systems. Rather, she used the term *gyn/ecology* to expand this limited perspective to recognize the importance of women's involvement in the health issues and care of their own bodies. This expanded view mandated that the context of women's health be investigated with women central rather than peripheral to the investigation. This broader view incorporates methods that extend beyond simple quantitative documentation of phenomena. Qualitative investigation is a valuable addition to women's health scholarship, by either free-standing or mixed-methods reports, in order to fully capture and interpret women's experience.

Conducting science in partnership with women further advances the contribution of women's health research to women's well-being. Engaging women in all phases of a research project, from conceptualization and planning to interpretation of results, is essential to advance authenticity, validity and emancipatory goals.

Sex Differences Are an Essential Predictor of Health Outcomes

As discussed earlier, prior to the paradigm shift, the prevailing clinical model for testing the therapeutic impact of drugs or devices was a 150-pound White male. Male physiology and behavior served as the standard, with differences demonstrated among women (e.g., higher rates of depression and greater susceptibility to Alzheimer's) characterized as deficits attributed to their failure to adapt normal life demands. The absence of women (and marginalized minorities) in randomized clinical trials generated results that were scientifically generalizable to less than 50% of the population of the United States. Moreover, sex bias fueled the privileging of conditions affecting men and disproportionately placed less interest and value on investigating conditions that predominantly affected women. Extrapolation of this phenomenon explains the comparatively few women scientists that were historically invited to participate in review sections, thus diminishing the likelihood that the scientific imperative to study factors primarily affecting the health of women would be persuasive and competitive in the funding decision process.

Awareness of the importance of sex differences and the necessity of including them in research is growing within the scientific community. A report by the Institute of Medicine (IOM) released in 2001, titled *Exploring the Biological Contributions to Human Health: Does Sex Matter?*, converged with earlier research and concluded that biological and physiological differences can explain the differential way illness affects men in comparison to women (IOM, 2001). Molecular research has uncovered the ubiquity of a sex genotype (XX in female, XY in male) in every cell that explains some differences in risk (e.g., an X-linked genetic disease). Other differences, such as women's greater language recovery following a left-hemisphere stroke as compared to men, are less apparent until it is recognized that women use both sides of the brain for language, whereas men rely more heavily on the left hemisphere. Greater sensitivity to pain in women versus men is an emerging difference. These examples highlight the need for stronger data that will enable us to answer the following questions initially posed by the 2001 IOM report: "1) How can information on sex differences be translated into preventative, diagnostic, and therapeutic practice? and 2) How can the new knowledge about and understanding of biological sex differences and similarities most effectively be used to positively affect patient outcomes and improve health and health care?"

The recognition that sex differences are an essential component not only to answering these questions but also to the wider realm of gyn/ecology is also critical. An important contributor to the wider "ecology of women" is the fact that gender is socially constructed—that is, sex is ascribed with physical, biological, hormonal, and anatomical attributes, whereas gender is determined in response to cultural and social interpretations of sex.

There are behavioral expectations of socially appropriate gender behavior. As these expectations play out, men and women typically have very different experiences of the same environment. This can be characterized in the saying "Men look at women; women watch themselves being watched." This notion captures concisely the reality that culture imposes very different developmental experiences on male and female children. Girls are taught from an early age that their appearance is a vital component of their value to society, with considerably less attention given to their achievements. In fact, it is not unusual for girls and women to minimize or not disclose personal accomplishments because they are concerned that this might detract from their social desirability. This practice exerts considerable influence on girls' developing self-esteem. It further encourages girls and women to turn themselves into an object to be observed—that is, self-objectification with socially imposed standards of beauty that are impossible to attain. Boys, on the other hand, develop in an environment where they are taught to aim for and celebrate the accomplishment of their physical and intellectual goals. The power ascribed to men as the watcher of women carries with it the privilege of deciding who or what to watch, as well as their value as determined by their accomplishments. The male/female power differential is a social and economic reality. Work that is socially attributed as women's work, for example, domestic activities or caregiving, is not valued at levels comparable to "real work" (i.e., men's work) nor is it taken into account in calculations of gross domestic product.

There is no question that eliminating sex bias in research is necessary to answer critical questions that will benefit the health of women. But if we are to attain the emancipatory goals for women's health research that Woods (1994) outlined more than a decade ago, it is essential that the broader ecology that women navigate also be investigated and taken into account.

The Fit and Contribution of UMSN Women's Health Faculty Research to Women's Health Scholarship

Women's health research at UMSN has built on the efforts of respected scientists who pioneered early pathways and provided pivotal role models for those who followed. Drs. Deborah Oakley, Nancy Reame, and Thelma Wells were the earliest UMSN recipients of NIH funding that pertained to women's health concerns: Wells from the National Institute on Aging in 1982 to study urinary incontinence, Reame from the Center for Nursing Research in 1987 to study premenstrual syndrome, and Oakley from the Center for Nursing Research in 1987 to study nursing care for contraceptive use. Dr. Wells provided a milestone contribution to nursing science in her service as a charter member of the first nursing study section. Dr. Reame was an original contributor to the groundbreaking publication *Our Bodies, Ourselves* (Boston Women's Health Book Collective, 1973). Although these scientists did not ground their research in feminist thought, the research questions they investigated were unequivocally intended to better the health and lives of women.

Increasingly stronger links with feminist theory and praxis, the Women's Studies department, and the Institute for Research on Women and Gender emerged throughout the 1990s and have continued to the present time. The Women in Society and Health (WISH) Research Interest Group was established to serve as an incubator for nursing research that embodied feminist principles such as gender equity, societal value, and personal sovereignty (Sampselle, 1990). WISH met regularly, providing a community that nurtured the fledgling programs of research (PORs) of junior faculty and doctoral students alike. Not surprisingly, many WISH members over the years held joint appointments in the Women's Studies department (Boyd, Kane Low, Sampselle, Seng). Dr. Carol Boyd successfully served as director of the Institute for Research on Women and Gender from 2005 to 2011. Likewise, many UMSN women's health faculty have served as members of the Women's Studies department or the executive committees of the Institute for Research on Women and Gender.

Women's Studies faculty ties with the Obstetrics and Gynecology department have been equally productive, with many women's health faculty holding joint appointments in that department or conducting collaborative research and training projects (Kane Low, Lori, Miller, Sampselle, Seng). The Specialized Center of Research (SCOR) project focused on birth, muscle injury, and pelvic floor disorders and was led by John DeLancey of the University of Michigan Medical School in collaboration with UMSN women's health faculty. Most notably, Janis Miller has led one of the three required R01-level projects for each cycle of the SCOR project's existence; the other two R01s are headed by John DeLancey and James Ashton-Miller. First funded in 2002 and continuously funded since then, the SCOR exemplifies interdisciplinary collaboration and productivity and serves as a training ground for the next generation of team scientists.

Each of the women's health POR briefs presented with this chapter constitutes evidence of successful interdisciplinary collaboration. This collaboration encompasses extensive coauthored publications, shared funding, numerous awards, and effective mentorship of doctoral and postdoctoral students. Women's health nurse scientists have provided a viable bridge between traditional medicine and feminism that has given rise to novel avenues of research, important changes in clinical practice, and policies that will have lasting impacts on women's health and women's studies. There is growing evidence of the global impact that women's health faculty efforts are generating. Their influence can be found on virtually every well-populated continent. The PORs are organized as follows: health of the pelvic floor (Sampselle, Miller, Kane Low), gender and gender bias in drug abuse (Boyd), maternal and newborn health in low-resource countries (Lori and Boyd), posttraumatic stress disorder effects on women's health (Seng), and advocating cultural and gender-sensitive policy in women's health (Lu). Although these PORs span a wide range of physical and psychological arenas, they are united in their application of feminist principles; their affirmation of women as partners, not subjects, in research; their determination to better women's lives; and their recognition that a paradigm shift is required in order to accomplish these research aims.

Collectively, women's health faculty productivity has clearly contributed to the larger women's health literature. This is particularly true for areas that shifted from a focus on treatment to prevention and for the growing recognition that team science is critical to advancing the frontiers of knowledge. It is striking to note how well aligned women's health faculty PORs are with the first four goals of the recently published Office of Women's

Health Research document *Moving Into the Future With New Dimensions and Strategies: A Vision for 2020 Women's Health Research* (Office of Women's Health Research, NIH, 2015).

The *first goal* is to increase sex-differences research in basic science studies. Often women's health nurse scientists focus on more advanced points of the translational research trajectory, testing the value of evidence demonstrated at a more basic science point. This is true of Dr. Boyd's pioneering work about the differences between males and females in the misuse, nonmedical use, and abuse of prescription drugs. Much of the explanation of those differences can be found in gender role enactment, but the differences she described open a potentially valuable path for the exploration of a molecular explanation.

The *second goal* is to incorporate findings of sex/gender differences in the design and application of new technologies, medical devices, and therapeutic drugs. The ongoing contributions that Drs. Kane Low, Miller, Sampselle, and Seng have made to the more than 15-year record of the ORWH-initiated Specialized Center of Research has advanced the goal of incorporating sex/gender differences into research in multiple ways.

The *third goal* is to actualize personalized prevention diagnostics and therapeutics for girls and women. All seven of the women's health PORs have advanced this goal: Drs. Sampselle, Miller, and Kane Low did so via their cumulative research informing prevention of urinary incontinence, and Drs. Miller and Kane Low did so in their newly funded project on the prevention of lower urinary tract symptoms (LUTS) in women across the life-span; Dr. Boyd's research established the role that incest and sexual abuse played in women's crack cocaine use and led to the institution of routine sexual violence screening by women's drug treatment programs; Dr. Seng found that depression in pregnancy is usually comorbid with posttraumatic stress disorder (PTSD; most powerfully due to childhood maltreatment) and that PTSD is the biggest predictor of postnatal depression, both of which undergirded her development of the "Cycles-Breaking" theoretical framework, which has the potential to change perinatal mental health service delivery from a nearly exclusive attention to mood and thought disorders to a primary focus on trauma-induced disorders; Dr. Lori demonstrated the value of maternity waiting homes in reducing maternal and neonatal complications and death, which has led to the incorporation of maternity waiting homes as a key component of the Liberian Ministry of Health and Social Welfare's Accelerated Action Plan to Reduce Maternal and Neonatal Mortality; and Dr. Lu found that the use of low-dose hormone replacement therapy in conjunction with folk regimens such as soy isoflavones enhanced menopausal women's agency and capacity for wellness behavior. The fourth goal is to create strategic alliances and partnerships to maximize the domestic and global impact of women's health research. As discussed above, women's health faculty have established strategic national network and are increasingly exerting beneficial influences in the global arena.

Future Projections for Women's Health Research at the UMSN

The recent shift in the national research agenda to embrace in-depth knowledge of effective prevention is affirming to the women's health scientific community. Indeed the increased resources provided by initiatives such as the Prevention of LUTS in Women bode well for the much-needed incorporation of preventive measures earlier in the life-span so that lifestyle behaviors can be used to prevent the development of pathology, thereby reducing increased health care costs.

The greater role that women's health faculty are playing in various global health initiatives positions them to use their expertise to better the lives of many women beyond the borders of the United States. As individual women's health researchers move their PORs along the translational research trajectory, they will find opportunities to conduct the practical clinical trials needed to demonstrate that their respective interventions are ready to be scaled up. This final phase of translation will propel their science to have a profound and far-reaching impact on global women's health.

References

Boston Women's Health Book Collective. (1973). *Our bodies, ourselves.* New York, NY: Simon and Schuster.

Daly, M. (1978). *Gyn/Ecology: The metaethics of radical feminism.* Boston, MA: Beacon Press.

Institute of Medicine. (2001). *Exploring the biological contributions to human health: Does sex matter?* Washington, DC: Author.

NIH Revitalization Act of 1993. *Clinical Research Equity Regarding Women and Minorities.* Bethesda, MD: National Institutes of Health.

Office of Women's Health Research, National Institutes of Health. (n.d.). What is women's health research? Retrieved from http://orwh.od.nih.gov/about/womenshealthresearch.asp

Office of Women's Health Research, National Institutes of Health. (2015). *Moving Into the Future With New Dimensions and Strategies: A Vision for 2020 Women's Health Research* (NIH Publication No. 10-7606).

Sampselle, C. (1990). The influence of feminist philosophy on nursing practice. *Image: The Journal of Nursing Scholarship, 22*(4), 243–247.

U.S. Department of Health and Human Services. (1985). *U.S. Public Health Service Task Force on Women's Health Issues Report, 100*(1). Washington, DC: Department of Health and Human Services.

Woods, N. (1994). The United States Women's health agenda: Analysis and critique. *Western Journal of Nursing Research, 16*(5), 467–479.

Gender, Health, and Drugs of Abuse

Carol J. Boyd, PhD, RN, FAAN

My program of research can best be described as focusing on drugs of abuse and the role that gender and gender bias play in drug-taking behaviors. As a feminist researcher, much of my early work focused exclusively on women; however, that has evolved in the past 15 years to a broader examination of the role gender plays in drug-taking behaviors and policy implications.

1983–1998

I began my research career in the early 1980s, focusing on women living in Detroit who injected either heroin or Talwin and pyribenzamine (Ts and Blues; a cheap substitute for heroin in the early 1980s). The women I worked with were not in drug treatment; in fact, they did not want to quit their drug use, but they wanted to be understood. Using feminist and psychological theories to guide my field-based studies, I was one of the first to examine women's opposite-sex relationships and the role these relationships played in women's use of heroin and Ts and Blues. By 1985, freebase cocaine (crack) had entered urban areas, and crack was changing the demographic character of street drug users. Funded by a branch of the National Institute of Justice in 1988 and the National Institute on Drug Abuse (NIDA) in 1989, my research established the role that incest and sexual abuse played in women's crack cocaine use, the role adult males played in women's initiation to crack cocaine, and the diathesis that leads to women's crack use. In 1993, I was one of the few nurse researchers to study women crack users in their communities (not in drug treatment).

Impact. This work led to an invitation to a meeting convened by the Institute of Medicine, where I presented "Assessing Future Research Needs: Mental and Addictive Disorders in Women." A year later, I was invited to serve on county-wide advisory boards such as the Genessee County Council for Chemically Dependent Pregnant Women and was invited to take a leadership role in national training workshops funded by the Center for Substance Abuse Prevention and NIDA. My early research and advisory roles were instrumental in advancing the need for gender-sensitive drug treatment programs. Indeed, it is now routine for women's treatment programs to assess for past sexual violence.

2000–2005

I have always been interested in women's cigarette smoking, particularly the gendered and cultural aspects of the behavior as well as the role it plays in polydrug use. In 1997, the Robert Wood Johnson Foundation funded Professors Cynthia Pomerleau, Abigail Stewart, and I as co–principal investigators. I collaborated with this team, which included my postdoctoral trainee Dr. Alyssa Zucker. I received funding in 2001 from the University of Michigan and the University of Miami to study cigarette advertising and young women's cigarette smoking.

Impact. Our research established (a) the role thinness pressures play in women's cigarette smoking (b) the role discrimination plays in girls' cigarette smoking, and (c) that resistance to tobacco advertising messages is a protective factor in reducing cigarette smoking.

1999–2016

In 1999, there was growing public awareness that college campuses were sites of increasing drug and alcohol use. With funding from the University of Michigan, I was the first to develop a web-based survey of undergraduate drug and alcohol use—the Student Life Survey (SLS)—and used the SLS with a representative sample of undergraduates. We continue to focus on subgroups of undergraduates: women, LGBT students, athletes, and students of color. This study was the first to alert the field to the growing prescription drug problem, and we were the first researchers to publish these data on college students.

Impact. Funded by NIDA and the National Institute of Alcohol Abuse and Alcoholism, my team was the first to establish the heterogeneity of prescription drug users, the benefits of living-learning communities on college campuses in reducing alcohol abuse, and the protective effects of same-sex living arrangements for reducing women's binge drinking. I developed categories based on motives and published a typology of prescription drug use that NIDA has used in its program announcements (distinguishing between misuse and nonmedical use). Further, this typology has helped inform the new questions added to the annual National Study of Drug Use and Health survey funded by NIDA. My work established (a) that web-based technologies produce valid and reliable data on substance use behaviors at a much lower cost, (b) that motives to engage in prescription drug abuse are associated with different risk profiles, and (c) that college campus administrators are more aware of the abuse of prescription medications and have instituted preventative strategies. I consult often on this topic.

2001–2016

In 2001, the superintendent of a Detroit-area school district serving three cities on Detroit's northern border was concerned about a federal mandate to desegregate schools and the impact of desegregation on student behaviors. My research team initiated a community-based participatory action research (CBPR) program that is ongoing to the present. This CBPR was initially funded by the University of Michigan and later by NIDA for a prospective study of adolescents' prescription drug abuse. This work demonstrated that CBPR yields important collaborations and benefits the community and researchers alike. We learned about gender differences in the misuse, nonmedical use, and abuse of prescription drugs, including the diversion and risks of these controlled substances. We also learned that the student survey was cost effective and could be adapted to younger respondents.

Impact. In 2007, I was invited to be the lead consultant on a new media campaign launched by the Office of National Drug Control Policy with the goal of reducing prescription drug abuse by adolescents. Because of my research with adolescents, on April 14, 2011, I was invited to provide congressional testimony on the growing problem of prescription drug abuse by adolescents. That same year, I joined the Surgeon General's expert panel on prescription drug abuse among youth. I have served in important consulting roles on scientific advisory panels for postmarketing surveillance and risk management studies (mandated by the Food and Drug Administration) of controlled medications. My work on adolescent drug abuse has led to new prevention efforts and social marketing messages to reduce the problem of prescription drug abuse. In 2013, studies showed that for the first time, adolescents' abuse of opioid analgesics was declining, and my colleagues and I believe that this is due in part to these media campaigns.

Problems Encountered During Program of Research

Despite a well-established program of research (POR), the biggest problem is obtaining funding for my research program. In the substance abuse field, researchers often "follows the drugs"—that is, we must study the new, emerging drugs of abuse and then focus our studies on the populations most at risk for abusing the emerging drugs. For instance, methamphetamine (crystal meth) is not used much in southeastern Michigan; thus when the National Institutes of Health or the Centers for Disease Control and Prevention want studies of methamphetamine, that poses a problem for researchers working in southeastern Michigan. In order to stay funded, I had to move from studying women who smoke crack to an adolescent and emerging adult population that uses pills. Each time I change drugs and populations, I must "retool"; however, I always use feminist processes and research strategies to work with my research team and expand our research programs.

Anticipated Future Progression

One of the best funding strategies for researchers is to keep their POR relevant to the health of the public. In the future, I will focus on medical marijuana and e-cigarettes because we know little about the consequences of adolescents' use of either. I remain committed to understanding the "gendering" of drug abuse.

Lessons Learned

I tell my postdoctoral fellows the following: (a) diversify your research portfolio and seek funding from multiple sources (e.g., foundations, state contracts, National Institutes of Health, etc.); (b) never give a presentation that cannot be turned into a published paper, and have the paper ready to submit immediately after the presentation; (c) do not take rejection (whether it's your R01 proposal, your manuscript, or an idea put forth in a workshop) personally—constructive critiques are a *gift*, and the men and women who critique your work are colleagues who want you to succeed; and (e) finally, move early in your career to embrace colleagues from other disciplines who will join your research team.

Key References

1983–1998

Boyd, C. J., Guthrie, B., Pohl, J. M., Whitmarsh, J., & Henderson, D. (1994). African-American women who smoke crack cocaine: Sexual trauma and the mother-daughter relationship. *Journal of Psychoactive Drugs, 26*(3), 243–247.

Boyd, C. J., & Mieczkowski, T. (1990). Drug use, health, family and social support in "crack" cocaine users. *Addictive Behaviors, 15*(5), 481–485.

2000–2005

Boyd, C. J., McCabe, S. E., & d'Arcy, H. (2003a). Ecstasy use among college undergraduates: Gender, race and sexual identity. *Journal of Substance Abuse Treatment, 24*(3), 209–215. PMID: 12810141

Boyd, C. J., McCabe,. S. E., & d'Arcy, H. (2003b). A modified version of the CAGE as an indicator of alcohol abuse and its consequences among undergraduate drinkers. *Substance Abuse, 24*(4), 221–232. PMID: 14574088

2001–2016

Boyd, C. J., Austic, E., Epstein-Ngo, Q., Veliz, P. T., & McCabe, S. E. (2015). A prospective study of adolescents' nonmedical use of anxiolytic and sleep medication. *Psychology of Addictive Behaviors, 29*(1), 184–191. PMCID: PMC4388758

Boyd, C. J., McCabe, S. E., Cranford, J. A., Morales, M., Lange, J. E., Reed, M. B., . . . Scott, M. S. (2008). Heavy episodic drinking and its consequences: The protective effects of same-sex, residential living-learning communities for undergraduate women. *Addictive Behaviors, 33*(8), 987–993. PMCID: 2528065

Boyd, C. J., McCabe, S. E., Cranford, J. A., & Young, A. (2006). Adolescents' motivations to abuse prescription medications. *Pediatrics, 118*(6), 2472–2480. PMCID: PMC17853

Boyd, C. J., Young, A., Grey, M., & McCabe, S. E. (2009). Adolescents' nonmedical use of prescription medications and other problem behaviors. *Journal of Adolescent Health, 45*(6), 543–550. PMCID: PMC2784421

Improving Maternal and Newborn Health in Low-Resource Countries

Jody Lori, PhD, RN, FAAN

My key contributions are in the design and testing of innovative models of care to improve maternal and newborn health in areas of the world challenged by a lack of human resources, long distances to care, and socioeconomic and cultural barriers. The design of the interventions utilizes a human rights framework to tackle the intractable problems of preventable maternal and newborn mortality. My research approach has contributed to the development of models of care for improved maternal and newborn health through a program of participatory action research in low-resource countries.

2004–2009

I began my research career as a member of an interdisciplinary team involving 18 schools across the University of Michigan campus. This research was funded by a National Institutes of Health Roadmap Initiative Grant (P20) and focused on disparities in rates of preterm birth between Blacks and Whites living in the greater Detroit area. Using this research as a springboard, colleagues and I from the medical school successfully submitted a BlueCross and BlueShield Foundation proposal to expand the work to examine how medical liability was affecting this crisis. Additionally, I was awarded a grant by MESA (Michigan En San Antonio) Center for Health Disparities (a P20 center in the School of Nursing funded by National Institute of Nursing Research [NINR]) as principal investigator (PI) to develop an event history calendar for use in the prenatal care assessment of women at high risk for preterm births. This P20 initiative, funded by NINR, was designed to support investigators in research related to health disparities.

Impact. A key outcome of this research was the development of an event history calendar that provides obstetric care providers with an easy visualization of how psychosocial risk behaviors and factors interact over time to influence a woman's pregnancy (Lori, Yi, & Martyn, 2011). This event history calendar was then expanded upon by other faculty and doctoral students in the School of Nursing.

During this same period, I also launched my global health research career in sub-Saharan Africa. Despite worldwide efforts, nearly 300,000 women die from preventable causes related to pregnancy and childbirth each year. I work independently and within interdisciplinary groups to bring the unique perspective of nursing and midwifery to the research design and to the development of policies at a national level to improve maternal and newborn health. In 2004, in collaboration with the American College of Nurse-Midwives, I conducted an implementation and evaluation of a community-based strategy, Home Based Life Saving Skills, in Ethiopia and subsequently in Liberia to increase access to basic life-saving measures in the community and decrease delays in reaching referral facilities (Lori, Majszak, & Martyn, 2011). This fieldwork led to my dissertation research and cemented my program of research firmly in the arena of addressing disparities in maternal and newborn health globally. My earliest contributions to the science focused on the cultural and sociopolitical issues surrounding maternal and newborn mortality in sub-Saharan Africa (Lori & Boyle, 2011).

Impact. Publications and presentations provided a deeper understanding, through a wide lens, into the vulnerability of women living in rural and remote locations on the margins of society. An overarching cultural theme was developed that provides the basis for an evolving interpretive theory of maternal mortality and morbidity in Liberia. Findings from the earliest studies conducted in Liberia were translated into a maternal mortality review protocol for the Ministry of Health and Social Welfare that was implemented by county health teams, thus providing the ministry with data for targeted programs to reduce maternal mortality (Lori & Starke, 2012).

During this same period, I joined an interdisciplinary team of collaborators from two continents to examine the maldistribution of the health care workforce in Ghana. Highlighted by the lack of progress on the Millennium Development Goals, there was a growing awareness of how the acute shortage of health care workers was impacting the global poor. This work was among the first to examine the drivers for rural postings among future members of the midwifery profession.

Impact. In rural Ghana, translation of my research has helped inform the development of retention schemes for nursing and midwifery by the Ghana Health Service. Findings from this research have been used to expand and improve the delivery of evidence-based midwifery care, ultimately improving patient outcomes in women's reproductive health (Lori, Rominski, et al., 2012).

2010–2016

In 2010, I was awarded (as PI) one of six innovation grants by U.S. Aid for International Development's (USAID) Child Survival and Health Grants Program for a 4-year project in Liberia, West Africa. Innovation, Research, Operations, and Planned Evaluation for Mothers and Children (I-ROPE) examined maternity waiting homes (MWHs) as an intervention to reduce maternal and neonatal complications and death by overcoming the critical barrier of distance to accessing safe delivery services at a health facility (Lori et al., 2013). The study incorporated the novel and innovative use of cell phones to collect real-time data from rural and remote areas within Liberia (Lori, Munro, Boyd, & Andreatta, 2012).

Impact. Based on the outcomes of this research, the Liberian Ministry of Health and Social Welfare recently included MWHs as a key component of their Accelerated Action Plan to Reduce Maternal and Neonatal Mortality. It also contributed to the growing field of mHealth (mobile health) research—the use of mobile devices such a cell phones to improve public health.

In 2011, I was awarded (as PI) a K01 from the International Fogarty Center at the National Institutes of Health. This funding expands my research to focus on prenatal care in Ghana. The focus has been to develop and test a manualized prenatal care program designed to improve health literacy and increase facility delivery.

Impact. The results of this study contribute to identifying new approaches for improved communication in prenatal care in order to increase health literacy, improve care, and increase facility delivery. This study is one of the first to examine maternal health literacy in a low-resource setting. I developed a manualized intervention and, building on the interpretive theory of my earlier work, utilized the beginnings of the Maternal Health Literacy Skills Framework as a basis for future large-scale studies examining maternal health literacy (Lori, Dahlem, et al., 2014; Lori, Munro, & Chuey, 2015). The manual is currently being translated into Spanish. Findings from the research were presented to the larger global community at the Maternal and Newborn Conference in Mexico City in 2015, sponsored by USAID, the Bill and Melinda Gates Foundation, and several agencies of the United Nations, among others.

Problems Encountered During the Development of Programs of Research

Initially, the biggest challenge I faced was discouragement from peers and mentors for doing global research. The funding streams for global research at that time were sparse and not often applied for by nurse researchers. This drew cautious concern from mentors about my ability to continue a program of research that would be difficult to fund. However, with support and encouragement from Dr. Shaké Ketefian and by looking outside the usual channels for funding, I was able to overcome this obstacle. Additionally, nursing research is frequently undervalued in areas of the world where I conduct my studies. Research in the global arena is dominated by public health and medicine. By engaging with interdisciplinary teams, I believe I have helped break down silos and have offered a distinctive lens to global research.

Anticipated Future Progression

My ability to conduct robust clinical studies has contributed to the development of the science of sustainable community-driven, community-based models of care and has influenced policy and practice. I have strived to serve as a role model for a form of participatory research that is culturally relevant, community-based, and collaborative and that creates a sustainable environment that enhances the role of nursing research.

Based on the success of the I-ROPE study in Liberia, our research team has been awarded Phase I (completed) and Phase II (2015–2018) funding from Merck Sharp & Dohme, a subsidiary of Merck, through its Merck for Mothers program to study the operational and financial sustainability of an entrepreneurial model of MWHs in Zambia.

My future work will focus on the continued development of an interpretive theory of maternal mortality and morbidity in sub-Saharan Africa. I am dedicated to improving maternal health.

Lessons Learned

My experience in sub-Saharan Africa in the first decade of this century has afforded me a depth of understanding, a network of local partners, and the ability to conduct rigorous research within the cultural context of rural and remote locations. My advice to junior colleagues is to (a) listen more often than you speak when working in cultures outside your own, (b) work with colleagues from other disciplines both within and outside of health care—this has been a great gift and has taught me the value of diversity, (c) never stop listening and learning, and finally, (d) follow your passion.

References

Lori, J. R., & Boyle, J. S. (2011). Cultural childbirth practices, beliefs and traditions in postconflict Liberia. *Health Care for Women International, 32*(6), 454–473. PMID: 21547801

Lori, J. R., Dahlem, C. H. Y., Ackah, J. V., & Adanu, R. M. K. (2014). Examining antenatal health literacy in Ghana, *Journal of Nursing Scholarship, 46*(6), 432–440. doi:10.1111/jnu.12094. PMID: 24930782

Lori, J. R., Majszak, C. M., & Martyn, K. M. (2010). Home-based life-saving skills in Liberia: Acquisition and retention of skills and knowledge. *Journal of Midwifery and Women's Health, 55*(4), 370–377. PMID: 20630364

Lori, J. R., Munro, M. L., Boyd, C. J., & Andreatta, P. (2012). Cell phones to collect pregnancy data from remote areas in Liberia. *Journal of Nursing Scholarship, 44*(3), 294–230. doi:10.1111/j.1547-5069.2012.01451.x. PMCID: PMC3432659

Lori, J. R., Munro, M. L., & Chuey, M. R. (2015). Use of a facilitated discussion model for antenatal care to improve communication. *International Journal of Nursing Studies, 54*, 84-94. PubMed PMID: 25862409.

Lori, J. R., Munro, M. L., Rominski, S., Williams, G., Dahn, B. T., Boyd, C. J., . . . Gweigale, W. (2013). Maternity waiting homes and traditional midwives in rural Liberia. *International Journal of Gynecology & Obstetrics, 123*(2), 114–118. doi:10.1016/j.ijgo.2013.05.024. PMCID: PMC3795996

Lori, J. R., Rominski, S., Richardson, J. S., Agyei-Baffour, P., Kweku, N. E., & Gyakobo, M. (2012). Factors influencing Ghanaian midwifery students' willingness to work in rural areas: A computerized survey. *International Journal of Nursing Studies, 49*(7), 834–841. PMID: 22385911

Lori, J. R., & Starke, A. (2012). A critical analysis of maternal morbidity and mortality in Liberia, West Africa. *Midwifery, 28*(1), 67–72. PMID: 21232836

Lori, J. R., Yi, C. H., & Martyn, K. M. (2011). Provider characteristics desired by African-American women in prenatal care. *Journal of Transcultural Nursing, 22*(1), 71–76. PMCID: PMC3277208

Labor Care Practices for Optimal Health Outcomes for Childbearing Women

Lisa Kane Low, PhD, RN

My program of research is centered on labor care practices that promote optimal health outcomes for the more than 4 million U.S. women who give birth annually. I work to advance the state of science related to labor care practices that support physiological birth while reducing untoward complications and the need for surgical birth by focusing on three integrated areas: (a) labor care practices that promote optimal health outcomes for marginalized populations of childbearing women, (b) labor care during the second stage, and (c) the implementation of evidence-based practices to improve the quality and safety of maternity care.

1996–2001

I entered the University of Michigan School of Nursing's (UMSN) doctoral program in women's health and graduate certificate in women's studies with a background of more than 15 years of practice, first as a staff nurse in labor and delivery, then as a certified nurse midwife, and eventually as director of the nurse-midwifery service at Hutzel Hospital in Detroit, Michigan. My doctoral dissertation, titled *Adolescents' Experience of Childbirth: Nothing Is Simple*, was cochaired by professors Carolyn Sampselle (nursing and women's studies) and Karin Martin (sociology and women's studies) and defended in 2001 (Kane Low et al., 2003). I then joined the UMSN faculty as research assistant professor, with a joint appointment in the Department of Women's Studies as a lecturer. This appointment coincided with being accepted as a Building Interdisciplinary Research Careers in Women's Health (BIRCWH) scholar. I was awarded this fellowship in 2001 as one of the first two nurses appointed nationally to this competitive interdisciplinary research development program.

2002–2007

As a BIRCWH Scholar, I continued to focus on the promotion of optimal outcomes for childbearing women and applied for a W. K. Kellogg Foundation grant to explore the value of a community-based doula care program for vulnerable populations of women and adolescents. A component of this work included the development of a program model for doula services using a community partnership with the Doulas Care program. The model development was funded by multiple foundations including the Pfizer Foundation, Michigan March of Dimes, Blue Cross Blue Shield of Michigan, and the Knight Foundation. Dissemination of the model occurred through publications and presentations (Kane Low, Moffatt, & Brennan, 2006). During this time, I expanded my focus on maternity care experiences to include pelvic floor health and the impact of childbirth. I was pleased to be invited by John DeLancey (University of Michigan Medical School) to be co–principal investigator (PI) on the Special Center for Research (SCOR) program he was leading, titled Sex and Gender Factors Affecting Women's Health, Birth, Muscle Injury, and Pelvic Floor Dysfunction. My role was to participate in and lead studies exploring women's experience of pelvic muscle dysfunction and childbirth, adding midwifery clinical insights to a team comprising obstetricians, bioengineers, and nursing colleagues Janis Miller and Carolyn Sampselle. The SCOR project was awarded initial funding in 2002 through 2007 and has been continuously funded as of 2016. During this period, I was also invited to serve as co-PI on a project led by Julia Seng, the Psychobiology of Post-Traumatic Stress Disorder and Adverse Outcomes of Childbearing (STACY Project). My role in this project was to coordinate recruitment in the Detroit area and provide expertise for assessing and measuring the intrapartum experience.

Impact. My involvement in these respective research projects contributed to my interest and understanding of optimal outcomes of childbirth and its measurement. I was honored to be part of the development and validation of the Optimality Index with nurse-midwifery colleagues Patricia Murphy and Judith Fullerton (Kane Low, Seng, & Miller, 2008). This new instrument and the work I have participated in as a member of the national Optimality Work Group has been recognized with a national research award from the Lamaze association, and the Optimality Index has now been translated for use in three countries.

2008–2013

The rich interdisciplinary climate at the University of Michigan fostered a productive working relationship with James Ashton-Miller (Bioengineering). We developed methods to better measure the pelvic floor demands of normal delivery, Developing Measures of Normal Delivery (the DiMEND project), and successfully applied for funding from local sources such as the Michigan Center for Health Intervention and the Michigan Center for Clinical and Translational Research to support this initiative. In 2011, I was awarded a National Institutes of Health R03 grant for my project Spontaneous vs. Directed Pushing: Analysis of Audiotapes of 2nd Stage Labor and Associated Outcomes, which built on prior work conducted at UMSN on incontinence risk due to childbirth (Kane Low, Miller, et al., 2012). Expanding the prior focus from incontinence to exploring women's experiences of pelvic floor changes secondary to childbirth, including the translation of evidence into practice to support optimal management of second-stage labor, was my contribution to improving maternity care practice.

Impact. Having served as PI on a series of three independently funded studies that focus on identifying the high-risk events for pelvic floor trauma has led to the identification of interventions that can be tested to reduce that risk. The state of science related to second-stage management is conflicted between recommendations to reduce the duration of the second stage and those that allow for a passive descent without time constraints. My research seeks to change the paradigm from focusing solely on global time or duration of the second stage to instead focus on the specific events that occur during that time that may create risk for negative pelvic floor outcomes. Two completed investigations demonstrate this line of investigation is promising and offers opportunity to develop interventions to improve outcomes. In my R03 investigation, nonphysiological pushing during the second stage of labor significantly increases risk for incontinence at 1 year postpartum and in the Evaluating Maternal Recovery From Labor and Delivery study (Miller, PI) study, prolonged active pushing explained increased risk of levator ani muscle tears more than total time in the second stage (Kane Low et al., 2014). These investigations provide a foundation to change the labor care practices we employ, such as directed pushing or rapid end-stage pushing, in an attempt to reduce the risks of negative outcomes.

2013–2016

As an extension of my focus on labor care practices, I have lead research projects in low-resource maternity care settings to address improving the quality of maternity care services. I led a team of nurse-midwives, including UMSN graduate Dr. Joanne Motino Bailey, and other public health professionals and women's studies scholars in an examination of maternal health in rural Honduras. We explored workforce capacity and transitions in maternity care services as well as the prevention of postpartum hemorrhages (Low et al., 2012). This work had an extended impact beyond dissemination as we developed a service learning experience for students to participate in the provision of maternity care and the conduct of clinical research in low-resource settings. Numerous students from this project went on to enroll in advanced practice nursing programs or pursue doctoral degrees and research in global health.

I have continued as an active member of the interdisciplinary Pelvic Floor Research Group for more than 15 years. Given the strong interests of the group in the factors that increase women's risk of pelvic floor dysfunction, it should not be surprising that my research interests have grown to encompass the multiple lower urinary tract symptoms (LUTS) that compromise the health of women across the life-span. Hence when Carolyn Sampselle was asked to serve at the National Institute of Nursing as senior advisor to the director, I was pleased to step in and assume the responsibilities on her projects. These projects included incontinence for childbearing women and a multisite study that is using group biobehavioral education to treat urinary incontinence in women above the age of 55. This work has informed a recent award from the National Institutes of Health for Prevention of LUTS in Women: Bladder Health Clinical Center, with Janis Miller as PI and me as coinvestigator. This is a transdisciplinary project that will focus on the promotion of healthy bladder status across the life-span. Nationally, I have also participated in the development of evidence-based guidelines for optimal maternity care practice. This work explores overused technologies that negatively affect childbirth outcomes (Moore, Kane Low, Titler, Dalton, & Sampselle, 2014) and care practices to reduce maternal morbidity and mortality (Main et al., 2015)

Future Directions

Future directions include exploring labor care practices that can serve to improve health outcomes for women, specifically reducing the risk of pelvic floor injury and promoting evidence-based practices to improve quality and safety during the maternity care cycle. This trajectory can reduce risks that result in more than 300,000 surgeries annually. I have also developed an application for funding that explores barriers to the translation of evidence-based strategies that promote the physiological management of second-stage labor across four health systems in Michigan and another proposal exploring the non-evidence-based use of electronic fetal monitoring across four health systems nationally. As a member of interdisciplinary scientific teams comprising scholars from nursing, midwifery, medicine, women's studies, bioengineering, sociology, and psychology, I am poised to continue moving my program of work forward by taking advantage of the privilege I have in experiencing the value of interdisciplinary team science with exceptional colleagues.

References

Kane Low, L., Martin, K., Sampselle, C., Guthrie, B., Stewart, A., & Oakley, D. (2003). Adolescents' experiences of childbirth: Contrasts with adults. *Journal of Midwifery and Women's Health, 48*(3), 192–198. doi:10.1016/S1526-9523(03)00091-6

Kane Low, L., Miller, J., Gao, Y., Ashton-Miller, J., DeLancey, J. O. L., & Sampselle, C. (2012). Spontaneous pushing to prevent postpartum urinary incontinence: A randomized, controlled trial. *International Journal of Urogynecology, 24*(3), 453–760. doi:10.1007/s00192-012-1884

Kane Low, L., Moffatt, A., & Brennan, P. (2006). Doulas as community health workers: Lessons learned from a volunteer program. *Journal of Perinatal Education, 15*(3), 25–33.

Kane Low, L., Seng, J., & Miller, J. (2008). Use of the optimality index-United States in perinatal clinical research: A validation study. *Journal of Midwifery and Women's Health, 53*(4), 302–309. doi:10.1016/j.jmwh.2008.01.009

Kane Low, L., Zielinski., R., Tao, Y., Galecki, A., Brandon, C., & Miller, J. (2014). Predicting birth-related levator ani tear severity in primiparous women: Evaluating maternal recovery from labor and delivery (EMRLD Study). *Open Journal of Obstetrics and Gynecology, 4*, 266–278. doi:10.4236/ojog.2014.46043

Main, E., Goffman, D., Scavone, B., Low, L. K., Bingham, D., Fontaine, P., . . . Levy, B. (2015). National partnership for maternal Safety: Consensus bundle on obstetric hemorrhage. *Obstetrics and Gynecology, 126*(1), 155–162. doi:10.1097/AOG.0000000000000869

Moore, J., Kane Low, L., Titler, M., Dalton, V., & Sampselle, C. (2014). Moving toward patient centered care: Women's decisions, perceptions, and experiences of the induction of labor process. *Birth, 41*(2), 138–146.

Advocating Cultural and Gender-Sensitive Policies in Women's Health Through Research

Zxy-Yann Jane Lu, PhD, RN

My program of research has focused on the menstrual health of Taiwanese women using a feminist perspective. My studies have demonstrated that bodily experiences in menstruation have produced and have been reproduced by the culturally specific womanhood. Menstrual attitudes tend to be natural and to emphasize regularity in nature, while practices of regulating menstruation such as taking folk medicine (*Syh-Wu Tang*) optimize female reproduction and also reveal the responsibility of motherhood in Taiwanese society (Cheng, Lu, Su, Chiang, & Wang, 2008; Chou, Lu, Wang, Lan, & Lin, 2008; Lu, 2001).

A feminist approach found that Taiwanese women experienced their menopausal bodies with less symptoms (i.e., hot flashes) and with more liberating attitudes than medical professionals who framed menopause as hormone deficiency disease and advocated hormonal replacement therapy (HRT) (Chou, Lu, & Pu, 2013; Lu & Yen, 2000; Yang & Lu, 2000). While the advanced medical technologies that infiltrate our everyday lives have been viewed as scientific achievements in Taiwanese society, my research indicated that menopausal bodies might be conceptualized as osteoporotic in medical discourse; a quantitative ultrasound osteoporosis screening test has been advocated as a preventive regimen for healthy bones and as reducing the social burden for ethically responsible aging bodies (Lu & Chen, 2007). However, how menopausal women incorporated medical technologies into their aging processes represented local biologies with diverse embodiments. New identities with sexual attraction have been empowered by medical technologies (Yang, Chu, & Lu, 2015), while using low-dose HRT and folk regimens (e.g., soy isoflavones) represented not only women's agency in the resistance of aging but also the transformation of self-sacrifice to independent wellness (Lu & Lin, 2012).

My research results have been translated into social policy through several actions: I was appointed to the Women's Rights Committee at the central government level from 2008 to 2009 to participate in gender equality policy making. Specific health-related impact includes Article 14 in the Gender Work Equality Act passed in 2002, which provides 1 day of menstrual leave each month; the law was further amended in 2014 to grant half pay for menstrual leave and for at least 3 days a year that do not count toward sick leave.

As a member of the Women's Rights Committee at the Executive Yuan (the executive branch of the central government) as well as the Gender Equality Committee at the Ministry of Health from 2008 to 2011, I had the opportunity to oversee all annual strategic health programs and policies to be examined for gender assessment. As the result of implementing gender mainstreaming policy, the widely distributed "Menopausal Health Promotion" pamphlet, compiled by the Obstetric and Gynecological Medical Association, was required to recognize the empowered agency of menopausal women and to include alternative folk medicine and health promotion activities (Chen & Lu, 2009).

The contribution of my research to education includes establishing the Program for Gender studies for both undergraduate and graduate students in 2008 at the National Yang-Ming University, in collaboration with faculty members from related disciplines, and developing and teaching two courses, Gender, Body, & Ethics and Women's Health and Health Care Technology, emphasizing the translation of my research results into pedagogical materials. Moreover, in 2012, I edited *Nursing and Society: Transdisciplinary Dialogue and Innovation* (Lu, Chiang, & Lin, 2012), a pedagogical textbook to facilitate teaching and learning in women's health that embodies a gendered perspective.

References

Chen, H.-C., & Lu, Z.-Y. J. (2009). Hormone replacement therapy as a disciplining power of menopausal women. *Journal of Chang Gung Institute of Technology, 10*, 115–122. [In Chinese].

Cheng, J.-F., Lu, Z.-Y. J., Su, Y.-C., Chiang, L.-C., & Wang, R.-Y. (2008). Traditional Chinese herbal medicine used to treat dysmenorrhea among Taiwanese women. *Journal of Clinical Nursing, 17*, 2588–2595.

Chou, Y.-C., Lu, Z.-Y. J., & Pu, C.-Y. (2013). Menopause experiences and attitudes in women with intellectual disability and in their family carers. *Journal of Intellectual & Developmental Disability, 38*(2), 114–123.

Chou, Y.-C., Lu, Z.-Y. J., Wang, F. T. Y., Lan, C.-F., & Lin, L.-C. (2008). Meanings and experiences of menstruation: Perceptions of institutionalized women with an intellectual disability. *Journal of Applied Research in Intellectual Disabilities, 21*(6), 575–584.

Lu, Z.-Y. J. (2001). The relationship between menstrual attitudes and menstrual symptoms among Taiwanese women. *Journal of Advanced Nursing, 33*(5), 621–628.

Lu, Z.-Y. J., & Chen, H.-C. (2007). Osteoporosis screening policy for menopausal women: Risk and discipline. *Journal of Nursing, 54*(2), 23–28. [In Chinese].

Lu, Z.-Y., Chiang, H.-H., & Lin, Y.-P. (2012). *Nursing & society: The transdisciplinary dialogue & innovation.* Taipei: Socio Publishing. [In Chinese].

Lu, Z.-Y. J., & Lin, H.-K. (2012). Disciplined body by quantitative ultrasound Osteoporosis screening test. In J. Z.-Y. Lu, H.-H. Chiang, & Y.-P. Lin (Eds.), *Nursing & society: The transdisciplinary dialogue & innovation* (pp. 85–108). Taipei: Socio Publishing. [In Chinese].

Lu, Z.-Y. J., & Yen, W.-K. (2000). Comparison of menopausal attitudes between Taiwanese midlife women and health professionals. *Tzu-Chi Medical Journal, 12*(4), 267–275. [In Chinese].

Yang, S.-C., Chu, C.-H., & Lu, Z.-Y. J. (2015). Sexual attraction: A concept analysis using an evolutionary perspective. *Journal of Nursing, 62*(1), 76–86. doi:10.6224/JN.62.1.76. [In Chinese].

Yang, S.-C., & Lu, Z.-Y. J. (2000). The politics of the menopausal body among Taiwanese women. *Journal of Nursing Research, 8*(5), 491–502. [In Chinese].

Understanding, Mitigating, and Eliminating Lower Urinary Tract Symptoms

Janis Miller, PhD, RN

My practice and research endeavors aim to understand the underlying pathology and how to best mitigate or eliminate lower urinary tract symptoms, such as incontinence and prolapse. My research contributes to literature that illuminates and individualizes treatment options.

1986–1990

Thelma Wells, now famous as a pioneer of nursing research, was at the University of Michigan School of Nursing when she conducted a major program of research on urinary incontinence in older women. Her writings, along with a presentation by gerontologist Joe Ouslander, inspired me to conduct my master's degree thesis on incontinence in the nursing home setting. I established instrument reliability and validity for recording incontinence patterns. My research showed that individuals' experiences with lower urinary tract symptoms differed widely. Despite this reality, all women were being treated essentially the same way; I wanted to individualize their care.

1991–1996

I was accepted as a doctoral student at the University of Michigan, and although I missed the chance to study directly under Thelma Wells, I was matched with Carolyn Sampselle. She had studied under Thelma Wells and as a junior faculty member, she had already received National Institutes of Health (NIH) funding. I recall (now with amusement) my angst at being matched with a mentor who was an obstetrics nurse. Obstetrics seemed far distant from my target population of older adults. How little did I know! I learned that the childbearing years frame much of what we now know about how pelvic floor disorders evolve over the life-span and into old age.

In 1990, Dr. Sampselle had formed a unique interdisciplinary research team that included James Ashton-Miller (engineer) and John DeLancey (urogynecologist). I joined the team as a graduate student research assistant. As the data collector, I became the "face of the studies" to women participating in our research. While these women told me their stories, I was also learning the scientific process of invention and refinement of a variety of new tools for quantifying the ancient problems of urine leakage and displaced pelvic organs. Objective measures became a hallmark of our team's work, including my own development of the "standing stress paper towel test" for quantifying the extent of leakage and the quantified speculum for quantifying Kegel muscle strength. The speculum design was led by James Ashton-Miller, with conceptualization contributions from John DeLancey as anatomy specialist, and I implemented real-world testing and refinement in the clinic.

During an independent study with James Ashton-Miller, I began to question the standard practice of prescribing pelvic floor rehabilitation as 100, or up to 300, contractions (Kegels) per day. My first publication as a doctoral student was a new protocol of graduated strength training that was more in line with muscle physiology principles.

Impact. New instruments and new protocols developed within an interdisciplinary team set the stage for 25 years of publishing new insights on incontinence and prolapse.

1997–1999

At the time of my postdoctoral work, it was thought that the effects of Kegel exercises could only be seen after 3 months. Therefore, when a research participant said I "cured [her] overnight" by teaching her to contract her pelvic floor muscles at the right moment, I took her comment seriously and tested the efficacy of this simple maneuver, which was later coined the "Knack maneuver." Its biomechanical properties (volitional lift and close of the urethra) translated into immediacy of objectively documented reduced urine leakage volume. Originally published during my postdoctoral training, the Knack maneuver is now named in more than 250 publications about pelvic muscle training.

Impact. To my knowledge, this was the first time that an engineer (James Ashton-Miller) was a formal mentor in postdoctoral training to a nurse. We used carefully designed experiments to chart mechanistic effects and explained the physiological reasons for the Knack's immediacy of symptom reduction.

2000–2016

During this time, I went back to school at the University of Michigan (UM) in the advanced practice nurse practitioner program and began a clinical practice at the UM health system outpatient urogynecology clinic with John DeLancey.

Impact. This practice environment solidified the sharing of ideas and a collaboration between John DeLancey, James Ashton-Miller, and myself that eventually garnered more than $15 million and 15 years of continuously funded NIH research. As coinvestigators on a Specialized Center of Research (SCOR) launched by the NIH Office of Women's Health, we led nine R01-scope projects packaged together with shared SCORs for synergistic potential. I was the lead of three projects and one core. Our team is a leader in productivity and is the only team to include a nurse as principal investigator (PI).

I served as the PI for a series of NIH studies that quantified the severity of birth-related injury of the levator ani (Kegel muscle) using magnetic resonance imaging. This work showed partial or full Kegel tears in select high-risk women. The impact of this work relates to whether Kegel exercises are appropriate for the more than 15% of women who have a Kegel muscle tear (a lifelong injury) since the muscle does not reattach and is rendered unable to contract. The tear is a key indicator for future prolapse. Future work is related to predictive factors for tear to move toward prevention.

In addition to my work in the United States, I am one of three founders of the International Center for Advanced Research and Training in Bukavu, Democratic Republic of Congo. This center is dedicated to supporting the research of both local and international researchers. A primary focus for the center is a unique hospital-based data repository on gynecological patients at Panzi Hospital, which is internationally renowned for its care of women with extreme pelvic fistulas and women who have experienced gender-based violence in times of war or conflict. I was the PI of the Global Challenges Third Century grant that launched the research center in 2013 and the initiation of the fistula data repository, which now has records of more than 1,000 women with documented fistula. The first manuscript from this repository is under review. The research center has garnered additional grants and interest, including from the Bill and Melinda Gates Foundation.

Problems Encountered During Program of Research Development

Status and power differentials on interdisciplinary teams are recognized as one of the most difficult problems to overcome, and with nursing as a gendered profession, these issues are very real. Time and conscious awareness are needed for addressing interdisciplinary work, elements needed in my own endeavors.

Anticipated Future Progression

All of my research work has been interdisciplinary; I formed bridges that undergird my newest role as PI for a U-grant funded by NIH. This grant is known as the Preventing Lower Urinary Symptoms (PLUS) grant. Michigan's site was chosen for its strong contributions to nursing (Janis Miller PI; Lisa Kane Low, coinvestigator) and its uniquely innovative environment for developing instruments and novel interventions. This newly funded grant also marks recognition by NIH of my mentor Carolyn Sampselle's lifelong work. I hope to carry forward her legacy.

Lessons Learned

My mentor James Ashton-Miller once told me, "Let the work speak for itself. Over time, it does." I believe he is right about this. Another mentor, John DeLancey, taught me this: "Quality work can only find its audience if you present and write the new findings such that the audience can see the conclusion before you ever tell it to them. If you can do this, you have succeeded." I believe he too was right. These are the things I strive for.

Selected Publications

Ashton-Miller, J., Zielinski, R., DeLancey, J., & Miller, J. M. (2014). Validity and reliability of an instrumented speculum designed to minimize the effect of intra-abdominal pressure on the measurement of pelvic floor muscle strength. *Clinical Biomechanics., 9*(10), 1146–1150. PMID: 25307868. PMCID: PMC4372800

Brandon, C., Jacobson, J., Low, L., Park, L., DeLancey, J. O., & Miller, J. (2012). Pubic bone injuries in primiparous women: Magnetic resonance imaging in detection and differential diagnosis of structural injury. *Ultrasound in Obstetrics and Gynecology, 39*(4), 444–451. doi:10.1002/uog.9082. PMID: 21728205

Miller, J. (2002). Criteria for therapeutic use of pelvic floor muscle training in women. *Journal of Wound Ostomy & Continence Nursing, 29*(6), 301–311. PMID: 12439454

*Miller, J. M., Guo, Y. S., & Becker-Rodseth, S. (2011). Cluster analysis of intake, output, and voiding habits collected from diary data. *Nursing Research, 60*(2), 115–123. PMCID: PMC3140406. PMID: 21317828

Miller, J. M., Perucchini, D., Carchidi, L. T., DeLancey, J. O., & Ashton-Miller, J. (2001). Pelvic floor muscle contraction during a cough and decreased vesical neck movement. *Obstetrics & Gynecology, 97*(2), 255–260. PMID: 11165591

Miller, J., Sampselle, C., Ashton-Miller, J., Son, G., & DeLancey, J. (2008). Clarification and confirmation of the Knack maneuver: The effect of volitional pelvic floor muscle contraction to preempt expected stress incontinence. *International Urogynecology Journal and Pelvic Floor Dysfunction, 19*(6), 773–782. PMCID: PMC2757097

*Miller, J. M., Low, L., Zielinski, R., Smith, A., DeLancey, J., & Brandon, C. (2015). Evaluating maternal recovery from labor and delivery: Bone and levator ani injuries. *American Journal of Obstetrics & Gynecology*, 213(2), 188. e1–188.e11. doi:10.1016/j.ajog.2015.05.001

Prevention of Urinary Incontinence in Women

Carolyn Sampselle, PhD, RN, FAAN

When I began my program of research (POR), the standard treatment for urinary inconti-nence (UI) in women was drugs or surgery. Both have adverse effects. Respecting the value of women's engagement in their health care, I focused on behavioral self-management, with UI prevention as the ultimate goal. My POR is now at the translational stage and has helped shift the research goal from treatment to the prevention of lower urinary tract symptoms in women.

1985–1989

During this time, I was invited to join Thelma Wells's research team, an opportunity that led to long-lasting interdisciplinary collaborations with respected colleagues such as John DeLancey, a urogynecologist, and Ananias Diokno, a urologist. With colleagues from the Wells team and small local grant support, I conducted a series of promising instrument development and pilot studies that supported applying for a National Center for Nurs-ing Research grant (NCNR; predecessor to the National Institute of Nursing Research [NINR)] and a First Individual Research Support and Transition (FIRST) Award for new investigators. As is not uncommon, that initial application was not funded—nor was my first revision. Steadfast support from team colleagues led to success with my second revi-sion and a key lesson in perseverance!

Impact. A pivotal outcome of this early period was the development of the Brink Digital Measure of Pelvic Muscle Strength, which I have used in every subsequent UI study (Brink, Sampselle, Wells, Diokno, Gillis, 1989). My early study findings identified reduced pelvic muscle strength following vaginal birth and suggested a strengthening ben-efit through pelvic muscle exercise.

1990–1994

The NCNR first award funding required that the PI devote 50% of his or her effort to research. This freed precious time for research at a critical point in my POR. Janis Miller, a doctoral student interested in UI, joined the project team and conducted her dissertation, comentored by DeLancey; James Ashton-Miller, a biomedical engineer; and me. Janis eventually joined the UM faculty and has become a valued colleague.

Impact. The results of the FIRST Award, which was conducted with childbearing women, demonstrated the capacity of pelvic floor muscle training in preventing birth-related UI (Sampselle et al., 1998). The project used Clinical Research Center resources, greatly expanding interdisciplinary opportunities. Parallel collaboration occurred with the Women's Studies department, substantially enhancing my feminist philosophy of health care. Building on early research results, I applied for an R01 during the final year of my FIRST Award.

1995–1999

The R01 application, UI Prevention: Reducing Birthing Risk, with DeLancey and Ashton-Miller as coinvestigators, was funded. I was also invited to serve as coinvestigator on an R01 awarded to DeLancey, What Damage Does Vaginal Birth Cause That Results in Stress UI, and a second R01 awarded to Diokno, Behavioral Modification to Prevent UI in Older Women. This continuous, often concurrent funding enabled me to leverage projects with colleagues in medicine, bioengineering, sociology, and epidemiology.

Impact. Taken together, this research yielded insights into the effects of pregnancy, childbirth, and menopause on women's risk of UI (Sampselle, Miller, Herzog, Diokno, 1996; Sampselle et al., 1998). Self-efficacy was shown to affect the capacity to adopt and sustain self-management for UI prevention (Sampselle, 2000). We showed lower UI risk with the adoption of behavioral self-management practices (Diokno et al., 2004).

2000–2004

Research accumulated supporting UI prevention with self-management. During this period, the Association of Women's Health, Obstetric, and Neonatal Nurses invited me to lead a national research utilization project, Continence for Women, to prepare clinicians to teach self-management practices to women in ambulatory care centers. Project results showed that adopting these practices reduced UI, increased quality of life, and decreased use/expense of absorbent pads (Sampselle et al., 2000).

Impact. POR results showed improved pelvic muscle strength, healthier voiding patterns, and 50% reduced risk of developing UI in older women assigned to behavioral self-management instruction (Diokno et al., 2004). The Continence for Women project showed that nonexpert clinicians could successfully deliver effective instruction in behavioral self-management (Sampselle et al., 2000).

2005–2016

Results supporting the benefits of self-management for UI prevention have continued to accumulate. We demonstrated that up to 55% of childbearing women can prevent UI by using a preemptive pelvic muscle contraction (Miller, Sampselle, Ashton-Miller, Hong, DeLancey, 2008) that at 12-months postintervention 58%–68% of women are still using the recommended practices to prevent UI (Messer et al., 2007), and that self-efficacy predicts adherence to UI self-management practices at 4-years postintervention (Messer et al., 2007). These findings are included in practice recommendations issued by the Association of Women's Health, Obstetric, and Neonatal Nurses (Association of Women's Health, Obstetric and Neonatal Nurses, 2000), the Cochrane Database of Systematic Reviews (Hay-Smith, Herbison, & Mørkvel, 2007), and the International Consultation on Incontinence/International Continence Society (Abrams, Cardozo, Khoury, & Wein, 2013).

After more than 20 years developing my POR on UI prevention, I was invited to spend a year at NIH as senior advisor to the director of the National Institute of Nursing Research. In order to do this, it was necessary to cut formal ties with NIH-sponsored research. Fortunately two able colleagues, Miller and Lisa Kane Low, a nationally respected nurse midwife and former doctoral student, were willing to assume research commitments I had to divest. This underscores the valuable collegiality and shared knowledge that are the fruits of an established research team! The NINR opportunity coincided with an initiative under way at the National Institute of Diabetes and Digestive and Kidney Diseases. Building compelling evidence supporting the benefit of behavioral self-management for UI prevention, Dr. Tamara Bavendum was focusing on the prevention of lower urinary tract symptoms (LUTS) in women and invited my participation. Her leadership and workshop results yielded the foundation for the initiative: Prevention of LUTS in Women: Bladder Health Clinical Centers (RFA-DK-14–004).

Impact. My POR, plus those of many others, has shifted the established NIH focus from the treatment of LUTS in women to one of prevention. The request for applications aims "to establish the knowledge . . . base necessary (for) prevention of LUTS." (NIH, 2014), knowledge that will guide future practices.

Problems Encountered During the Development of Programs of Research

During my 25 years of leading a POR, the greatest challenge has been to maintain a clear focus. In a research-intense environment, there are multiple opportunities to engage, some of which are more tangential to my primary focus than others, for example, those led by my strong feminist philosophy, I was drawn to study violence against women early in my career. Although I continue to affirm that line of investigation as critical to the health of women, I was unable to sustain two dissimilar areas of research and realigned my efforts to focus on UI prevention. Later in my career, I was given the opportunity to lead the Community Engagement component of the University of Michigan Clinical and Translational Award (CTSA). Although there was potential to divert my energy, I saw an opportunity to use feminist methods that I have consistently embraced. As my own research was advancing to a translational focus, I was able to establish sufficient overlap that the added focus did not diminish productivity. In fact, CTSA resources supported two recent R01s.

Anticipated Future Progression

I formally retired in 2014 and am completing my final translational project, which examines the comparative effectiveness of a small group bladder health class that provides women with essential knowledge about behavioral self-management to prevent UI and a DVD that delivers similar content in a one-on-one venue. I am pleased to note that Kane Low will continue her role as PI on the project Group Learning to Decrease Incidents of Lower Urinary Symptoms, which is one of three sites in a multisite study to determine the effectiveness of the behavioral self-management program. Janis Miller learned recently that she has received the NIDDK Prevention of Lower Urinary Tract Symptoms in Women: Bladder Health Clinical Centers Award with Lisa Kane Low as coprincipal investigator. It has been my great good fortune to work with the talented investigators who have studied this issue over the years; this recent development feels very much like passing the baton to a winning team!

Lessons Learned

1. Respect your colleagues and know that if you are fortunate, they will become long-standing colleagues as time passes; hence don't burn bridges, and keep relationships cordial.
2. Work smart by keeping your research focused, and maintain that focus even when you take on responsibilities that are essential to being a good citizen in the academic community, such as supervising students who share your research interest.
3. Enjoy the ride! There are times when it feels like you have overcommitted, but aim for dual mileage from your efforts. Celebrate the positive outcomes, whether it is a newly funded grant, an important publication, or a student's (or former student's) success.

References

Abrams, P., Cardozo, L., Khoury, S., & Wein, A. (Eds.). (2013). *Incontinence*. Paris: International Consultation on Incontinence. Retrieved from http://www.ics.org/Publications/ICI_5/INCONTINENCE.pdf

Association of Women's Health, Obstetric, and Neonatal Nurses. (2000). *Evidence-based clinical practice guideline: Continence for women*. Washington, DC: Author.

Brink, C., Sampselle, C., Wells, T., Diokno, A., & Gillis, G. (1989). A digital test for pelvic muscle strength in older women with urinary incontinence. *Nursing Research, 38*(4), 196–199.

Diokno, A., Sampselle, C., Herzog, A., Raghunathan, T., Hines, S., Messer, K. C., & Leite, M. (2004). Prevention of urinary incontinence by behavioral modification program: A randomized, controlled trial among older women in the community. *Journal of Urology, 171*(3), 1165–1171.

Hay-Smith, J., Herbison, P., & Mørkvel, S. (2007). Physical therapies for prevention of urinary and faecal incontinence in adults. *Cochrane Database of Systematic Reviews, 2007*(4). Retrieved from http://www.ncbi.nlm.nih.gov/pubmed/17943783

Messer, K., Hines, S., Raghunathan, T., Seng, J., Diokno, A., & Sampselle, C. (2007). Self-efficacy as a predictor to PFMT adherence in a prevention of urinary incontinence clinical trial. *Health Education & Behavior, 34*(6), 942–952.

Miller, J., Sampselle, C., Ashton-Miller, J., Hong, G., & Delancey, J. (2008). Clarification and confirmation of the Knack maneuver: The effect of volitional pelvic floor muscle contraction to preempt expected stress incontinence. *International Urogynecology Journal, 19*(6), 773–782. doi:0.1007/s00192-007-0525-3

National Institutes of Health. (2014). Prevention of LUTS in Women: Bladder Health Clinical Centers. Retrieved from http://grants.nih.gov/grants/guide/rfa-files/RFA-DK-14-004.html

Sampselle, C. (2000). Behavioral intervention for urinary incontinence in women: Evidence for practice. *Journal of Midwifery & Women's Health, 45*(2), 94–103. doi:10.1016/S1526-9523(99)00016-1

Sampselle, C., Miller, J., Herzog, A., & Diokno, A. (1996). Behavioral modification: Group teaching outcomes. *Urologic Nursing, 16*(2), 59–63.

Sampselle, C., Miller, J., Mims, B., DeLancey, J., Ashton-Miller, J., & Antonakos, C. (1998). Effect of pelvic muscle exercise on transient incontinence during pregnancy and after birth. *Obstetrics & Gynecology, 91*(3), 406–412.

Sampselle, C., Wyman, J., Thomas, K., Newman, D., Gray, M., Dougherty, M., & Burns, P. (2000). Continence for women: A Test of AWHONN's evidence-based protocol in clinical practice. *Journal of Obstetric, Gynecologic, Neonatal Nursing, 29*(1), 18–26.

Effects of Posttraumatic Stress Disorder on Women's Health

Julia S. Seng, PhD, RN, FAAN

The overarching research question I study is an interdisciplinary one in the domain of women's health: How does posttraumatic stress disorder (PTSD) affect women's health across the life-span, including childbearing outcomes? Answers to that initial outcomes research question have led to two new streams of research: (a) focusing on biological mechanisms of adverse outcomes, and (b) developing and testing interventions.

When I began studying the effects of PTSD as a University of Michigan School of Nursing doctoral student in the women's health concentration in 1999, it was an entirely novel research question because we had only learned in 1995 the extent to which women suffered from PTSD. My doctoral dissertation was the first study ever published to link PTSD with pregnancy complications (Seng et al., 2001).

The Stress, Trauma, Anxiety, and the Childbearing Year (STACY) Project (NIH R01 NR008767) was the first outcomes study anywhere in the world adequately powered to demonstrate the effects of PTSD on childbearing. Our 2009 report on prevalence showed that the rate among diverse women in early pregnancy was twice as high as for non-pregnant women and that childhood maltreatment trauma conveyed a 12-fold risk for meeting PTSD diagnostic criteria. In terms of perinatal outcomes, we reported in 2011 a half-pound (283 gram) decrement in birth weight, and our stratified analyses demonstrated that this adverse outcome was observed primarily among women whose PTSD was from childhood maltreatment (Seng, Kane Low, Sperlich, Ronis, & Liberzon, 2011; Seng, Kane Low, Sperlich, Ronis, & Liberzon, 2009). In terms of mental health outcomes, we reported in 2013 entirely new and extremely solid findings that depression in pregnancy was usually comorbid with PTSD and that PTSD during pregnancy was the biggest predictor of postnatal depression (Seng et al, 2013). This has the potential to change the focus of perinatal mental health service delivery from nearly exclusive attention to mood and thought disorders (i.e., depression, anxiety, and psychosis) to a primary focus on trauma-related disorders, including PTSD, comorbid depression, and dissociation. Our work affirmed that a mother's postnatal depression does indeed increase the risk of delayed or impaired bonding with her infant. However, our study's design allowed us to clearly demonstrate that this is the case only when the mother also has PTSD; depression alone during the postnatal period is not associated with impaired bonding. We have attended to structural inequalities and health disparities throughout this work and have demonstrated that women in public sector clinics have vastly higher rates of PTSD in pregnancy (13.9% vs. 2.7%) and that when PTSD is taken into account in models predicting gestational age, African American race is no longer an independently significant predictor of shorter gestation.

Our biological data also strongly support the need to focus future research and clinical attention on the traumatic stress sequelae of childhood maltreatment (i.e., PTSD and the complex form of PTSD that is characterized by dissociation).

The STACY Project's perinatal, psychological, developmental, and biological findings point strongly toward new interventions to improve such childbearing outcomes as prematurity, birth weight, postnatal depression, and attachment disorders. *Addressing PTSD and dissociation* before or during pregnancy and *preventing childhood maltreatment* are likely means toward improving population health.

Now that we know how toxic PTSD is to childbearing women, we are working hard to provide an evidence-based intervention. We collaborated with research participants and drew from our book, *Survivor Moms* (Sperlich & Seng, 2008), which was honored as the American College of Nurse Midwives' Book of the Year, to create a psychoeducation program called The Survivor Moms' Companion to address the needs of women with PTSD related to childhood maltreatment. We have completed pilot work showing the intervention is feasible to deliver in low-resource settings and very well liked by the women who use it, in addition to showing promise for improving outcomes (Seng et al., 2011). One goal of intervention in pregnancy is to improve the woman's mental health, childbearing experience, and her start in mothering. But we also aim to determine whether the Survivor Moms' Companion can contribute to *disrupting the intergenerational cycles of abuse and psychiatric vulnerability* that intersect during the childbearing year.

This intervention work rests on a transdisciplinary "Cycles-Breaking" theoretical framework that undergirds the work of an international group of researchers that I lead, known as the CASEY (Child Abuse, Stress, and the Early Years) Collaboration. The Cycles-Breaking theoretical framework is the result of empirical theory testing during the STACY Project R01 study and an integration of literature from numerous disciplines, including nursing, midwifery, psychology, psychiatry, infant mental health, child welfare, social work, and neuroscience (Seng et al., 2013). It is a contribution to health and social science to have integrated attention to theoretical propositions across the particular, but delimited, field of vision of each of these respective professional and scientific domains. In the past, psychiatric problems and violence have been addressed and studied separately. The last 20 years have seen a narrowing of this gap. But transdisciplinary work has not yet become a norm. As a nurse and midwife, I have developed expertise that includes feminist views of violence and childhood maltreatment, their psychiatric sequelae and impacts on the body, and the importance of social context. I have been able to call for—and provide empirical support for—*integration* of what we know about how the intergenerational "cycle of abuse" and "cycle of psychiatric vulnerability" intersect during the childbearing year, from pregnancy into early parenting. This transdisciplinary framework has provided an essential foundation for team science.

The "Cycles-Breaking" framework (however awkward the name) has been a locus around which to assemble a strong international team to conduct an efficacy-to-effectiveness program of research. The CASEY Collaboration includes child welfare research and policy experts from the University of Edinburgh, Scotland; parenting and perinatal psychology researchers from Monash University, Melbourne, Australia; and a nursing, midwifery, infant mental health, and statistics team from the University of Michigan. This work is aligned with calls from the U.S. Substance Abuse and Mental Health Services Administration's National Center for Trauma-Informed Care for trauma-informed health services delivery and evidence-based front-line, trauma-specific treatment. During my sabbatical leave in 2015, I led the CASEY Collaboration in producing a book for child welfare and maternity professionals titled *Trauma Informed Care in the Perinatal Period* (Seng & Taylor, 2015).

Problems Encountered

One of the biggest problems I have encountered is obtaining funding for psychoeducation intervention research in an era when high-tech studies focusing on "omics," such as genomics, metabolomics, and proteomics, seem favored by National Institutes of Health (NIH). Without sufficient funding, it has been difficult to produce the evidence base needed to translate the intervention into clinical use. A second challenge has always been bridging the "mind-body" divide in academic disciplines. Often as a nurse-midwife, my expertise on PTSD is not respected in the mental health disciplines. Conversely, my perinatal colleagues often are not interested in PTSD, even though we are demonstrating how very important it is to health. Being a professor of women's studies, as well as nursing and obstetrics, helps me stand my ground and draw determination and persistence from knowing that this research can make a difference in the lives of women and their children into the future.

Anticipated Future Progression

I look forward to next steps in this program of research that are responsive to the needs of the world, locally and globally. The Survivor Moms' Companion was first piloted in Michigan and has since been piloted in Melbourne, Australia. It is currently being studied as part of a major maltreatment-prevention initiative in the city of Blackpool in the United Kingdom and as a perinatal mental health intervention in Cyprus. We are using cutting-edge, hybrid effectiveness-implementation science projects to study the outcomes for the women and the organizations. We hope this front-line trauma-informed intervention is a high-impact idea whose time has come.

Lessons Learned

Being well-schooled as a scientist is an excellent starting point. My greatest satisfaction and perhaps greatest "edge" as a researcher is continuing to learn every day on the job. It's not always a pleasure, since much of what I learn comes from critique and rejections. Bouncing back and problem solving almost always lead me to find new ideas and new techniques that make my work better. I learn from teaching too—the effort to stay up to date bears fruit for my science.

Selected References

Seng, J. S., Kane Low, L. M., Sperlich, M. I., Ronis, D. L., & Liberzon, I. (2009). Trauma history and risk for PTSD among nulliparous women in maternity care. *Obstetrics & Gynecology, 114*, 839–847. PMCID: PMC3124073

Seng, J. S., Kane Low, L. M., Sperlich, M., Ronis, D. L., & Liberzon, I. (2011). Posttraumatic stress disorder is associated with lower birth weight and shorter gestation. *British Journal of Obstetrics and Gynaecology, 118*, 1329–1339. PMCID: PMC3171570

Seng, J. S., Oakley, D. J., Sampselle, C. M., Killion, C., Graham-Bernmann, S., & Liberzon, I. (2001). Posttraumatic stress disorder and pregnancy complications. *Obstetrics and Gynecology, 97*(1), 17–22.

Seng, J. S., Sperlich, M., Kane Low, L., Ronis, D., Muzik, M., & Liberzon, I. (2013). Childhood abuse history, posttraumatic stress disorder, postpartum mental health, and bonding: A prospective cohort study. *Journal of Midwifery and Women's Health, 58*, 57–68. PMCID: PMC3564506

Seng, J. S., & Taylor, J. (2015). *Trauma informed care in the perinatal period*. Edinburgh, Scotland: Dunedin Academic Press.

Sperlich, M., & Seng, J. S. (2008). *Survivor moms: Women's stories of birthing, mothering, and healing after sexual abuse*. Eugene, OR: Motherbaby Press.

Nursing and Health Care Systems

CHAPTER 9

Nursing and Health Care Systems at the University of Michigan

Richard W. Redman, PhD, RN

SHORT PAPERS SUBMITTED FOR THIS CHAPTER

Carol S. Brewer

Sung-Hyun Cho

Christopher Friese

Ada Sue Hinshaw

Beatrice J. Kalisch

Shaké Ketefian

Milisa Manojlovich

Richard W. Redman

Ann E. Rogers and Linda D. Scott

Anne Snowdon

Marita G. Titler

Huey-Ming Tzeng

One of the hallmarks of the University of Michigan School of Nursing's (UMSN) PhD program has been the offering of research in nursing science concentrations as an integral part of the curriculum. The opportunity for students to examine knowledge development, analytic methods, and substantive issues in significant areas of nursing science through the program concentrations has been unique among most PhD programs in nursing nationally. The nursing systems concentration, which examines nursing health services research, was developed formally in 1990 and has prepared a number of PhD graduates since then. Given the nature of nursing systems research, it should be pointed out that students and faculty at UMSN were involved in nursing systems research before the formal approval of the nursing systems concentration.

One reason nursing systems as a concentration has been unique in UMSN's PhD program is the long-standing national debate over whether nursing systems research is, in fact, research contributing to nursing science. Because of the nature of the questions addressed in nursing systems research—and the fact that by definition, health services research is inherently interdisciplinary—faculties nationally have sometimes felt that nurses who want to conduct this type of research could obtain their research training more appropriately in a program in public health or one of the social sciences. To the credit of UMSN's faculty, they saw the distinct components that a nursing perspective brings to health services research and proudly offered this concentration in the PhD program. To this day, UMSN's program is still one of the few in which doctoral students can focus on the conduct of nursing systems research in a curriculum with advanced course work in substantive areas related to their interests in nursing systems and under the guidance of well-qualified mentors who, themselves, are conducting nursing systems research.

This chapter examines major contributions to nursing systems research and knowledge development made by UMSN faculty and PhD graduates. First, definitions and elements of nursing and health services research are reviewed briefly to provide the context and framework for reviewing UMSN's contributions. Next, the research briefs submitted by faculty and PhD alumni will be placed within the framework, their research reviewed, and the impact of their work highlighted. Finally, an assessment of the impact of the reviewed programs of research and a look to the future of nursing health services research will be offered.

Nursing and Health Services Research

Providers and officials in health care have been examining issues such as access, cost, and quality of health care since the 1800s. It is important to note that one of the early health service researchers was Florence Nightingale, who used data and graphs to examine hygiene and infection control. Since then, a variety of disciplines have engaged in what we call health services research. In the early to mid-20th century, when social and political conditions prompted policy development to deal with health care delivery and insurance to pay for services, it was recognized that health services research frequently provided insights about the types of services needed and how they best could be provided to meet growing demand. At the federal level, as National Institutes of Health (NIH) developed, there were study sections devoted to health services research as well. In 1968, the National Center for Health Services Research and Development was founded to support research and related training for the improvement of the organization, staffing, delivery, and financing of health care. This agency evolved into the Agency for Health Care Policy and Research in the 1980s and eventually into the Agency for Healthcare Research and Quality (AHRQ) (Langley, 2009). Of note is the fact that the development and expansion of doctoral education in nursing paralleled this growth in health services research.

Health services research is defined as

the multidisciplinary field of scientific investigation that studies how social factors, financing systems, organizational structures and processes, health technologies, and personal behaviors affect access to healthcare, the quality and cost of healthcare, and ultimately our health and well-being. Its research domains are individuals, families, organizations, institutions, communities, and populations. (Lohr & Steinwachs, 2002, p. 7)

This definition has formally been adopted by AcademyHealth, the professional association for health services researchers. AcademyHealth also offers the following guiding questions for the science of health services: What works? For whom? At what cost? Under what circumstances? (AcademyHealth, 2015).

In 2004, an invitational conference was held to examine the intersection of nursing and health services research. Invited papers from prominent interdisciplinary health services researchers were presented and a research agenda for nursing health services research was developed by participants. The agenda focused on key contributions in health services research made by nurse researchers and identified ongoing gaps where the contributions of nurse researchers are essential (Jones & Mark, 2005).

A Framework for Examining Nursing Systems Research at Michigan

Using the classic definition of health services research presented earlier, and integrating that with the essential research questions generated in the 2004 invitational conference on nursing health services research, a framework was developed. The intent was to provide a framework for examining the many contributions made by nursing systems researchers, both faculty and PhD alumni, from UMSN.

The briefs on programs of research submitted for inclusion in this volume describe the research programs and the impact of the work submitted by current and former faculty and graduates of the PhD program. Last names of investigators in that area of research have been placed in the framework to illustrate the array of contributions addressing essential elements in the nursing health services framework (see Table 9-a).

Table 9-a. Nursing Systems Research Contributions by Faculty and PhD Alumni at the University of Michigan School of Nursing[a]

Classic Health Services Research	Substantive nursing systems research focus	Level or focus of research/scholarship			
		Microsystems	Macrosystems	Synthesis	Policy
Access to Care	Practice environments	Brewer; Friese; Kalisch; Manojlovich; Redman & Ketefian	Redman		Friese
	Staffing and utilization of nursing care	Cho; Brewer; Redman & Ketefian	Brewer; Cho	Brewer	Cho
	Provider behaviors	Brewer; Friese; Manojlovich; Rogers & Scott	Brewer; Redman		Friese; Kalisch; Rogers & Scott
Health & Well-Being	Health status	Snowdon			
	Technology innovations	Snowdon; Tzeng	Redman		
	Structure/process/outcomes of nursing care	Cho; Friese; Manojlovich; Redman & Ketefian; Titler; Tzeng			
Quality	Evidence-based practice	Ketefian; Titler	Titler	Titler	Titler; Hinshaw
	Safety	Brewer; Kalisch; Manojlovich; Rogers & Scott; Snowdon; Titler			
	Ethical frameworks & decision making	Ketefian	Tzeng	Ketefian	
Cost of Health Care	Cost of nursing care	Titler			
	Cost-effectiveness	Snowdon; Titler		Titler	

[a] Adapted from Jones and Mark, 2005; Steinwachs, 2009.

The categorizations illustrated within the framework are from the perspective of the author(s) and are not intended to be mutually exclusive. As is often the case, the focus of a given research project might be viewed from several emphases and is subject to interpretation. For example, research on a particular aspect of the nursing practice environment might focus on the influence of organizational culture on both nursing performance and clinical outcomes. Rather than placing the same projects or investigators in multiple cells in the framework, the individuals are placed in the cell that best conveys the primary emphasis in their work.

The following sections of this chapter discuss the highlights and the impact of each researcher's work. The intent is not to repeat the extensive contributions and details of each research program submitted for this volume; rather, it is my hope that the extent of the contributions and their impact on knowledge development and the shaping of policy to guide nursing practice and health care delivery will be readily apparent from this brief review. More detail on a given individual's research program can be found in the research briefs, which follow this chapter.

Highlights of Research Contributions by PhD Alumni and Faculty

Access to Care, Staffing, and Provider Behaviors

Extensive research contributions are noted by PhD alumni and faculty as they examined different aspects of nursing practice at the interface of patient care delivery. Some of the research has focused on patient care units or microsystems of care and the impact these practice environments have on nurse performance and patient care. Another major trajectory has been the supply and demand of nursing resources, ranging from the microsystem on through to policy levels. Finally, several scientists have investigated different aspects of provider behavior, in nurses and physicians, and how these impact performance and outcomes.

Dr. Carol Brewer (PhD alumna) has an extensive research portfolio in addressing nursing workforce issues, primarily focusing on the supply of nurses and ranging from the micro to macro levels and including synthesis. She began this work in her dissertation, which was supported by a National Services Research Award funded by NIH. She conducted economic analyses of the influence of wages on the cyclical shortages of nurses. Throughout her career, she has focused on examining the relationship of different variables that influence nurses' work decisions. These have included market characteristics, such as percent of health maintenance organization competition in the market, and the personal characteristics of nurses themselves, such as nurses being married and how that relates to their decision whether to work full or part time. To this day, she is one of the few health services researchers in any discipline to focus on the econometrics of the supply of nurses and their participation in the workforce.

She extended her interests on nurses' decisions related to work beyond wages and demographic characteristics and also conducted various studies to examine how organizational commitment, intent to leave, and job satisfaction are related to why and how nurses make decisions to work. Additionally, she has conducted work on nurses' perceptions of their work environments and how these work environment factors are as important as wages in nurses' decisions whether to work. She developed predictive models of these relationships, which have increased our understanding of how work environments affect nurses' intent to stay, organizational commitment, and job satisfaction. While these have been key variables used in other industries by organizational researchers, Brewer has been one of the few researchers to use these variables consistently in examinations of the supply of nurses.

She also has examined staff nurse perceptions of incivility and verbal abuse in their work environments and how they influence their intent to stay. The negativity associated with high levels of verbal abuse, especially from physicians, has been consistently related to lower job satisfaction, higher turnover, and reduced commitment to the organization. These negative work environments, and the resulting increased turnover, create increased costs for the organization and have an impact on an organization's ability to attract and retain young nurses. Her economic perspective has consistently been integrated into her research, and the contributions have been noteworthy in this regard.

Dr. Christopher Friese (faculty) has examined nursing practice environments in several ways with a particular emphasis on ambulatory nursing in oncology settings. Part of this work has resulted in a major measure used to assess practice environments of nurses in ambulatory oncology settings. It has recently been used by the Dana-Farber Cancer Institute, one of the leading oncology centers in the United States. His research on the relationship of nurses' education and patient outcomes has had considerable impact nationally and has been cited in the Institute of Medicine's (IOM, 2010) report *The Future of Nursing*, policy briefs, and strategic plans of major nursing organizations and groups. His current work is addressing the increased risk for adverse health outcomes among oncology nurses due to the suboptimal use of protective equipment. He is currently conducting a randomized controlled trial to test interventions that can improve the use of protective equipment by nurses and reduce hazardous drug exposure in ambulatory settings. He also has conducted extensive research in the quality of care domain, and the significance of that work will be discussed later in this chapter.

Dr. Beatrice Kalisch (faculty) has made extensive contributions toward our understanding of the image of nursing and the impact that has had on professional advancement, nurses' involvement in shaping health policy, and practice-environment concepts related to missed nursing care (i.e., standard required nursing care that is not being provided) and nursing teamwork. In the 1970s, she received NIH funding to examine the impact of federal funding on nursing practice, education, and research. That work resulted in the landmark work around the engagement of nurses in health policy and the history and image of nursing, six books, and an increased involvement of nurses in lobbying and the shaping of health policy. One outcome of the increased awareness of the importance of nurses becoming politically active was the appointment of Carolyne Davis, former dean of UMSN, as director of the Health Care Financing Administration (HCFA), the predecessor of the current Centers for Medicaid and Medicare Services (CMS).

More recently, Kalisch's work has focused on missed nursing care and the errors of omission that can result. She has documented the extent to which missed care may exist and the development and testing of an instrument to measure missed care. Concurrent with this work, she has examined teamwork in nursing and its relationship to nurse staffing outcomes and the quality and safety of care. This important work has extended into the international arena and has resulted in several major publications.

Dr. Milisa Manojlovich (PhD alumna and faculty) has conducted several studies examining the contextual factors in practice environments that influence nurse-physician communication and, in turn, the clinical outcomes of patients. She began in this domain with her dissertation, and over the course of multiple studies, she has examined variables such as nurses' self-efficacy for professional practice and the strength of nursing leadership in the workplace as important predictors for professional practice behaviors and job satisfaction. She has extended her methods to examine nurse-physician communication over time, beginning with nurse-centric measures and moving on to focus on both parties in the communication equation. She also has used a number of different innovative methods to study communication. Her current research is examining the effect of health information technology on nurse-physician communication to describe how communication technologies facilitate or hinder communication. Her work has contributed important insights on how these communication patterns can have an impact on not only nurses and their practice but also clinical outcomes.

Dr. Sung-Hyun Cho (PhD alumna) has developed a well-recognized program of research addressing nurse staffing and patient outcomes. Her research was funded by a Health Services Dissertation Research grant from AHRQ, the first student in UMSN's PhD program to receive one and only the second to date of all PhD students UMSN. The publication from her dissertation is consistently included in meta-analyses of the staffing literature and has had a significant impact in international literature, with more than 200 citations. She has conducted multiple studies examining different aspects of nurse staffing and its relationship to job satisfaction and turnover, quality of care, and mortality in intensive care units. She has examined the impact of reduced lengths of stay in hospitals on nursing workloads. Her research on staffing has informed the development of policy at medical centers in Korea, the Korean Hospital Nurses Association, and the National Assembly of Korea.

Drs. Anne Rogers (former faculty member) and Linda Scott (PhD alumna) have conducted seminal research on hours worked by nurses and the effects of those hours on patient safety. Through their Staff Nurse Fatigue and Patient Safety Program, they have made a major impact on increasing our understanding of the importance of nurse fatigue and its relationship to errors and adverse events. Their research has been used by the Institute of Medicine to recommend that nurses should not be allowed to provide patient care for more than 12 hours in a 24-hour period nor should they work more than 60 hours in 7 days. The U.S. Congress used this research to mandate a similar recommendation in all Veterans Health Administration facilities. Their research has been widely disseminated in high-impact interdisciplinary journals. The significance of their research findings generated global media attention that was recognized by the American Academy of Nursing. Several professional nursing organizations in the United States and Canada have developed policy and position statements based on this research program. Their work has had global impact in clinical settings as well as the policy arena.

Drs. Richard Redman and Shaké Ketefian (both former PhD program directors and faculty), in collaboration with directors of nursing at the University of Michigan Health System, conducted a major longitudinal study to investigate the effects of work and role redesign on nurses and patients in acute care and ambulatory settings. This research was one of the first, and one of only a few, to examine the major changes that were under way nationally due to a nursing shortage and rapid changes in hospital reimbursement. In addition to wide dissemination of the results, the data from the project supported three dissertations and 12 master's theses.

Redman continued this work with colleagues in several other private health systems, examining the roles of patient care technicians or multiskilled workers on nurses, managers, and other health professionals. Overall, the new types of roles on the nursing care team resulted in positive outcomes. The expanding roles and responsibilities of the nurse manager under these new models of care often resulted in increased stress for managers, and this research is still relevant today.

Health Status and Technology Innovations

While there have been fewer research programs in this domain, the work by two PhD alumnae provides important insights that could serve as exemplars for future research in this area. Given the increased integration of technology in health care, the applications of innovations in technology can be expected to increase in the years to come.

Dr. Anne Snowdon (PhD alumna) has conducted work in health and health status assessment that has resulted in technologic innovations in Canada. In the area of cognitive assessment, she worked with a team to develop and test an electronic version of the Montreal Cognitive Assessment Tool, a standardized paper-and-pencil measure used extensively in primary care. The assessment tool has been designed and tested for use by individuals and families to reduce the stress of this type of assessment for people with changes in cognitive function and to engage them directly in the assessment process in the primary care setting. It offers an important opportunity for individuals and families to directly engage in their health in an area of growing concern. In addition, it enhances the productivity of primary care providers. Incorporating this type of digital assessment into primary care as a means to assess the area of cognition and its potential decline is timely and innovative.

Snowdon also has made substantive contributions in the design and use of child safety seats for children traveling in vehicles. A multimedia educational intervention was designed and tested to increase parental knowledge and understanding of the proper use of child safety seats, including measures to ensure correct seat size as the child grows. This program was tested in five provinces in Canada, with significant increases in parent knowledge and use of safety seats for children. The work has been cited as one of the few national intervention studies in child injury prevention in Canada. It also has been recognized with awards by the Canadian Institutes of Health Research. The work in child safety also has led to the design of an innovative safety latch for fastening child seats to the vehicle, which offers greater stability and safety. This has led to a strategic partnership with industry and an entire line of safety products available commercially in 15 countries.

As part of the data collection in this study, Snowdon and colleagues used smartphones to collect data. This software application, using Blackberry devices for data collection, was profiled by Research in Motion, the developer of Blackberry technology, as a global case study for innovative solutions. This type of application has now been extended to include multiple applications for navigating data in a variety of health decision support systems.

Dr. Huey-Ming Tzeng (PhD alumna) has incorporated the use of technology into her ongoing program of research in care quality and patient safety. Focusing on falls prevention of adult patients in hospitals, she developed the first use of archived hospital call-light data to monitor and predict the falls of inpatients. Building on this, she collaborated with computer scientists and engineers to design and test a prototype sensor device that measures hospital bed height and generates computerized reminders to maintain beds at the lowest levels. This work led to the development of a web-based falls prevention application that engages patients to take an active role in preventing falls during hospitalization. This cutting-edge work has resulted in an innovative application of technology that engages patients in focusing on their safety and health status.

Quality Dimensions of Nursing and Health Care

The University of Michigan and the School of Nursing are well known for their quality of health and nursing care in terms of conceptualization, measurement, and knowledge development. This work has been going on for decades, so it is not surprising that the majority of faculty and alumni who submitted research briefs report on programs of research in this domain. Dr. Avedis Donabedian, the architect of the structure-process-outcome model for the conceptualization and measurement of quality in health care, was a long-standing member of the School of Public Health faculty. He came to the University of Michigan in 1961 and did all his work on quality over the course of his career at the university (National Library of Medicine, 1998). His model is referred to as the Donabedian model, and his groundbreaking work in that realm led to decades of research at the university across all health disciplines on different aspects of quality of care. That work continues today.

In UMSN, a major project titled Conduct and Utilization of Research in Nursing (CURN) was conducted beginning in the late 1970s. The CURN project was funded by the Division of Nursing at the Department of Health, Education, and Welfare (predecessor of the Department of Health and Human Services). The purpose of the project was to develop and implement a model for the use of scientific nursing knowledge in clinical practice. The project was based on the supposition that conducting research and utilizing the results of that research in practice are both essential to improving nursing practice. The project was conducted in 34 different hospital nursing departments and resulted in an 11-volume set of booklets that provided guidance on research utilization and the implementation of change in the clinical setting (Horsley, Crane, Crabtree, & Wood, 1983). This early project on research utilization and evidence-based practice may have been the first of its kind and serves as a good example of the type of work going on at the university in the area of quality of care. The CURN project began around the time the PhD program was implemented, and some of the faculty and PhD students at that time were involved in the project.

The research programs of nursing faculty and PhD students have frequently addressed the assessment of quality of care and its different dimensions. Many of the programs of research highlighted in the section on access to care, practice environments, and staffing also can be highlighted in this section on quality. The programs of research have addressed the full continuum of the Donabedian model of structure, process, and outcome variables. They also have addressed more contemporary elements of quality that focus on the translation and utilization of evidence to guide practice or safety in health care delivery. The contemporary emphasis on safety in health care, with preventing errors and adverse events, is an essential component in many of the programs of research represented in this volume. The programs of research of faculty and alumni highlighted earlier will be acknowledged here from the perspective of quality and safety. In addition, several additional faculty and alumni programs of research will be discussed here.

Several programs of research have included clinical outcomes as a dependent variable when examining nursing care delivery. Cho has demonstrated over time that better nurse staffing was associated with a decrease in the occurrence of pneumonia after surgery. She also has demonstrated the relationship of nurse staffing levels and patient mortality in intensive care units. This work, in part, has shaped policy at the hospital and governmental levels in Korea. Friese characterizes his entire program of research within the quality of care framework. His current intervention work in ambulatory oncology nursing resulted from fundamental work in examining the knowledge gap in quality of care and identifying high-priority targets for intervention work. His work examining patient outcomes and nurses' education levels has had a major impact at the state and federal levels. His work on the value of performing baseline flow cytometry to confirm the diagnosis of chronic lymphocytic leukemia patients has lead the National Quality Forum and the American Society of Hematology to adopt this as a quality of care indicator. Manojlovich has examined the nurse-physician communication relationship to clinical outcomes. Her work found that the timeliness of communication was a predictor of pressure ulcer prevalence and that variability in communication was inversely related to ventilator-associated pneumonia. Tzeng has examined effective interventions to prevent the falls of adult patients in hospitals, and her work in this area has been replicated in hospitals across the United States and in countries in Asia.

The engagement of patients in evaluating the quality of the care they receive as well as the providers who deliver that care is an important outcome variable that has been examined in several of the research programs reported in this volume. Redman and Ketefian developed an instrument to assess patient satisfaction with nursing care in hospital and ambulatory settings. This assessment is different from the ones found in many patient satisfaction measures, which focus more on the hotel-like aspects of health care in hospital and ambulatory settings. Additionally, Redman reconceptualized patients' assessment of their care experience by engaging them to identify expectations for their care experiences and designing and testing an instrument to assess patient care experiences from the perspective of whether expectations were met. Tzeng now describes her focus as patient-centric, in keeping with the current emphasis on patient- and family-centered care.

Building on the strong foundations for evidence-based practice established in the CURN project, several researchers have reported on their work in this domain. Ketefian was at the forefront of this movement in the early 1970s, conducting her dissertation on the extent to which nursing research was being used to improve practice. She extended this work to examine how nurses in practice were following research evidence in taking the temperature of patients. This work resulted in several publications in nursing at a time when most of the literature on research utilization was found primarily in the social sciences.

Dr. Marita Titler (faculty) has centered her program of research on the utilization of research and on outcomes effectiveness and acknowledges the influence of the CURN project on her early work in these domains. Titler has participated in the development and dissemination of more than 30 evidence-based practice guidelines for the care of older adults. These are included in the National Guideline Clearinghouse, a repository of validated practice guidelines. As part of her work, she developed and tested the translating research into practice (TRIP) model, one of the most widely used models for translation and implementation science globally. She and colleagues have developed and tested two measures to assess the amount of evidence-based care patients receive when experiencing either acute or cancer pain. Findings from her work in translation and implementation science have influenced regulatory standards of the Joint Commission (formerly the Joint Commission on Accreditation of Hospitals) and of CMS at the federal level.

Titler has had a long-standing role in the evidence-based practice movement in nursing and health care delivery. She and colleagues developed the Iowa Model of Evidence-Based Practice to Improve Quality of Care, a model that is used nationally and internationally. She founded and directs the National Nursing Practice Network, a learning collaborative designed to advance professional nursing practice through the application of evidence in care delivery. This network has more than 100 hospitals and health systems participating in its work. She is sought extensively as an expert consultant in evidence-based practice and as of 2016 has served as guest editor of six special journal issues focused on evidence-based practice.

In outcomes effectiveness research, Titler has conducted multiple research projects, all with national funding. These projects have examined the unique contributions of nursing interventions in patients with heart failure and hip fractures as well as hospitalized older adults at risk for falls. She has published extensively in highly recognized journals on the unique contributions of nursing interventions to a variety of patient outcomes such as adverse events, cost, failure to rescue, and discharge disposition. The impact of her work has been substantial and recognized through major awards from NIH, Sigma Theta Tau International, and the American Organization of Nurse Executives.

Dr. Ada Sue Hinshaw (dean emerita) has had a long-standing career as a nurse scientist, which culminated in several key leadership appointments during her career. She was the inaugural director of the National Center for Nursing Research and, subsequently, the National Institute of Nursing Research at NIH. She has had a long-standing program of research examining factors associated with the impact of nursing research results on shaping health policy at the organizational, state, national, and international levels. She has studied the processes through which nursing research can inform policy and has identified important characteristics, barriers, and successful strategies for informing and shaping health policy. This work has been reported in a landmark book that is widely used by scientists and in schools of nursing.

Another essential dimension of quality of nursing care is ethical decision making and practice in accord with professional ethical standards. Ketefian has had a long-standing program of scholarship and research in examining how professional work environments are related to ethical practice. She has investigated the concept of moral reasoning and the measurement of ethical practice, as well as the interrelationship between the two constructs. This work led to a synthesis of the literature examining the relationship between moral reasoning and ethical practice, published as a book by the National League for Nursing. Similar work resulted in a meta-analysis conducted under the aegis of the Midwest Nursing Research Society. Her work extended into an examination of scientific integrity in research and scholarship. As part of this examination, she developed and published a list of scientific integrity guidelines, which is now in its second edition.

Tzeng examined ethical issues rooted in providers' concerns and fears about caring for patients during the severe acute respiratory syndrome (SARS) epidemic in Asia that began in 2004. The fears of a pandemic and of human-to-human transmission of SARS created fear and panic in both health professionals and the general public. Her work brought attention to the importance of developing infection control measures based on scientific evidence and the importance of providing up-to-date information about the emerging disease.

Cost and Cost-Effectiveness of Nursing Care

While interest and concern over the cost of health care have been growing since the 1960s, it has been slowly incorporated as a variable in health services research. It presents measurement challenges and, until recently, has not been part of the education of clinicians and, in turn, researchers. While evident in a small part of the research reviewed here, it is present in ways that will likely grow in the future.

Titler has examined the costs of adverse events, such as falls and medication errors, in many of her projects. A number of her projects have demonstrated the cost-savings of the type and dose of nursing interventions on patient outcomes. In her use of the TRIP intervention to improve processes of care for hospitalized older adults with hip fractures, results demonstrated a net cost savings of $1,500 per patient. Her work in this realm is unique to date.

Snowdon has developed a conceptual model for examining the adoption and scalability of innovations in health care, balancing key stakeholders and their assessment of the value proposition of multiple innovations. She envisions proof of value and reimbursement (as related to cost) as fundamental components in the adoption process. She is in the process of testing the impact of this framework to achieve value for patients with multiple comorbidities and high rates of health services utilization. She also is leading a Canadian program of research on supply chain innovation in health systems, recognizing that supplies are an important component in any cost equation. She is involved in investigating key aspects of innovation adoption that are essential to achieve value and cost-effective care for patients and families.

Coda

This brief review of the programs of research of PhD program faculty and alumni in nursing systems exemplifies the substantive contributions to knowledge and practice that have been made since the program's inception. The scope and depth of scholarship across the continuum of health services research is noteworthy. The scholarship over the years has been conceptual and empirical. A variety of methodologies have been used, ranging from quantitative to qualitative, including newer mixed methods approaches. Designs have included panel studies, randomized controlled interventions, and repeated measures. Data collection methods have ranged from primary to secondary analyses of existing large data files. Some work has resulted in the development and psychometric assessment of new measurement tools. Foci of the projects have been at the microsystems level as well as across health delivery systems. Syntheses of existing research and meta-analytic studies have also been conducted.

Equally as important have been the significance and the impact of the research by these scientists. Over the years, the contributions and findings of these faculty and alumni have shaped health policy at the local, state, federal, and international levels. They have resulted in changes in professional practice and health delivery system standards in professional organizations and governmental agencies, including internationally. The extensive publications, including scientific articles and books, have shaped and extended the respective research domains in nursing systems in ways that are in keeping with the best University of Michigan traditions, preparing the "leaders and best" in nursing and health services research. Perhaps most important, the research of these scientists has made an impact in the quality and safety of health care delivered to patients and families, both directly and indirectly.

As of 2016, there has not been a national dialogue within the community of nursing science to examine the quality and direction of nursing PhD programs. The rapid advances in all sciences and technology, as well as in society's needs, are stimulating this in-depth examination. This examination of nursing PhD programs is being directed by the Council for the Advancement of Nursing Science (Breslin, Sebastian, Trautman, & Rosseter, 2015). Out of this dialogue comes the recommendation for a renewed vision for the preparation of nurse scientists in emerging areas of science and technology (Henly et al., 2015). There also is a call for retaining the substantive content and methods that have long been part of nursing PhD programs (Villarruel & Fairman, 2015). As the results of this dialogue are reviewed, it becomes clear that the University of Michigan's preparation of nurse scientists has been and continues to be at the forefront. Many of the recommended areas for inclusion in the future preparation of nurse scientists have already been included in the programs of research reviewed in this chapter. And some of the areas under recommendation for inclusion in PhD programs have already been emphasized in UMSN's PhD program concentration in nursing systems for years. The talent and vision of the faculty and students in UMSN's PhD program in nursing science have been a hallmark of the program, and there is every reason to expect this will continue in the future.

References

AcademyHealth. (2015). What Is HSR? Retrieved from https://www.academyhealth.org/About/content.cfm?ItemNumber=831&navItemNumber=514

Breslin, E., Sebastian, J., Trautman, D., & Rosseter, R. (2015). Sustaining excellence and relevance in PhD nursing education. *Nursing Outlook, 63*, 428–431. doi:10.1016/j.outlook.2015.04.002

Henly, S. J., McCarthy, D. O., Wyman, J. F., Stone, P. W., Redeker, N. S., McCarthy, A., & Conley, Y. P. (2015). Integrating emerging areas of nursing science into PhD Programs. *Nursing Outlook, 63*, 408–416. doi:10.1016/j.outlook.2015.04.010

Horsley, J. A., Crane, J., Crabtree, M. K., & Wood, D. J. (1983). *Using research to improve nursing practice: A guide.* New York, NY: Grune & Stratton.

Institute of Medicine. (2010). *The future of nursing: Leading change, advancing health.* Washington, DC: National Academies Press.

Jones, C. B., & Mark, B. A. (2005). The intersection of nursing and health services research: An agenda to guide future research. *Nursing Outlook, 53*(6), 324–332. doi:10.1016/j.outlook.2005.09.003

Langley, K. (2009). Health services research, origins. In R. M. Mullner (Ed.), *Encyclopedia of Health Services Research* (vol. 1, pp. 544–549). Washington, DC: Sage Publications.

Lohr, K. N., & Steinwachs, D. M. (2002). Health services research: An evolving definition of the field. *Health Services Research, 37*(1), 15–17.

National Library of Medicine. (1998). History of Health Services Research Project: Interview with Avedis Donabe-
    dian. National Information Center on Health Services Research and Health Care Technology (NICHSR).
    Retrieved from https://www.nlm.nih.gov/hmd/nichsr/donabedian.html
Steinwachs, D. M. (2009). Health services research, definition. In R. M. Mullner (Ed.), *Encyclopedia of Health
    Services Research* (vol. 1, pp. 539–544). Washington, DC: Sage Publications.
Villarruel, A. M., & Fairman, J. A. (2015). The Council for the Advancement of Nursing Science, Idea Festi-
    val Advisory Committee: Good ideas that need to go further. *Nursing Outlook, 63,* 436–438. doi:10.1016/j
    .outlook.2015.04.003

Highlights From a Program of Nursing Workforce Research

Carol S. Brewer, PhD, RN, FAAN

A quantitatively adequate and high-quality supply of nurses is the backbone of our health care system's workforce, but this cannot be achieved in the midst of frequent nursing short-ages. Understanding the cyclical nature and impact of nursing shortages and the result of work environments on nurse outcomes has been the continuing motivation of my research since my dissertation.

A central concern in the economics of shortages is the role of wages, as wages typically rise during a shortage and draw new entrants into the profession. In one of my stud-ies (Brewer et al., 2006), we used a large nationally representative sample (N = 25,471) from the 2000 National Sample Survey of Registered Nurses to show the impact of wages on nurses' work decisions. By 2000, a smaller overall percentage of nurses were employed in nursing. I showed in this economic analysis that wages were not related to work partici-pation but that they were negatively related only to whether single or married registered nurses (RNs) worked full time.

Several market-level variables (e.g., index of competition among health maintenance organizations [HMOs], percentage of HMO hospital services paid through a fee sched-ule) also had an impact on whether RNs worked full time or at all, particularly for mar-ried RNs. Additional other income also negatively influenced whether RNs worked and reduced the full time work of married RNs. This responsiveness to other family income and market variables now helps explain the responsiveness of RNs to the 2008 recession—when spouses lost jobs, nurses stayed in their jobs longer and postponed retirement. However, this study was unique compared to other economic approaches in that we also examined job satisfaction. Satisfaction was significant and positive for married female

RNs. Thus it was clear that economic variables are not the only determinants of work decisions for nurses and that wage increases alone will not solve workforce shortages. The purely economic approach to nursing shortages using wages and demographic data does not adequately explain *why* RNs respond to wages as they make employment decisions or what their work environments are like. This finding led me to consider turnover theories that explain nurses' decision to leave an employer.

Two issues were important in connecting economic models to nurses' work decisions and nurse outcomes such as turnover, intent to leave, and job satisfaction. The first is the availability of longitudinal data. Turnover, a RN-level measure of nurses leaving employers, has been known to be related to satisfaction and other work environment attitudes for a long time. However, turnover cannot be measured directly unless follow-up data confirming the RN left the employer becomes available. The second issue is the availability of economic and demographic data as well as data about nurse outcomes of the work environment (e.g., intent to stay, satisfaction, organizational commitment, with predictors such as autonomy, promotional opportunities, or quantitative workloads). As principal investigator (PI) in a series of grants and associated papers, I developed studies for assessing nurse perceptions of the work environment. My research showed that work environment factors are as important as wages in explaining the work decisions of nurses.

Nurse outcomes such as turnover, organizational commitment, and satisfaction have important cost and quality implications for the U.S. health care system. Our landmark longitudinal study of early career RNs was funded by the Robert Wood Johnson Foundation for more than 10 years; our work has included six repeated surveys with a panel of new graduate nurses (the sixth survey was completed in 2015) and three additional comparison cohorts (to be completed in 2016). These surveys have been unique in the breadth of economic and attitudinal work environment variables included and the longitudinal aspects of the samples.

One purpose of this longitudinal study was to determine the actual turnover rate of new graduates over time and the factors that impact their intent to stay and turnover. For example, we determined that of new RNs, 14.0% who responded to our first survey in 2006 left their first job by the second survey 1 year later, but up to 56% of RNs (unpublished data) had left their first job by the fifth survey in 2013, indicating that over time there is considerable employer churning among new graduates, in spite of the recession during the later surveys. A large proportion remain employed in hospitals as the rate dropped from 87.2% in the first survey to 66.0% in the sixth survey (unpublished data). The implication of our work is that employers who design and maintain high quality-work environments should be able to slow the movement of early career nurses out of hospitals.

Another major focus of my work has been to examine the theoretical relationships among the major turnover predictors to clarify the important role of intent to stay, organizational commitment, and satisfaction as well as predictors specific to turnover (Brewer,

Chao, Colder, Kovner, & Chacko, 2015; Brewer, Kovner, Greene, Tukov-Shuser, & Djukic, 2012). Using a probit regression model (Brewer et al., 2012), we found that in the presence of intent to stay, most economic and demographic factors were not significant nor, surprisingly, were satisfaction and organizational commitment, although intent to stay did negatively predict turnover. However, satisfaction and organizational commitment were only significant if intent to stay was dropped from the model. In a later study (Brewer et al., 2015), using fours of the panels of data, we focused on just the key terminal variables of intent, search, job satisfaction, and organizational commitment using a structural equation approach, which confirmed the causal relationships suggested in the earlier study. We also carefully controlled for potential history and attrition biases. In the earlier (Brewer et al., 2012) study, most of the work environment attitudes (e.g., autonomy, quantitative workload, organizational constraints, supervisor support, and promotional opportunities) only indirectly influenced turnover and intent to stay through satisfaction and organizational commitment. The only other independent positive predictor of turnover in this study was injury. The implication of this study was the importance of organizational leaders creating policies that foster safe, high-quality work environments, which in turn avert costly turnover. My work has also shown that excluding organizational commitment is a serious methodological omission. Many nursing studies do not include either organizational commitment or injuries, instead focusing primarily on job satisfaction as a predictor of intent to leave and turnover.

One important feature of work environments is the level of incivility nurses must tolerate. We examined verbal abuse among nurses only and also among nurses and physicians in relation to the work environment and intent to stay. I showed in two papers (Brewer, Kovner, Obeidat, & Budin, 2013; Budin, Brewer, Chao, & Kovner, 2013) that verbal abuse among nurses as well as by physicians is strongly related to job characteristics such as the overall quality of the work environment and intent to stay, as well as the degree of verbal abuse by physicians. Verbal abuse by physicians is significantly associated with poor workgroup cohesion, lower supervisory and mentor support, higher workloads, higher organizational constraints, and nurse-colleague abuse. Among nurses, higher verbal abuse was also associated with lower levels of autonomy, supervisory support, mentor support, workgroup cohesion, distributive justice, procedural justice, and promotional opportunities. In both studies, nurses experiencing high verbal abuse from physicians or other nurses were more likely to work in hospitals, or nonmagnet hospitals, and work daytime or 12-hour shifts. In both studies, work environments tolerating higher verbal abuse are strongly associated with nurses experiencing lower job satisfaction, organizational commitment, and intent to stay. This important nursing leadership policy issue raises the question of whether a negative work environment creates/allows verbal abuse or verbal abuse emanates from the "bad apple" and then spreads to the whole "barrel." Turnover is costly in both economic and human terms, but it is avoidable if work environments are positive; the implication is that organizational leadership must take action to create these environments.

When nurses are easy to replace because of an adequate supply, leaders might be less motivated to make positive work environments a priority. Under shortage conditions with high turnover, there is both more strain and job dissatisfaction among the existing staff, and they are harder to replace. A positive environment with elements such as supervisor support, promotional opportunities, and minimal organizational constraints might be harder to maintain but is essential if employers want to attract and retain new nurses. Important strategies for proactive leaders maintaining a positive environment include setting zero-tolerance policies, including for physicians; assessing for problem areas; developing interprofessional communication strategies; avoiding denial; and dealing with problematic employees.

This brief summary has indicated a few of the areas in which my research has contributed to health systems research: identifying major predictors of turnover, intent to stay, organizational commitment, and job satisfaction and their relationships using advanced analytical strategies and providing a greater understanding of positive work environments for nurses.

References

Brewer, C. S., Chao, Y. Y., Colder, C. R., Kovner, C. T., & Chacko, T. P. (2015). A structural equation model of turnover for a longitudinal survey among early career registered nurses. *International Journal of Nursing Studies, 52*(11), 1735–1745. doi:10.1016/j.ijnurstu.2015.06.017

Brewer, C. S., Kovner, C. T., Greene, W., Tukov-Shuser, M., & Djukic, M. (2012). Predictors of actual turnover in a national sample of newly licensed registered nurses employed in hospitals. *Journal of Advanced Nursing, 68*(3), 521–538. doi:10.1111/j.1365-2648.2011.05753.x

Brewer, C. S., Kovner, C. T., Obeidat, R. F., & Budin, W. (2013). Positive work environments of early career RNs and the correlation with physician verbal abuse. *Nursing Outlook, 61*(6), 408–416. doi:10.1016/j.outlook.2013.01.004

Brewer, C. S., Kovner, C. T., Wu, Y. W., Greene, W., Yu, L., & Reimers, C. (2006). Factors influencing female RN's work behavior. *Health Services Research, 41*(3), 860–886.

Budin, W., Brewer, C. S., Chao, Y. Y., & Kovner, C. T. (2013). Verbal abuse from nurse colleagues and work environment of early career registered nurses. *Journal of Nursing Scholarship, 45*(3), 308–316. doi:10.1111/jnu.12033

A Workforce Policy to Highlight the Contribution of Nurses

Sung-Hyun Cho, PhD, RN

My program of research was shaped initially during my doctoral study at the University of Michigan School of Nursing (UMSN). Prior to admission to UMSN, I had worked as a staff nurse on a neonatal intensive care unit, a pediatric ward, and the quality improvement department of the Seoul National University Hospital, South Korea. Through my clinical experiences, I observed that nurses made a difference and that understaffing could threaten patient safety; however, nurses were not very good at demonstrating their roles and contributions to the improvement of patient outcomes and quality of patient care. My doctoral courses, especially on research methodology and patient outcomes research, enabled me to conduct my doctoral research on nurse staffing and adverse patient outcomes.

My doctoral research was funded by the Agency for Healthcare Research and Quality (Health Services Dissertation Research Grants). Using California hospital databases, I reported that better nurse staffing was associated with a decrease in the occurrence of pneumonia after surgery and that the occurrence of adverse events was associated with a significantly prolonged length of stay (LOS) and increased medical costs. The study findings were published in *Nursing Research* (Cho, Ketefian, Barkauskas, & Smith, 2003). This article has been cited more than 200 times in academic journals and was selected as one of most-cited (top 1%) papers by the National Research Foundation of Korea in 2013.

After returning to my country, I continued my research on nurse staffing and patient outcomes. Analyzing nurse surveys and national health insurance data, I reported through several publications that nurse staffing was associated with quality of care, nurse job outcomes, and patient mortality in intensive care units (Cho, Hwang, & Kim, 2008). I was interviewed on television just after my study was published and thus given a great opportunity to disseminate publicly the study finding of the inverse relationship between nurse staffing and patient mortality in intensive care units. This publication has been utilized as scientific evidence that supports the significance of nursing care to patient outcomes. I also believe that my study drew public attention to nurse staffing issues and encouraged nurse researchers to conduct additional studies on nurse staffing and patient outcomes.

Another study on nurse staffing issues examined the impact of reduction in hospital LOS on nursing workloads. I observed a dramatic decrease in LOS in acute care hospitals in Korea and reported that a shorter LOS was associated with higher work demands, and higher work demands were associated with worse nurse outcomes (Cho, Park, Jeon, Chang, & Hong, 2014). I also served as an advisory committee member in the Seoul

Medical Center, which implemented a new policy of increasing nurse staffing in inpatient units. I collaborated with the nursing director of the medical center to evaluate the policy impact on nursing care quality and disseminated the study finding of the effect of increasing nurse staffing on missed nursing care through an academic conference and a publication (Cho, Kim, Yeon, You, & Lee, 2015). This is a good example of how my research can contribute to society by suggesting a new model of nursing services that improves nursing care quality.

My research interests have expanded to other issues related to the nursing workforce, including the turnover of newly licensed nurses, nurse migration and geographic imbalances, and work environment (e.g., workplace violence against nurses). I conducted survival analysis as a new statistical methodology to analyze nurse turnover and reported low survival rates of newly licensed nurses in their first job (Cho, Lee, Mark, & Yun, 2012). In another study of the globalization of the nurse workforce, I addressed policy and ethical issues from the perspective of a researcher in a middle-income country, which I believe might be different from that in high-income countries (Cho, Lee, Mark, & Jones, 2014).

Recently I started collaboration with the Korean Hospital Nurses Association to produce evidence of nurses' contribution to higher quality care and better patient outcomes. This collaboration is very important because the government plans to change the nursing workforce by introducing a new type of licensed nursing personnel, and there are continuing debates among interest groups, including professional nursing organizations. I have given lectures to various audiences, including members of the National Assembly as well as nurse leaders, to address the roles of nurses in the future health care system based on my research findings.

In conclusion, my doctoral study at UMSN provided me with a sound foundation for my program of research. After graduation, I was able to develop my program of research on the basis of research experience I gained while at the university. I hope to continue my research on nurse workforce issues and contribute to enriching national and international evidence that nurses make a difference and that high-quality nursing care improves patient outcomes.

References

Cho, S. H., Hwang, J. H., & Kim, J. (2008). Nurse staffing and patient mortality in intensive care units. *Nursing Research, 57*, 322–330.

Cho, S. H., Ketefian, S., Barkauskas, V. H., & Smith, D. G. (2003). The effects of nurse staffing on adverse events, morbidity, mortality and medical costs. *Nursing Research, 52*, 71–79.

Cho, S. H., Kim, Y. S., Yeon, K. N., You, S. J., & Lee, I. D. (2015). Effects of increasing nurse staffing on missed nursing care. *International Nursing Review, 62*, 267–274.

Cho, S. H., Lee, J. Y., Mark, B. A., & Jones, C. B. (2014). Geographic mobility of Korean new graduate nurses from their first to subsequent jobs and metropolitan-nonmetropolitan differences in their job satisfaction. *Nursing Outlook, 62*, 22–28.

Cho, S. H., Lee, J. Y., Mark, B. A., & Yun, S. C. (2012). Turnover of new graduate nurses in their first job using survival analysis. *Journal of Nursing Scholarship, 44*(1), 63–70.

Cho, S. H., Park, M., Jeon, S. H., Chang, H. E., & Hong, H. J. (2014). Average hospital length of stay, nurses' work demands, and their health and job outcomes. *Journal of Nursing Scholarship, 46*, 199–206.

The Opportunity and Obligation to Improve Care Delivery

Christopher Friese, PhD, RN, FAAN

The Problem

Despite the astounding volume of cancer care delivered in this country, very little is known about the quality of care delivered. Evaluating the quality of care delivered to high-risk populations—such as patients with a cancer diagnosis or undergoing major surgery—is a crucial ingredient to optimal patient, system, and financial outcomes.

A Program of Research

My research program evaluates the quality of care delivery as perceived by patients and providers. There are two connected components to the research program. First, I study the structure, process, and outcomes of care delivered to patients. Second, I evaluate the quality of care delivered from the perspective of providers, most often nurses. My novel approach to study both patient and provider perspectives enables me to triangulate findings and identify high-priority topics for future research, intervention, and policy development. The primary methods to advance this research program include (a) secondary analysis of existing datasets and (b) surveys to patients and/or providers. More recently, I have conducted practice-based intervention studies focused on nurses.

Measurement Advances

I recognized a glaring omission in instruments used to measure the practice environments of nurses who are employed in ambulatory oncology settings. My K99/R00 award funded a series of focus groups, cognitive interviews, and pilot surveys that yielded a revised set of items derived from the Practice Environment Scale of the Nursing Work Index. In 2012, I published the 23-item instrument and demonstrated its validity and reliability in *Oncology Nursing Forum* (Friese, 2012). In 2015, this measure was used by the Dana-Farber Cancer Institute to measure the practice environments of nurses and nurse practitioners in ambulatory oncology settings. That work was accepted for publication in *Cancer Nursing* (Friese, Siefert, Thomas-Frost, Walker, & Ponte, 2015). I hope to test the measure in nononcology settings in future work.

Current Intervention Work

My research program has bridged the knowledge gap surrounding the quality of care delivered to oncology patients by identifying high-priority targets for intervention. My efforts to highlight the issue of nurses' hazardous drug exposure has resulted in an R01 grant funded by the National Institute for Occupational Safety and Health (NIOSH) (Friese, Mendelsohn-Victor, et al., 2015). Oncology nurses are at an increased risk for adverse health outcomes due to suboptimal use of protective equipment. This cluster randomized controlled trial will increase our understanding of how an audit and feedback intervention can improve the use of protective equipment by nurses and reduce hazardous drug exposure in the chaotic ambulatory oncology setting.

Policy Impact

My research findings address the critical policy question "How do we deliver high-quality, affordable care to Americans with serious illnesses?" Publications describing results of my research have influenced clinical practice guidelines, as well as state and national policy. For example, my 2008 paper in *Health Services Research* (Friese, Lake, Aiken, Silber, & Sochalski, 2008), which examined the relationship between patient outcomes and nurses' education and practice environments, was cited in the Institute of Medicine report *The Future of Nursing (IOM, 2010)*, in a policy brief for the American Association of Colleges of Nursing, and in the strategic plans for the New York and North Carolina state boards of nursing. My papers in *BMJ Quality and Safety* (Friese, Himes-Ferris, Frasier, McCullagh, & Griggs, 2012) and *Cancer Nursing* (Friese, Siefert, et al., 2015), which examined hazardous drug exposure by ambulatory oncology nurses, renewed a national discussion on hazardous drug-handling policies (Friese et al., 2014; Friese et al., 2012). In 2015 and after my consultation, Senate Bill 237 was introduced in Michigan to require facilities that administer hazardous drugs to provide adequate personal protective equipment and training to reduce exposures.

My paper in *Cancer* (Friese et al., 2010), which identified the mortality benefit of performing baseline flow cytometry to confirm a diagnosis in patients with chronic lymphocytic leukemia, informed the National Quality Forum and American Society of Hematology endorsement of baseline flow cytometry performance as a quality of care indicator. My 2009 paper in *Cancer* (Friese, Neville, Edge, Hassett, & Earle, 2009) on breast biopsy patterns was cited by the American College of Surgeons "Choosing Wisely" campaign, which recommends the avoidance of surgical biopsy as the first diagnostic procedure for breast anomalies.

Future Directions

In addition to my current research topics, which have led to multiple publications and grant awards, I relish the opportunity to ask and answer new research questions that affect the quality of care delivered to high-risk populations. In February 2015, I submitted an R01 application to the National Cancer Institute to understand the patient, treatment, and practice-related factors that influence the risk of treatment-associated toxicities for women with breast cancer. During the first year of my R01 from NIOSH—which will end in June 2018—I planned (a) supplements or renewals on efficient methods to detect chemotherapy exposure and (b) the expansion of our work to other settings (e.g., inpatient settings, homecare) and populations (e.g., pharmacists and housekeepers).

References

Friese, C. R. (2012). Practice environments of nurses employed in ambulatory oncology settings: Measure refinement. *Oncology Nursing Forum, 39*(2), 166–172. doi:10.1188/12.ONF.166-172

Friese, C. R., Earle, C. C., Magazu, L. S., Brown, J. R., Neville, B. A., Hevelone, N. D., . . . Abel, G. A. (2010). Timeliness and quality of diagnostic care for Medicare recipients with chronic lymphocytic leukemia. *Cancer, 117*(7), 1470–1477. doi:10.1002/cncr.25655

Friese, C. R., Himes-Ferris, L., Frasier, M. N., McCullagh, M. C., & Griggs, J. J. (2012). Structures and processes of care in ambulatory oncology settings and nurse-reported exposure to chemotherapy. *BMJ Quality & Safety, 21*(9), 753–759. doi:10.1136/bmjqs-2011-000178

Friese, C. R., Lake, E. T., Aiken, L. H., Silber, J. H., & Sochalski, J. (2008). Hospital nurse practice environments and outcomes for surgical oncology patients. *Health Services Research, 43*(4), 1145–11463. doi:10.1111/j.1475-6773.2007.00825.x

Friese, C. R., McArdle, C., Zhao, T., Sun, D., Spasojevic, I., Polovich, M., & McCullagh, M. C. (2014). Antineoplastic drug exposure in an ambulatory setting: A pilot study. *Cancer Nursing, 38*(2), 111–117. doi:10.1097/NCC.0000000000000143

Friese, C. R., Mendelsohn-Victor, K., Wen, B., Sun, D., Sutcliffe, K., Yang, J. J., . . . DEFENS Study Investigators. (2015). DEFENS—Drug Exposure Feedback and Education for Nurses' Safety: Study protocol for a randomized controlled trial. *Trials, 16*(1), 171. doi:10.1186/s13063-015-0674-5

Friese, C. R., Neville, B. A., Edge, S. B., Hassett, M. J., & Earle, C. C. (2009). Breast biopsy patterns and outcomes in surveillance, epidemiology, and end results-Medicare data. *Cancer, 115*(4), 716–724. doi:10.1002/cncr.24085

Friese, C. R., Siefert, M. L., Thomas-Frost, K., Walker, S., & Ponte, P. R. (2015). Using data to strengthen ambulatory oncology nursing practice. *Cancer Nursing, 39*(1), 74–79. doi:10.1097/NCC.0000000000000240

Institute of Medicine. (2010). *The future of nursing: Leading change, advancing health.* Washington, DC: National Academies Press.

Nursing Research Shaping Health Policy

Ada Sue Hinshaw, PhD, RN, FAAN

Understanding how nurse scientists shape health policy with their research programs has been the focus of my scholarship since assuming the directorship of the National Institute of Nursing Research (NINR; formerly the National Center for Nursing Research [NCNR]) at the National Institutes of Health in 1987. The first priority of NINR was to amass the knowledge needed to provide evidence-based practice. As the institute approached its 25th anniversary, the influence of nursing research on health policy at the organizational, community, state, national, and international levels was becoming evident.

Focusing on the processes of how nursing research was influencing health policy and noting the successful strategies being used by nurse scientists was at the heart of my scholarship during my years as dean of the University of Michigan School of Nursing. This scholarly program culminated in a study conducted with senior nurse investigators who had pursued their research through multiple grants and whose programs had shown obvious evidence of being included in health policy at various levels. Ultimately, I coauthored *Shaping Health Policy Through Nursing Research* with Dr. Patricia A. Grady, which has been successful as a textbook for students in Doctor of Philosophy (PhD) and Doctor of Nursing Practice (DNP) programs (Hinshaw & Grady, 2011).

Appointment as Distinguished Scholar

Following my term as dean, I was privileged to be offered and supported for a year as a Distinguished Scholar (2007), jointly sponsored by the American Nurses' Foundation, the American Academy of Nursing, and the Institute of Medicine (renamed the National Academy of Medicine [NAM]). The study I carried out was titled Nurse Scientists Shaping Health Policy. The investigation utilized in-depth interviews of senior nurse researchers who had received one or two continuation grants from NINR. After two decades of stable financial support, four questions were asked of the senior nurse scientists in considering the influence of their research on health policy at the organizational, community, state, or national levels:

- What characteristics of their research helped shape health policy?
- What external factors assisted them in shaping health policy with their research?
- What were the barriers to using their research in shaping health policy?
- What were the successful strategies they had used to facilitate their research in shaping health policy?

The results were published in *Shaping Health Policy Through Nursing Research* (Hinshaw & Grady, 2011). The concepts listed below are those most frequently cited by the nurse scientists:

- Characteristics of nursing research shaping health policy; for example, studies focus on important public health issues and draw interest from and include multiple disciplines.
- External factors that support nursing research and health policy; for example, research programs were housed in strong research university environments, and the research was timely in terms of informing critical health issues.
- Barriers to nursing research informing health policy; for example, lack of interest by policy makers so that no "window of opportunity" and no economic data were included in the studies.
- Successful strategies used by nurse scientists; for example, studies informed national health guidelines and shaped policy through congressional testimony, NAM Roundtables, and reports.

In summary, through involvement at the national level in policy making and influencing organizations such as NINR and NAM, a strong interest was fostered in understanding how nursing research might shape health policy as well as health practice. This short paper provides documentation of the culmination of a program of scholarship that included active involvement in shaping health policy and in studying the processes through which nursing research can inform such policy at the organizational, community, state, national, and international levels.

Reference

Hinshaw, A. S., & Grady, P. (2011). *Shaping health policy through nursing research*. New York, NY: Springer.

From Policy/Politics to History
to Image to Nursing Studies

Beatrice J. Kalisch, PhD, RN, FAAN

I joined the University of Michigan School of Nursing (UMSN) in 1974 as professor and chair of Parent-Child Nursing. In that role, I led the establishment of the master's degree programs in women and children. Over my 40 years at UMSN, my key areas of research have been policy and politics; nursing history; the image of the nurse; and, since 2006, missed nursing care—a term I coined to describe standard required nursing care that is not being provided—and nursing teamwork.

Policy and Politics Studies

The policy and politics studies started with an R01 grant from the National Institutes of Health that was awarded to me and Philip Kalisch at our previous employment. We transferred it to the University of Michigan when we came here. This study involved an assessment of the impact of federal funding on nursing practice, education, and research from 1940 to 1985, such as Title VIII, U.S. Cadet Nurse Corps, and so on. Data gathering for this study involved reviewing extensive archival data and interviews with most of the senators and congressmen and key nurse leaders in education and practice during those years. This study resulted in numerous publications, including *Nursing Involvement in Health Planning* (Kalisch & Kalisch, 1978) and other books and articles.

This work also led to the study of nursing politics, which had not been explored before. Most nurses shunned politics, feeling it was "dirty" and something nurses should not be involved in. We wrote a first article on the subject of politics, and later a book, *Politics of Nursing* (*American Journal of Nursing* Book of the Year Award; Kalisch & Kalisch, 1982). We initiated the first courses on the subject, and several of our students over the years entered into the political world by becoming lobbyists, while others completed research on the subject. In 1979, the UMSN students organized a march on Washington to protest the recision of funds for nursing (Title VIII), gathering students from 22 other schools to participate and meet on the steps of the Capitol. They sat in the balcony of the House of Representatives, watching the legislation being enacted. Several key leaders emerged from this effort, including Carolyne Davis, who was appointed to head up Health Care Financing Administration (which became the Centers for Medicare and Medicaid Services).

Historical Studies

Started in the years prior to joining UMSN, my research partner and I completed a number of historical studies during our time at UMSN. The following studies are examples of this work:

- Kalisch, P., & Kalisch, B. (1979, 1986, 1994). *The advance of American nursing* (1st, 2nd, 3rd, and 4th eds.). Boston, MA: Little, Brown. (*American Journal of Nursing* Book of the Year Award for each edition.)
- Kalisch, B., & Kalisch, P. (1976). Is history of nursing alive and well? *Nursing Outlook, 24*, 362–369.
- Kalisch, P., & Kalisch, B. (1976). Untrained but undaunted: The women nurses of the blue and the grey. *Nursing Forum, 15*(1), 4–33.
- Kalisch, P., & Kalisch, B. (1976). Nurses under fire: The World War II experience of nurses on Bataan and Corregidor. *Nursing Research, 25*, 409–429.
- Kalisch, B. (1975). Of half-gods and mortals: Aesculapian authority. *Nursing Outlook, 23*, 22–28.
- Kalisch, B., & Kalisch, P. (1975). Slaves, servants, or saints? An analysis of the system of nurse training in the United States, 1873–1948. *Nursing Forum, 14*(3), 222–226.

Image of Nurses and Nursing Studies

Based on the interviews we conducted with senators and congressmen as part of the above studies, we realized the profound inaccuracy of the image of the nurse (e.g., when asked about why there was not an institute for nursing research, they responded that they thought physicians did research, not nurses). This finding led us to applying for and being awarded several R01s to study the public image of nursing from 1900 to the present. These studies involved identifying and collecting media depictions with one or more nurse characters from all forms of media. We then completed a content analysis of 1,843 novels, 403 motion pictures, 875 television shows, and 20,000-plus newspaper articles The results of this study were published in articles and several books, among them *Images of Nurses on Television* (Kalisch, Kalisch, & Scobey, 1983) and *The Changing Image of the Nurse* (Kalisch & Kalisch, 1987; recipient of the *American Journal of Nursing* Book of the Year Award).

Missed Nursing Care

Since 2006, I have conducted 15 studies on missed nursing care or errors of omission. The public tends to think of medical errors as actions a provider did to a patient that caused harm; however, a common type of medical error is the error of omission. Errors of omission happen when something should have been done for the patient to reduce the risk of harm but was not done. The first study of missed nursing care employed focus groups with nursing staff to identify the scope of care missed in the acute care setting. Findings revealed nine areas of missed care (ambulation, turning, delayed or missed feedings, patient teaching, discharge planning, emotional support, hygiene, intake and output documentation, and surveillance). Based on this work, a quantitative survey tool to measure missed nursing care (The MISSCARE Survey) was developed and tested. Findings identified a substantial amount of missed care in 14 hospitals and 124 patient care units involving more than 4,500 nursing staff. Survey respondents indicated missing a great amount of care—for example, ambulation (84%), assessing of the effectiveness of medications (83%), turning (82%), and mouth care (82%). Part 2 of the MISSCARE Survey measured reasons for missing nursing care (labor resources, material resources, and teamwork/communication). Both the elements of missed care and reasons were similar across hospitals.

Nursing Teamwork

My research in nursing teamwork showed that when people work on high-performing teams, they are more satisfied, more productive, and less stressed; consequently, the quality of the care they deliver is higher, there are fewer errors, and patients are more satisfied. The use of the Salas model in explaining nursing teamwork was substantiated by a qualitative study. The next step was the development and testing of the Nursing Teamwork Survey (NTS).

Other studies included examining the relationship between teamwork and staffing, missed nursing care, and electronic health records. I also developed several interventions including "Teamwork Tactics."

International Studies

Finally, I have studied missed nursing care and teamwork in seven countries (Australia, Iceland, Italy, Lebanon, South Korea, Turkey, and the United States). The MISSCARE Survey has been translated into Icelandic, Italian, Korean, and Turkish using a step-by-step process. There were significant differences in the total amount of missed nursing and teamwork among the seven countries. The NTS has been translated into Korean, Turkish, and Portuguese.

References

Bragadóttir, H., Kalisch, B., Jónsdóttir, H. H., & Smáradóttir, S. (2015). Translation and psychometric testing of the Icelandic version of the *MISSCARE Survey. Scandinavian Journal of Caring Sciences, 29*(3), 563–572.

Kalisch, B., Aebersold, M., Tschannen, D., McLaughlin, M., & Lane, S. (2014). An intervention to increase nursing teamwork using virtual media. *Western Journal of Nursing Research, 37*(2), 164–179.

Kalisch, B., & Kalisch, P. (1974). *From training to education: The impact of federal aid on schools of nursing in the United States in the 1940s.*

Kalisch, P., & Kalisch, B. (1978). *Nursing involvement in health planning.* Washington, DC: U.S. Department of Health, Education and Welfare.

Kalisch, B., & Kalisch, P. (1982). *Politics of nursing.* Philadelphia: J. B. Lippincott.

Kalisch, P., & Kalisch, B. (1987). *The changing image of the nurse.* Menlo Park, CA: Addison-Wesley

Kalisch, P., Kalisch, B., & Scobey, M. (1983). *Images of nurses on television.* New York, NY: Springer.

Kalisch, B., & Xie, B. (2014). Missed nursing care. *Journal of Nursing Science in China, 29*(9), 1–4.

Kalisch, B., Xie, B., & Ronis, D. (2013). Train-the-trainer intervention to increase nursing teamwork and decrease missed nursing care in acute care patient units. *Nursing Research, 62*(6), 405–413.

An Intellectual Journey

Shaké Ketefian, EdD, RN, FAAN

My program of research and scholarship has been guided by a number of concerns, the two most important being (a) how knowledge is being produced and used in nursing, in the United States and, in the past two decades, internationally, and (b) how work environments can be organized so that they are more conducive and supportive of practice and/ or scholarship that are of high quality and high ethical standards? Furthermore, given the status of nursing and health care in other countries, and the historical leadership of U.S. nursing, how might I make a difference, using teaching/learning opportunities to make a positive impact in selected countries and settings? In view of my academic leadership roles in graduate education in the United States and internationally, it is important that I stay engaged and produce relevant scholarship.

How Is Knowledge Developed and Used?

During my doctoral study, nursing science was a very new field: the journal *Nursing Research* had been in publication for less than 20 years, and research, which was generally about nurses, was frequently carried out by social scientists. Thus, given how little research there was, I became interested in finding out to what extent the results of nursing research were being used to improve practice or education or whatever domain the results were relevant to. This theme became the central question of my dissertation and my research thereafter. The question was investigated within the nursing education realm, using educational innovations and the extent to which those innovations were based on research-based knowledge. I found that some innovations were based on sound science, whereas for others innovations the science was less clear and based primarily on common sense, logic, and reasoning.

In my first faculty position, I carried out a research study to investigate the extent to which research-based knowledge undergirded nursing practice—a negligible extent, as the results showed.

In 1995, the University of Michigan hosted the then annual Doctoral Forum held nationally. For the first time, we focused on international doctoral education and knowledge development issues and invited international speakers and attendees. In a revised conference format, we prepared several papers in advance so participants could read prior to attending and then discuss them during the conference. My colleague Professor Richard Redman and I wrote one of the papers (Ketefian & Redman, 1997). We did an analysis of knowledge development from a global perspective using three approaches: *contextual*, which deals with the U.S. social environment and how it influences our knowledge and theory; *quantitative*, which considers rapid developments of our doctoral programs and increases in our journals and our scientists; and *qualitative*, which deals with the ways in which our values affect our theory development and our science. We concluded that at that time, Western perspectives and values heavily influenced our science; that while admired and emulated worldwide, our science lacked global characteristics; and further, that our doctoral programs might be producing scientists who do not challenge Western perspectives and assumptions in our science. In order to promote multicultural knowledge development and make our science globally relevant, we made a number of recommendations. The paper has been read extensively worldwide and was the lead article in the redesigned *Journal of Nursing Scholarship* (Ketefian & Redman, 1997).

In the recent past, universities around the world have been looking for ways to encourage faculty to engage in research while also finding ways to evaluate that research; this is the case for countries that are new to science production. Thus universities are requiring that their faculty publish in journals with a high impact factor (IF) and see this as a measure of quality of the faculty's work. Working with a team of nurse scientists representing five countries, I organized and led a study that investigated the scholarly environments of their countries. Three of the countries had policies that required faculty to publish in high-IF journals (Brazil, Taiwan, and Thailand; Group A countries), and the other two countries (United Kingdom and United States; Group B countries) did not have such policies, although implicitly they encouraged such policies. We asked highly engaged scholars in all five countries to provide their perceptions on specific topics with regard to the research question. We concluded that requirements to publish in high-IF journals did not make a significant difference, as Group B countries and one country in Group A continued to do so regardless of such policies. Rather, we speculated that other factors needed to be present as well, such as the resource base of the country, qualified nurse scientists, and other types of facilitation (Ketefian, Dai, Hanucharurnkul, Mendes, & Norman, 2010).

How Can Work Environments Be Made Conductive to Ethical Practice?

Early in my career, I served on ethics committees of the New York State Nurses Association and the American Nurses Association (ANA). In the case of ANA, the goal was to revise and update the *Code for Nurses* (1976). I began considering the ways in which research questions can be framed so that they can be empirically investigated, since value questions inherent in ethics cannot be answered through empirical research. I came across the work of Laurence Kohlberg, who was developing the concept of moral reasoning (or moral judgment) and its measurement. This construct addressed the way we reason about moral choice but not the content of the moral choice. In this sense, cognitive processes are at work, and moral reasoning is a necessary but insufficient condition for moral action. Kohlberg discussed two modes of cultivating moral education—moral discussion and the creation of a moral atmosphere—demonstrating how these work in shaping educational environments and prison systems.

I embarked on a multiyear project of developing an instrument to measure moral behavior in nursing work environments and conducted a series of studies investigating personal and environmental factors that influence moral behavior (see Ketefian, 1981).

Subsequent to these studies, I carried out a literature synthesis with one of my doctoral students, Dr. Ingrid Ormond (Venohr), published as a book by the National League for Nursing (Ketefian & Ormond, 1988). We specifically examined the relationship between moral reasoning and ethical practice; however, given that the majority of the studies were qualitative, we could not arrive at a definitive conclusion. We made recommendations regarding questions that needed to be investigated and emphasized the importance of methodological rigor. Ten years later, the literature seemed to have become much more focused, with greater attention to methodologic issues. We were able to carry out a formal meta-analysis, which I led, with the participation of the ethics research section of the Midwest Nursing Research Society (MNRS). This study tested some of the same hypotheses the 1981 study. We found that while moral reasoning and ethical practice were related, a number of studies for testing this latter hypothesis had to be eliminated, drastically reducing the sample size. More research is indicated in this area (Ketefian, 2001).

Over the years, my ethical practice interests evolved to include scientific integrity concerns and how we could teach scientific integrity in doctoral education and practice it in our own research. I collaborated with a colleague on several studies (e.g., Ketefian & Lenz, 1995) and subsequently, chaired a committee of the Midwest Nursing Research Society that developed scientific integrity guidelines, the first of its kind by a major professional nursing organization; this document use extensively by scientists in the region (MNRS, 2002).

I collaborated with nursing service colleagues, along with Professor Redman, on a work redesign project that lasted for 4 years in the 1990s. He describes the nature of this project and the scholarly yield in his brief, "Care Quality, Safety, and Clinical and Organizational Outcomes."

Other Avenues of Contribution and National/International Impact

In the mid- to late 1990s, I became involved in international doctoral education and colead the formation of the International Network for Doctoral Education in Nursing (INDEN), along with professors Hugh McKenna (United Kingdom) and Afaf Meleis (United States). On short order, members (doctoral students and doctoral faculty) joined from nearly 40 countries. It was an exciting time of extensive international interactions, learning, and collaborations that led to wide-ranging scholarship in the area of doctoral education around the world. Several noteworthy initiatives were undertaken during my presidency at INDEN (serving as founding president) (http://nursing.jhu.edu/excellence/ inden/index.html). First was the development of standards, criteria, and indicators for doctoral education, which are now used worldwide, Second, was a collaboration with Sigma Theta Tau International, the nursing honor society, to offer short-term postdoctoral fellowships to international scholars from middle- and low-resource countries, which continues today and has benefited many scholars and contributed to advancing nursing research and doctoral education worldwide, And third was a volume on international doctoral education spearheaded and edited by me and Dr. Hugh McKenna (2005). In addition, numerous collaboratively prepared papers were published in various nursing journals around the world (see Ketefian, Davidson, Daly, Chang, & Srisuphan, 2005).

I was invited to edit an issue of the *Journal of Nursing Science*, a Thai journal on doctoral education in several Asian countries, and also provided a synthesis (Ketefian, 2013;

see last chapter for synthesis); this widely read document represented the state of affairs in doctoral education in Asia at the time.

I recently collaborated with teams from seven countries to evaluate doctoral education. This team was led by Professor Mi Ja Kim, who had used the INDEN standards, criteria, and indicators to design an instrument for the evaluation of doctoral programs (Kim et al., 2015).

My publications are numerous and are widely read and cited around the world. My tool of ethical practice has been translated into Chinese and Korean, and the MNRS scientific integrity guidelines have been translated into Spanish (Mexico) and Chinese (Taiwan).

References

Ketefian, S. (1981). Moral reasoning and moral behavior among selected groups of practicing nurses. *Nursing Research, 30,* 171–176.

Ketefian, S. (2001). The relationship of education and moral reasoning to ethical practice: A meta-analysis of quantitative studies. *Scholarly Inquiry for Nursing Practice, 15*(1), 3–18.

Ketefian, S. (Guest Ed.). (2013). Doctoral nursing education in Asia: Current challenges and Future directions. *Journal of Nursing Science, 31* (Suppl.).

Ketefian, S., Dai, Y. T., Hanucharurnkul, S., Mendes, I. A. C., & Norman, I. J. (2010). Environments for scholarship and journal impact factor in five countries. *International Nursing Review, 57,* 343–351.

Ketefian, S., Davidson, P., Daly, J., Chang, E., & Srisuphan, W. (2005). Issues and challenges in International doctoral education. *Nursing and Health Sciences, 7*(3), 150–156.

Ketefian, S., & Lenz, E. R. (1995). Promoting scientific integrity in nursing research, part II: Strategies. *Journal of Professional Nursing, 11*(5), 263–269.

Ketefian, S., & McKenna, H. P. (Eds.). (2005). *Doctoral education in nursing: International perspectives.* London: Routledge.

Ketefian, S., & Ormond, I. (1988). *Moral reasoning and ethical practice in nursing: An integrative review.* New York, NY: National League for Nursing.

Ketefian, S., & Redman, R. (1997). Generating nursing science in the global community. *Journal of Nursing Scholarship, 29*(1), 11–15.

Kim, M. J., Park, C. G., McKenna, H., Ketefian, S., Park, S. H., Klopper, H., Lee, H., . . . Khan, S. (2015). Quality of nursing doctoral education in seven countries: Online survey of faculty and students/graduates. *Journal of Advanced Nursing, 71*(5), 1098–1109.

Midwest Nursing Research Society. (2002). *Guidelines for scientific integrity* (2nd ed.). Wheat Ridge, CO: Author.

Rethinking Communication for Improved Patient Outcomes

Milisa Manojlovich, PhD, RN

The Problem

Poor communication between physicians and nurses is one of the most common causes of adverse events for hospitalized patients (Leape & Berwick, 2005) and a major root cause of all sentinel events reported to the Joint Commission (Joint Commission, n.d.). There has been a general lack of progress in improving communication between nurses and physicians for several reasons. First, most studies have been cross-sectional, impeding the ability to establish the causes of poor communication. The lack of a causal connection limits the ability to develop effective interventions to improve communication. Second, quantitative methods have predominated, limiting our ability to understand the contextual elements that influence communication, as well as the perspectives of physicians and nurses themselves. Third, most studies have queried either physicians or nurses but rarely both. In those few studies that have investigated both groups, results have been consistent: physicians report good communication with nurses, while nurses report poor communication with physicians.

A Program of Research

My program of research explores how communication between physicians and nurses influences outcomes for hospitalized patients. Since communication interventions to date have had limited success, the ultimate goal of my research is to develop effective interventions to improve communication. Movement toward this goal is happening along empirical and conceptual paths. Empirically, I began studying communication with quantitative methods, but more recently, O have gravitated toward qualitative and mixed methods. Qualitative methods are superior to quantitative methods for exploring the meaning of effective communication as experienced by nurses and physicians themselves.

Conceptually, I am promulgating an uncommon definition of communication: the development of mutual understanding. The patient safety movement, borrowing heavily from the aviation industry, has promoted a definition of communication that emphasizes the transmission of information from sender to receiver. While this definition has merit, research that ignores the development of mutual understanding may be hampering efforts to improve communication between two health care disciplines steeped in different knowledge traditions.

Knowledge Gaps Filled Using Quantitative Methods

I began studying the subject of communication in the early 2000s by focusing on learning more about the *contextual* elements surrounding nurse-physician communication (i.e., the interrelated conditions in which communication occurs) and how these influence communication to contribute to adverse events. In my dissertation study. I approached the phenomenon of nurse-physician communication tangentially by examining work environment factors that may affect professional nursing practice behaviors, including communication. My research employed quantitative methods and included only nurse perceptions of their communication with physicians. Despite this "one sided" view of an interdisciplinary process, my findings were novel. This initial study found that a combination of workplace empowerment, nurses' self-efficacy for professional practice, and the strength of nursing leadership explained 46% of the variance in professional practice behaviors, extending our knowledge of the effect of the hospital practice environment on nurses' professional practice behaviors and communication (Manojlovich, 2005a).

Additional studies over the next few years continued to use self-reported, nurse-centric quantitative methods. I moved from an emphasis on contextual elements of communication to focus on the process of nurse-physician communication itself. One study demonstrated that work environment factors (both workplace empowerment and professional practice characteristics) and nurse-physician communication predicted 61% of the variance in nurses' job satisfaction. This study also demonstrated that communication is a process mediating the relationship between work environment factors and nurses' job satisfaction, a significant finding since process links between environmental structures and outcomes have rarely been identified (Manojlovich, 2005b).

I extended my work into environment-communication-outcome linkages with funding from the Blue Cross Blue Shield of Michigan Foundation. Study results indicated that workplace empowerment and professional practice characteristics together predicted 34% of the variance in nurse-physician communication; that the timeliness of communication was a predictor of pressure ulcer prevalence; and that variability in nurses' understanding of communication was inversely related to ventilator-associated pneumonia (Manojlovich & DeCicco, 2007). This study was significant because almost half of the variance in nurse-physician communication was explained by factors in the work environment, highlighting the importance of context to communication.

Knowledge Gaps Filled Using Qualitative Methods

With colleagues from the Veterans Health Administration, I began to use qualitative methods, including the perspectives of both physicians and nurses. I recognized that communication is a complex process not easily captured in its entirety by one methodological approach alone. We used mixed methods in a study conducted in three intensive care units of a single veterans hospital and discovered that nurses who reported having a weak safety culture on their unit also were the least satisfied with their communication with physicians (Manojlovich et al., 2011).

A qualitative study consisting of observation, shadowing, and focus groups of both physicians and nurses exposed many communication barriers, including a culture norm of nurses and physicians avoiding face-to-face communication. The sequential use of observation, shadowing, and focus groups was an innovative method that had not previously described in the literature but was powerful in its ability to capture the "what," "how," and "why" of communication events (Manojlovich et al., 2015).

Results from several of the studies described above were used as pilot data for a federally funded grant focusing on the effect of health information technology on health care provider communication. The purpose of this R01 study was to describe in detail how communication technologies facilitate or hinder communication between nurses and physicians with the ultimate goal of identifying the optimal ways to support effective communication. This study used a sequential mixed-methods design to generate a richer view of how physicians and nurses use communication technology to deal with patient care issues that are often ambiguous by their nature and require input from multiple disciplines for successful resolution.

Future Directions

Future work will continue to use qualitative methods to determine if effective communication (through the development of mutual understanding) between physicians and nurses can be identified and captured. How mutual understanding develops is poorly understood because little attention has been paid to it thus far. In an upcoming grant application, colleagues and I will determine if videotaping conversations between nurses and physicians can capture, measure, and characterize mutual understanding.

References

Joint Commission. (n.d.). Sentinel events. Retrieved from http://www.jointcommission.org/sentinel_event.aspx

Leape, L. L., & Berwick, D. M. (2005). Five years after To Err Is Human: What have we learned? *JAMA, 293*(19), 2384–2390. doi:10.1001/jama.293.19.2384

Manojlovich, M. (2005a). Predictors of professional nursing practice behaviors in hospital settings. *Nursing Research, 54*(1), 41–47. doi:10.1097/NNA.0b013e3181f37e7d

Manojlovich, M. (2005b). Linking the practice environment to nurses' job satisfaction through nurse-physician communication. *Journal of Nursing Scholarship, 37*(4), 367–373.

Manojlovich, M., & DeCicco, B. (2007). Healthy work environments, nurse-physician communication, and patients' outcomes. *American Journal of Critical Care, 16*(6), 536–543.

Manojlovich, M., Harrod, M., Holtz, B., Hofer, T. P., Kuhn, L., & Krein, S. L. (2015). The use of multiple qualitative methods to characterize communication events between physicians and nurses. *Health Communication, 30*(1), 61–69. PMID: 24483246.

Manojlovich, M., Saint, S., Forman, J., Fletcher, C. E., Keith, R., & Krein, S. (2011). Developing and testing a tool to measure nurse/physician communication in the intensive care unit. *Journal of Patient Safety, 7*(2), 80–84.

Care Quality, Safety, and Clinical and Organizational Outcomes

Richard W. Redman, PhD, RN

During my academic career (1979–2014), I have held a variety of leadership positions, ranging from program director to associate and interim dean. While my responsibilities were primarily administrative, I always strived to maintain a program of research and scholarship. I had the good fortune throughout the years to collaborate with a number of colleagues, conducting my research in interdisciplinary teams. I arrived at Michigan in 1988 and since then have been involved in a variety of projects.

My overall program of research has focused broadly on quality and patient safety in nursing practice environments and their impact on clinical and organizational outcomes. Sometimes I focused on the nursing care team, and at other times I focused on the broader patient care organizational environment. I have been involved in a number of projects within this broad focus, ranging from nurses and patients to organizational outcomes.

In 1990, I began working with a large team to investigate the effects of work redesign on nurses and patients in acute care and ambulatory settings. The team consisted of Professor Shaké Ketefian in the School of Nursing and several directors of nursing in the University of Michigan Health System (UMHS). The directors were Beverly Jones, Carol

Spengler, Joan Robinson, Debra Finch, and Sheri Dufek. This project lasted for 5 years, and in addition to several publications, the data from the project were used in 3 dissertations and 12 master's theses at the University of Michigan School of Nursing.

At that time, UMHS was facing environmental demands common across the U.S. health system: a nursing shortage in the marketplace, financial challenges due to prospective reimbursement and managed care, and increased needs for efficiency. Nursing, along with other health professions, was faced with demands to redesign the care system to improve both the quality and efficiency of its practice. The work redesign project at UMHS was developed to measure the effects of work and role redesign efforts undertaken by the nursing care team. A longitudinal design, with three major data collections over a 4-year period, was implemented using the job characteristics model (Hackman & Oldham, 1980) as the conceptual framework. A variety of standardized instruments were used to assess job characteristics, work roles and responsibilities, job satisfaction, ethical decision making, perceptions of organizational culture and values, and organizational commitment. In addition, institutional data were collected on unit- and organizational-level nursing turnover.

An instrument to measure patient satisfaction with nursing care was developed and tested as part of this project (Ketefian, Redman, Nash, & Bogue, 1997). Conceptual and methodological challenges in conducting this type of research were reported in the literature. The work redesign efforts were shown not to have a detrimental effect on nursing turnover (Redman, Cho, Ketefian, & Hong, 2000). Similar positive results were found on nursing and patient satisfaction (Tzeng, Ketefian, & Redman, 2002). Organizational culture and values were found to be directly related to work redesign outcomes (Tzeng, Redman, & Ketefian, 2000).

As work redesign efforts expanded nationally, many hospitals experimented with new roles on the nursing care team. Often these roles were referred to as patient care technicians or expanded roles for the traditional nursing assistant. I, along with several colleagues, undertook the evaluation of these roles in three private sector hospitals in Michigan. The evaluation was similar to the UMHS project, but the focus was more on the impact of these roles on nurses, managers, and other health disciplines. Qualitative data revealed positive data from the perspectives of managers and other health professionals such as pharmacists and respiratory therapists (Jones, Redman, VandenBosch, Holdwick, & Wolgin, 1999). Overall results of the new multiskilled workers were positive in terms of their contributions to the nursing care team (VandenBosch, Wolgin, Redman, Jones, 1997). Organizational culture was directly related to both positive and negative outcomes, depending on the particular organization. These changes in the nursing care team often resulted in an expansion of the responsibilities of the nurse manager and increased the stress on their roles.

My work with patient satisfaction as an outcome variable resulted in my rethinking about satisfaction from the patient's perspective. Most patient satisfaction instruments available at that time focused more on hotel-like aspects of the care experience and often did not consider necessarily what was important to the patient. Nationally, there was a renewed interested in patient-centered care, and the patient's perspective and preferences were being given more emphasis. My interest shifted to patient expectations and examining how these expectations influenced their assessment of the care experience. A discussion of the importance of patient-centered care based on patients' expectations for that care led me to an examination of the conceptual issues in patient-centered care and the development of an instrument to measure those expectations (Redman & Lynn, 2005). This model of expectations was used in a study to compare Mexican immigrant and second-generation Mexican American mothers' expectations for the care of their children. Findings supported a shared core of expectations for both immigrant and Mexican American mothers but also differences in health care access and financing, time spent in health care encounters, and cultural and linguistic expectations for care (Clark & Redman, 2007).

In the mid-2000s, colleagues and I conducted two national surveys of staff nurses to assess their perceptions of satisfaction with their career choice and their commitment to nursing as a career. Low-to-moderate levels of work satisfaction were documented along with moderate-to-high levels of career satisfaction, suggesting a number of important implications for employers of nurses in all sectors of the United States (Lynn & Redman, 2006; Lynn, Redman, & Zomorodi, 2006). The article in *Western Journal of Nursing* (Lynn & Redman, 2006) was among the top-10 downloads from that journal in 2006 and 2007.

In 2010, I became involved in a university-wide health initiative in Ghana. As a result, I became part of large interdisciplinary team comprising physicians and nurses from the University of Michigan and Ghana. This project, funded by the Fogarty International Center at the National Institutes of Health, consisted of a collaborative effort among Kwame Nkrumah University of Science and Technology, Komfo Anokye Teaching Hospital (KATH), and the University of Michigan's Department of Emergency Medicine and the School of Nursing. Two major goals of this project were to establish a certificate program and nursing baccalaureate specialization in emergency nursing and a residency program in emergency medicine. The nursing education programs have been established, and two cohorts have graduated successfully (Bell et al., 2014). The medical residency has also been successfully implemented, and two cohorts have completed training in emergency medicine. The focus of the project now is on ensuring quality and safe practice in the emergency department at KATH. Interdisciplinary team training of nurses and physicians in the emergency department, or the A & E as it is called in their setting, has been implemented. A longitudinal evaluation is now in process to measure the effects of this team training using the TeamSTEPPS curriculum and methodology developed by the Agency for Healthcare Research and Quality in the United States. The approach has been adapted to fit the Ghanaian culture and practice setting. The project continues as of this writing and will end in 2016.

References

Bell, S. A., Redman, R., Bam, V., Lapham, Tagoe, N., Yakubu, J., & Donkor, P. (2014). Development of an emergency nursing training curriculum in Ghana. *International Journal of Emergency Nursing, 22*(4), 202–207. doi:10.1016.jienj.2014.02.002

Clark, L., & Redman, R. (2007). Mexican immigrant mothers' expectations for children's health services. *Western Journal of Nursing Research, 29*(6), 670–690.

Hackman, J. R., & Oldham, G. R. (1980). *Work redesign.* Reading, MA: Addison-Wesley.

Jones, K. R., Redman, R. W., VandenBosch, T. M., Holdwick, C., & Wolgin, F. (1999). Evaluation of the multi-functional worker role: A stakeholder analysis. *Outcomes Management for Nursing Practice, 3*(3), 128–135.

Ketefian, S., Redman, R. W., Nash, M. G., & Bogue, E. L. (1997). Inpatient and ambulatory patient satisfaction with nursing care. *Quality Management in Health Care, 5*(4), 66–75.

Lynn, M., & Redman, R. W. (2006). Staff nurses and their solutions to the nursing shortage. *Western Journal of Nursing Research, 28*(6), 678–693.

Lynn, M., Redman, R. W., & Zomorodi, M. G. (2006). The canaries in the coalmine speak: Why someone should (and should not) become a nurse. *Nursing Administration Quarterly, 30*(4), 340–350.

Redman, R. W., Cho, S. H., Ketefian, S., & Hong, O. S. (2000). Predictors of nurse turnover: Model development and testing. *Journal of Korean Academy of Nursing, 30*(7), 1667–1678.

Redman, R. W., & Ketefian, S. (1995). Conceptual and methodological issues in work redesign. In K. Kelly & M. Maas (Eds.), *Series of nursing administration: Health care work redesign* (vol. 7, pp. 5–20). Thousand Oaks, CA: Sage Publications.

Redman, R. W., & Lynn, M. (2005). Assessment of patient expectations for care. *Research and Theory for Nursing Practice, 19*(3), 275–285.

Tzeng, H. M., Ketefian, S., & Redman, R. W. (2002). Relationship of nurses' assessment of organizational culture, job satisfaction, and patient satisfaction with nursing care. *International Journal of Nursing Studies, 39*, 79–84.

Tzeng, H. H., Redman, R. W., & Ketefian, S. (2000). Pocket effects within an organization's culture. *Tajen Journal, 18*, 237–252.

VandenBosch, T., Wolgin, F., Redman, R. W., & Jones, K. R. (1997). Evaluating the implementation of multi-skilled workers. *Journal of Nursing Staff Development, 13*(1), 51–55.

Staff Nurse Fatigue and Patient Safety Research Program

Ann E. Rogers, PhD, RN, FAAN

Linda D. Scott, PhD, RN, NEA-BC, FAAN

The Staff Nurse Fatigue and Patient Safety Program, developed by Dr. Ann E. Rogers, a former University of Michigan faculty member, and Dr. Linda D. Scott, an alumna of the University of Michigan School of Nursing, has had a major impact on policy, patient safety, nursing science, and organizational processes.

Although numerous studies documented the effects of resident work hours on patient safety, no one had systematically examined the hours worked by nurses and the effects of those work hours on patient safety until the early 2000s. Our seminal research was one of the first national efforts to quantify nurse work hours and their relationship to patient safety (Rogers, Hwang, Scott, Aiken, & Dinges, 2004). Combined with a replication of the parent study (Scott, Rogers, Hwang, & Zhang, 2006), we were able to describe the hours worked during a 1-month period by a representative sample comprising almost 900 hospital staff nurses. The findings generated more than 12 manuscripts and several book chapters. Furthermore, our data were used to develop a 2004 recommendation by the Institute of Medicine (IOM) that nurses should not be allowed to provide patient care for more than 12 hours in a 24-hour period nor should they work more than 60 hours in a 7-day period. Also that year, the U.S. Congress mandated that all Veterans Health Administration facilities limit the hours worked by registered nurses to no more than 12 hours in a 24-hour period.

These initial studies (R01 HS11963-01 and R01 HS11963-01S1), funded by the Agency for Healthcare Research and Quality, have served as the catalyst for numerous related studies of nurse work hours in the United States and throughout the world (Australia and Canada). Other researchers have discovered that 12-hour shifts and overtime are associated with altered vigilance and deficits in cognitive processing, as well as increases in iatrogenic infections, needle stick injuries, and adverse events, including increased patient mortality and decreased nurse retention.

Our research has been widely disseminated in national and international presentations as well as in top-tier nursing and interdisciplinary journals. This includes our first publication on work hours (Rogers et al., 2004), which was one of the 25 most-read papers in the high-impact journal *Health Affairs* for 4 consecutive years following its publication. It has been cited in more than 600 publications and professional papers, representing a broad audience with diverse foci including nursing, education, and public policy. The significance of these findings generated global media attention that was recognized by the American Academy of Nursing, which honored this research with a prestigious media award.

Findings from the Staff Nurse Fatigue and Patient Safety Research Program also triggered several professional organizations such as the Association of PeriOperative Registered Nurses (AORN), the National Association of Neonatal Nurses (NANN), and the Washington State Nurses Association to develop policy and position statements regarding overtime, shift duration, and duration between work shifts. More formal guidelines have also been published by the Registered Nurses Association of Ontario and the American Nurses Association (ANA). Dr. Rogers cochaired both the Registered Nurse Association of Ontario Expert Panel that wrote *Best Practices Guidelines: Preventing and Mitigating Nurse Fatigue in Healthcare* (2011) and the Steering Committee of the ANA Professional Issues Panel that issued guidelines related to nurse fatigue (ANA, 2014). Dr. Scott was also a member of the ANA Steering Committee. In December 2011, the Joint Commission

(2011) identified extended work hours and work-related fatigue as sentinel events and called for interventions to mitigate adverse patient outcomes, citing our research in *Sentinel Event Alert 48* (Joint Commission, 2011).

The Staff Nurse Fatigue and Patient Safety Program also found that sleep deprivation and fatigue are prevalent among hospital staff nurses. Nurses who worked more than 12.5 consecutive hours were more likely to struggle to stay awake at work. Additionally, the risk of falling asleep at work almost doubled when shifts exceeded 8 hours and increased even more when shifts exceeded durations of 12 or more consecutive hours. It was found that for each hour of sleep lost, the risk for error increased by 7%. Without fatigue management and intervention, patient safety will continue to be in jeopardy. Therefore, we tested the feasibility of a fatigue countermeasures program for nurses in Michigan. Funded by a substantial grant from the Blue Cross Blue Shield of Michigan Foundation, findings of this research provided preliminary data on the effects of fatigue management strategies on error reduction and their potential for use in the national health care arena. These results were not only used to support workplace initiatives, they provided evidence of the transferability of a human factors intervention normally used in the industrial section to the health care practice environment (Scott, Hofmeister, Rogness, & Rogers, 2010a, 2010b). Moreover, it addressed the IOM's recommendation to develop educational and interventional methods for fatigue reduction. Drs. Rogers and Scott have continued to examine the effects of fatigue and sleep deprivation of health outcomes of professional nurses and the patients in their care.

References

American Nurses Association. (2014). Addressing nurse fatigue to promote safety and health: Joint responsibilities of registered nurses and employers to reduce risks. Retrieved from http://nursingworld.org/Nurse-Fatigue-Panel

Joint Commission. (2011, December 14). Health worker fatigue and patient safety. *Joint commission sentinel event alert, 48.*

Registered Nurses Association of Ontario Expert Panel. (2011). *Best practices guidelines: Preventing and mitigating nurse fatigue in healthcare.* Toronto: Author.

Rogers, A. E., Hwang, W.-T., Scott, L. D., Aiken, L. H., & Dinges, D. F. (2004). The working hours of hospital staff nurses and patient safety. *Health Affairs, 23,* 202–212.

Scott, L. D., Hofmeister, N., Rogness, N., & Rogers, A. E. (2010a). An interventional approach for patient and nurse safety: A fatigue countermeasures feasibility study. *Nursing Research, 59,* 250–258.

Scott, L. D., Hofmeister, N., Rogness, N., & Rogers, A. E. (2010b). Implementing a fatigue countermeasures program for nurses: A focus group analysis. *Journal of Nursing Administration, 40,* 233–240.

Scott, L. D., Rogers, A. E., Hwang, W.-T., & Zhang, Y. (2006). The effects of critical care nurses' work hours on vigilance and patients' safety. *American Journal of Critical Care, 15,* 30–37.

From Health Promotion and Risk Reduction to Health System Entrepreneurship and Innovation

Anne Snowdon, PhD, RN

Health systems globally are challenged by increasing demands for services by populations that are aging and experiencing growing rates of chronic illness. The costs of health systems around the world are outpacing the gross domestic product (GDP) of most countries. The United States and Canada account for the highest per capita spending on health systems among all Organisation for Economic Co-operation and Development (OECD) countries. More than 17% of North America's GDP is spent on health care, yet rankings on health system performance are the lowest (ranked 10th for Canada and 11th for the United States) among the OECD group. Current health systems in North America are unsustainable financially, and performance ranks poorly; transformational change and innovation will be required in very aggressive timelines if health systems are to be able to deliver value to the populations they serve.

My doctoral work at the University of Michigan School of Nursing provided an important platform from which to become a leader in health system innovation, for the commercialization of research outcomes, and more recently, for Canada-U.S. collaboration to advance health system transformation toward sustainable, high-performing systems that offer value. My dissertation research focused on health promotion and risk reduction, which is a theme that traverses my scholarly work following the completion of my PhD. An overview of my research is described as it has evolved over time, including the following: (a) commercialization and product development; (b) injury prevention and evidence-informed policy; and (c) health system transformation to achieve sustainable, high performing health systems in North America.

Product Development and Commercialization

Four elements of product development and commercialization will be discussed.

Injury Prevention Safety Seat Education Program for Canadian families (2004–2006). Bobby Shooster Rides Safely in His Booster is a multimedia educational intervention for families that teaches parents and children about the importance of using child safety seats correctly while traveling in vehicles. The program engages all family members and includes a children's story book, a CD presentation for parents on how to safely install child seats in vehicles, a guide book for parents on the correct use of child seats, and a specialized "Car Seat Safety Chart" for families to measure the heights and weights of children to determine the correct seat as they grow and develop over time. The program was supported by Daimler Chrysler and AUTO21 and won the 2006 Canadian Institutes of Health Research Partnership Award.

Development of United Survey Management Information System Software (2010–2012). This system allows the collection of survey data, using smartphone to enter data digitally, for transcription onto data servers in real time. The system was the outcome of a partnership with Research in Motion (RIM), which supplied Blackberry devices for the national child seat survey with Transport Canada that was conducted in 2006 and 2010. The software was developed for all mobile devices and survey data were collected using the Blackberry devices for roadside and parking lot observations in 187 sites across Canada, collecting data on more than 10,000 parents across Canada. The successful software was profiled by RIM as a global case study for innovative solutions for Blackberry users.

Innovation in booster seat design and commercialization. Research outcomes describing children's use of child safety seats led to a strategic partnership with Magna International to design and commercialize a new booster seat product, now known as the Clek. The Clek offered an innovative latch feature that fastened the seat to the vehicle, offering greater stability of the seat in the event of a crash. Design features influenced by children's descriptions included specialized foam for greater comfort, smaller dimensions so that it could not be seen by peers outside the vehicle, and colorful covers inspired by children's drawings of their "ideal" booster seat. The new product was launched in Canada in September 2007 and in the United States in June 2008. The Clek booster seat won a number of awards including the Junior Products Manufacturing award and the iParenting award for innovation. Clek is now a very successful Ontario-based company with an entire line of safety products that are commercialized and marketed in 15 countries.

Development of a digital Montreal Cognitive Assessment Tool for primary care (2012). One of the challenges health systems face is the wait times for specialized assessment of brain health by specialists in neurology for people whose brain health is changing and may demonstrate early signs of dementia-related symptoms. This project developed and tested an electronic version of the Montreal Cognitive Assessment (MOCA) tool in primary care settings in Ontario. The digital tool enabled individuals and their families to self-administer the MOCA to reduce the stress of undergoing this assessment for people with changes in brain health and to engage people directly in the assessment process, enhancing productivity in primary care settings.

Health System Innovation Transformation Program of Research

Adoption of new, innovative models of care must overcome significant barriers—namely, challenges for entrepreneurs and industry in accessing health systems, difficulty accessing clinical leaders to support the adoption of technologies, challenging policy environments that may not enable the adoption of innovations, and limitations in the capacity to create the necessary evidence of impact of an innovation that is needed to support adoption and scalability. In order for companies to successfully demonstrate value to health system leaders, the evidence of impact and value must be established using empirical research.

In order for innovation adoption to be successful, the implementation of innovations in the health system must necessarily involve and deliver *value* to each of the key stakeholders (industry, policy makers, clinicians, health system leaders and organizations, patients/families, and academic teams). Defining and establishing the value proposition for all health system stakeholders is the fundamental basis for successful innovation adoption and scalability. If value is not achieved for just one of the stakeholders, adoption of the product(s) by a health system is jeopardized. Each of the stakeholder groups within health systems are participants in my innovation research program of work, which is designed to demonstrate the impact of innovative product(s) in a health system setting and to examine and design a pathway for innovation adoption and scalability within and across health systems. In order for an innovative product to be adopted, it must have evidence supporting proof of concept. To scale an innovation across a health system, evidence supporting proof of relevance and proof of value and reimbursement must be established.

The current innovation project work focuses on designing and testing the impact of integrated models of health care service delivery to achieve value for patients with multiple comorbidities and high rates of health services utilization. Integrated models for youth mental health services in communities are in development and will be implemented in four Canadian provinces (British Columbia in 2015, Alberta and Ontario in 2016). A large research grant ($3 million over a 3-year period) on innovative procurement is currently under way, funded by the Ministry of Government and Consumer Services, to complete a suite of 17 case studies examining how innovation unfolds in the Ontario health system and the barriers and enablers of innovation adoption, particularly relative to how products are procured in the Ontario health system. Finally, I am leading a national program of research on supply chain innovation in health systems. Supply chain of products from manufacturer to patient is currently not well developed in global health systems. This program of work maps out innovative supply chain pathways to enhance and strengthen patient safety and economic value for health systems.

The sustainability of global health systems will depend on transformational innovation that is scaled across the entire health care system. Scalability of innovation in health systems will depend on the capacity of health systems to engage industry partners, mobilize health leaders to drive forward on innovation adoption, work with clinicians to adopt new models of care, leverage technologies, and transform health services to achieve value for patients and families that is sustainable and cost effective. Scalability of innovations with a demonstrated value for health systems must be the central goal of any innovation strategy. My current program of work seeks to achieve the transformational change health systems require to become sustainable and high performing and to deliver value to the populations they serve.

Several references are provided below that exemplify Snowdon's work.

Selected Publications

Snowdon, A., Alessi, C., Bassi, H., & DeForge, R. T., & Schnarr, K. (2015). Enhancing patient Experience through personalization of health services. *Healthcare Management Forum, 28*, 182–185.

Snowdon, A. W., Hussein, A., Purc-Stevenson, R., Follo, G., & Ahmed, E. (2009). A longitudinal study of the effectiveness of a multi-media intervention on parents' knowledge and use of vehicle safety systems for children, *Accident Analysis and Prevention, 41*, 498–505.

Snowdon, A. W., Schnarr, K., & Alessi, C. (2015). Global trends in health system innovation. In V. K. Singh, & P. Lillrank (Eds.), *Innovations in healthcare management: Cost-effective solutions for developing and sustaining excellence* (pp. 100–117). Boca Raton, FL: CRC Press.

Snowdon, A. W., Schnarr, K., Hussein, A., Cramm, H., & Alessi, C. (2015). Global health innovation and performance outcomes: An empirical exploration of OECD Nations. In L. H. Friedman, J. Goes, G. T. Savage, S. Buttigieg, C. Rathert, & W. Eiff (Eds.), *Advances in Health Care Management, 17* (pp. 39–69). Bingley, UK: Emerald Group Publishing.

Research in Translation and Implementation Science

Marita G. Titler, PhD, RN, FAAN

My program of research is in outcomes effectiveness and implementation science. The following sections summarize major findings from my research with an explication of the impact on research, practice, education, and health policy.

Translation and Implementation Science

My research in translation and implementation science began as I directed for 15 years the Research Translation and Dissemination Core of the federally funded (National Institute of Nursing Research) Gerontology Nursing Intervention Research Center (P30). As part of this work, we developed and disseminated more than 30 evidence-based practice guidelines for the care of older adults that were published and included in the National Guideline Clearinghouse.

I have been principal investigator (PI) on three translation studies funded by the Agency for Healthcare Research and Quality (AHRQ) (R01) and the Robert Wood Johnson Foundation (RWJF); co-PI on one funded by the National Cancer Institute (R01); and coinvestigator on numerous others funded by the National Institutes of Health, AHRQ, the Department of Veterans Affairs, and the Centers for Disease Control and Prevention. The impact of my translation and implementation studies has demonstrated that a multifaceted translation research into practice intervention improves processes and outcomes of care for older adults with acute pain and cancer pain and those at risk for falls (Titler et al., 2009). This research resulted in the translating research into practice (TRIP) model, developed from Rogers's Diffusion of Innovations framework, to guide the development and testing of implementation interventions (Titler, 2010). The TRIP model is now used by other investigators testing implementation interventions in hospitals and community settings. We also developed, tested, and published two practice tools—the Acute Pain Management Summative Index and the Cancer Pain Practice Index—that measure the amount of evidence-based care the patient receives. We have demonstrated that the delivery of evidence-based care saves health care dollars (Brooks, Titler, Ardery, & Herr, 2009). These findings have impacted regulatory standards of the Joint Commission and the Centers for Medicaid and Medicare Services (Institute of Medicine, 2011). My program of research provides training for master's and doctoral (PhD/DNP) students and has resulted in more than 35 publications in research and practice journals. These studies have also resulted in methods papers (Newhouse, Bobay, Dykes, Stevens, & Titler, 2013) and have promoted the integration of this emerging area of science into PhD education (Henly et al., 2015).

Evidence-Based Practice

Complementary to my research in translation science is my long-standing commitment to improving care delivery and patient outcomes through evidence-based practice (EBP). Nursing has a rich history of using research in practice, pioneered by Florence Nightingale, who used data to change practices that contributed to high mortality rates in hospitals and communities. Today, EBP is defined as the conscientious and judicious use of current best evidence in conjunction with clinical expertise and patient values to guide health care decisions. In contrast, translation science is the investigation of methods, interventions, and variables that influence the adoption of EBPs by individuals and organizations to improve clinical and operational decision making in health care (Titler, 2010).

I started my work in EBP as an advanced practice nurse in the early 1980s, when the term "research utilization" was common in this field. I was mentored by several individuals whose work was highly influenced by the Conduct and Utilization of Research in Nursing (CURN) project housed at the University of Michigan School of Nursing and led by Drs. Joanne Horsely and Joyce Crane (Horsley & Crane, 1983). In this year of celebrations, it is important to acknowledge and recognize the CURN project, the investigators, and the students who set the stage for many who learned from their pioneering work. For example, Dr. Margaret Reynolds, a PhD student on the CURN project, went on to lead interdisciplinary EBP at the Trinity Health System as well as participate in my implementation research. It is with humility that I note many of us today who are dedicated to EBP strive to have the global and far-reaching impact demonstrated by these scholarly pioneers.

My contributions to EBP are informed by my program of research in implementation science. I am the principal author of the Iowa Model of EBP to Improve Quality of Care, which is used nationally and internationally. I have presented EBP workshops around the world to educate staff nurses and students about EBP and implementation. To extend my expertise in EBP, I direct the National Nursing Practice Network (NNPN), a learning collaborative of more than 108 hospitals and health systems across the United States. The mission of NNPN is to advance professional nursing practice through the application of evidence in care delivery, support nursing leadership development for EBP, and conduct multisite research to increase the understanding of mechanisms and strategies that foster the use of evidence by those delivering health care services (http://www.nnpnetwork.org). The impact of my work has helped transform nursing practice from a tradition-based practice to an evidence-based practice where delivery of evidence-based care is now the expectation of all clinicians. My work in this field has resulted in multiple publications, including serving as guest editor for six special journal issues on EBP.

Outcomes Effectiveness Research

Outcomes effectiveness research is the study of the effect of various health care treatments on patient outcomes (Titler & Pressler, 2011). As PI of an NINR-funded R01, I led a multidisciplinary investigative team in examining the unique contributions of nursing interventions to patient outcomes of three hospitalized older adult populations—those with heart failure or hip fractures and those at risk for falls. This study used 4 years of data from nine electronic repositories at a large Midwest medical center that included documentation of nursing interventions using the Nursing Interventions Classification.

From these nine electronic repositories, we built a large effectiveness research database to examine interventions that affect patient outcomes. We published more than 20 papers in refereed journals that demonstrated the unique contributions of nursing interventions to patient outcomes after controlling for medical and pharmacological treatments, context of care, severity of illness, and patient characteristics. The impact of this research is that it demonstrated the unique contributions of various nursing interventions to a variety of patient outcomes such as adverse events (e.g., falls, medication errors), cost, failure to rescue, and discharge disposition (Titler et al., 2008). These studies demonstrated methods for measuring nursing intervention dose and the effect of nursing intervention dose on patient outcomes. The impact includes an outcomes effectiveness research model and the use of propensity scoring methods in outcomes effectiveness research.

The impact of this research on students was inclusion as investigators and coauthors on papers, learning analytic methods, and using the dataset for their research, resulting in three PhD dissertations. Additional outcomes effectiveness studies, funded by the American Organization of Nurse Executives (AONE) and the Robert Wood Johnson Foundation (RWJF), have demonstrated the need for the education and mentorship of nurse managers in creating EBP environments and the insufficient evidence-based care provided to older hospitalized adults to prevent falls (Kueny, Shever, Lehan Mackin, & Titler, 2015).

Cost

My program of research also addresses health care costs. For example, not only did we demonstrate the effectiveness of the TRIP intervention in improving processes of care and patient outcomes for hospitalized older adults with hip fractures (Titler et al., 2009), we also demonstrated a net-cost savings of $1,500 per patient in a cluster randomized trial (Brooks et al., 2009). A number of our outcomes effectiveness studies have demonstrated the costs and cost savings by type and dose of nursing interventions (Titler et al., 2008).

Summary

In summary, my program of research has impacted practice, advanced the science in the field, and provided a robust training environment for doctoral students. In acknowledgement of my contributions, I have been awarded several national honors including election to the National Academy of Medicine, the President's Award in Translation Science from NINR, the Elizabeth McWilliams Miller Award for Excellence in Research from Sigma Theta Tau International (STTI), the National Nurse Researcher Award from AONE, and the Clinical Scholarship Award from STTI.

References

Brooks, J. M., Titler, M. G., Ardery, G., & Herr, K. (2009). Effect of evidence-based acute pain management practices on inpatient costs. *Health Services Research, 44*(1), 245–263.

Henly, S. J., McCarthy, D. O., Wyman, J. F., Heitkemper, M. M., Redeker, N. S., Titler, M. G., . . . Dunbar-Jacob, J. (2015). Emerging areas of science: Recommendations for nursing science education from the Council for the Advancement of Nursing Science Idea Festival. *Nursing Outlook, 63*(4), 398–407. doi:10.1016/j.outlook.2015.04.007

Horsley, J. A., & Crane, J. (1983). *Using research to improve nursing practice: A guide.* New York, NY: Grune & Stratton.

Institute of Medicine. (2011). *Clinical practice guidelines we can trust.* Washington, DC: National Academies Press. Retrieved from http://www.nap.edu/catalog/13058/clinical-practice-guidelines-we-can-trust

Kueny, A., Shever, L., Lehan Mackin, M., & Titler, M. G. (2015). Facilitating the implementation of evidence-based practice through contextual support for nursing leadership. *Journal of Healthcare Leadership, 7,* 29–39. doi:https://dx.doi.org/10.2147/JHL.S45077

Newhouse, R., Bobay, K., Dykes, P. C., Stevens, K. R., & Titler, M. G. (2013). Methodology issues in implementation science. *Medical Care, 51,* S32–S40.

Titler, M. G. (2010). Translation science and context. *Research and Theory for Nursing Practice, 24*(1), 35–55.

Titler, M. G., Herr, K., Brooks, J., Xie, X.-J., Ardery, G., Schilling, M., . . . Clarke, W. (2009). Translating research into practice intervention improves management of acute pain in older hip fracture patients. *Health Services Research, 44*(1), 264–287.

Titler, M. G., Jensen, G. A., Dochterman, J. M., Xie, X. J., Kanak, M., Reed, D., & Shever, L. L. (2008). Cost of hospital care for older adults with heart failure: Medical, pharmaceutical, and nursing costs. *Health Service Research, 43*(2), 635–655.

Titler, M. G., & Pressler, S. J. (2011). Advancing effectiveness science: An opportunity for nursing. *Research and Theory for Nursing Practice, 25*(2), 75.

A Shift From Being Clinician-Centric to Patient-Centric

Huey-Ming Tzeng, PhD, RN, FAAN

I have been conducting nursing systems research on *quality and patient safety* as my program of research since earning my PhD in 1997. Since that time, my journey has become "Uberized." I had my first Uber ridesharing experience in October 2014 in San Diego, California. The traditional taxicab model was built around the convenience and desires of taxi drivers and their affiliated companies rather than their customers. Uber has changed taxi transportation from being driver-centric to customer-centric (Karten, 2015). Uber has regulatory issues and has been legally challenged or even banned in some cities. However, the aspect people love about Uber is the customer-centric business model and the technology (Thompson, 2015).

The Uber customer-centric phenomenon is gradually filtering into health care. Our health care industry is in the throes of changing the health care model from that of being clinician-centric to being patient-centric. The "Uberization" of health care is occurring, as illustrated by movements to put the preferences of patients and their families first (Karten, 2015). Transforming the traditional health care model into an Uberized one requires getting patients and their families to become more engaged as partners in their care However, our society has not yet identified either the patient engagement behaviors or the patient technologies to support these changes through clinical practice and research. Research directions in health care and the role of researchers in health care and nursing systems are also being Uberized, with a shift toward greater emphasis on participatory action research. For example, patients and their families are being encouraged to actively engage in health care research. Their roles in research may range from providing data as study subjects to actually serving as members of a research team. Actively involving patients in research could lead to improvements in health care, such as greater patient-centeredness and better clinical adoptability of research findings.

My passion for nursing systems research led me to address pertinent issues in the context of *promoting care quality and patient safety for adult patients* in hospital settings, including the following four main areas: the relationship between patient satisfaction with nursing care and nurses' job satisfaction, clinicians' professional obligation and ethics related to newly emerging infectious diseases, patient falls, and patient engagement. My nursing systems research journey has shifted from being clinician-centric to becoming patient-centric and continues on that path today. My work has addressed some of the most critical areas of health policy changes, including the environment of care for acutely ill patients and others with restricted mobility, clinicians' actions for preventing hospital-based outbreaks of emerging and existing respiratory infectious diseases, patient roles in hospital fall prevention, gaps in service quality and patient-centered care, and avoidable rehospitalizations of "frequent fliers." Examples from each of these four issues follow.

Relationship Between Patient Satisfaction With Nursing Care and Nurses' Job Satisfaction

During my doctoral study at the University of Michigan School of Nursing (1994–1997), I investigated the association between staff nurses' job satisfaction and inpatients' satisfaction with nursing care in a U.S. teaching medical center. My enthusiasm for this line of research continued after I began my academic career in Taiwan, where I was able to document that nurses' job satisfaction is significantly correlated with inpatients' levels of satisfaction with nursing care. This study was the first to validate the common sense notion that more satisfied nurses foster more positive patient experiences (Tzeng & Ketefian,

2002). Further research is warranted on the notion that happier nurses foster better patient experiences and that happier patients in turn foster more positive nursing experiences, a virtuous cycle.

Clinicians' Professional Obligation and Ethics Related to Newly Emerging Infectious Diseases

I address issues as they surface in clinical settings, and this approach is exemplified by my journal articles and newspaper commentaries related to severe acute respiratory syndrome (SARS). The SARS outbreak occurred while I was working in Taiwan in 2004, and I was one of the first to study the pressing ethical issues that threatened the quality of patient care, with a focus on nurses' concerns and fears about caring for SARS-infected patients. In addition, I investigated individuals' (e.g., university students, nurses, and physicians) fear when faced with a possible H5N1 human-to-human pandemic, a newly emerging avian flu infectious disease, in Taiwan in 2005. For physicians and nurses, the perceived possibility of an avian flu outbreak and the belief that hospitals lacked sufficient infection control measures and equipment contributed to their personal fear of an avian flu epidemic. For university students, the perceived possibility of avian flu being a threat to humans contributed to their personal fear. Similar to the findings of my earlier SARS studies, unnecessary fear and/or panic can be avoided if the public and personnel working in health care institutions are provided with sufficient, up-to-date information about the emerging disease. Addressing pressing health care issues through research has become one of the ways I serve the nursing professional community as well as the "global village."

Patient Falls

Since 2006, I have made consistent and outstanding contributions on the important issue of falls prevention in adult populations in hospital settings. For example, my 2011–2012 multihospital nurse survey study (Tzeng & Yin, 2015) on effective interventions to prevent hospital falls in adults has been well received by nursing executives because of its significant impact on hospital policies and service delivery; yet the findings from this study challenged the status quo about best practices in fall prevention. Since publishing the first article of this study in April 2013 (Tzeng & Yin, 2013), the study has been replicated by other clinician scholars at nine health systems or hospitals located in United States and other countries (e.g., China and Taiwan).

Working in interdisciplinary research and embracing the participatory action research method by actively involving patients and clinicians in research designs has been rewarding for me and has led to innovative and cutting-edge outcomes. My collaboration with a nursing graduate student and a nursing informatics specialist marked the first use of archived hospital call-light tracking data to monitor and predict inpatient fall rates. Paired with a computer science and engineering team, we developed and tested a prototype network sensor device that measures bed height and generates computerized reminders to maintain beds in the lowest position. This research, extended by opinions received from clinicians, patients, community-dwelling residents, and application programmers, led to *iEngaging*, an innovative web-based fall prevention intervention application released in 2015 that engages patients aged 65 years and older and empowers them to take an active role in preventing a fall during hospitalization (http://www.acton-patientsafety .com). The user testing study assessed the feasibility of a functional prototype of *iEngaging* to engage patients in their own fall prevention care during hospital stays by interviewing older adults and health care providers. The *iEngaging* application was perceived by these older adults and health care providers as being easy to use, effective, and practical (Tzeng, Yin, CY, Fitzgerald, & Graham, 2015).

Patient Engagement

In early 2014, inspired by the Triple Aim of better care, better population health, and lower health care costs (Institute for Healthcare Improvement, 2014), I added a strong emphasis on patient engagement and care coordination to my program of research. Previous studies have found that nursing professionals serving as hospital-based, clinic-based, or community-based navigators or health coaches could help improve health care utilization (i.e., lower rehospitalization and emergency room use rates). However, the role of nursing professionals in motivating patients to participate in self-care and how nurses can work with patients in this way still need to be defined. A cultural change in health care systems toward being patient-centric and placing more value on patient engagement is warranted, and this change must come from health care providers. Research on optimum practice culture and infrastructure (e.g., staffing and policies) is needed to promote patient-centered care.

In summary, as the first author or coauthor, I have published my research in highly regarded peer-reviewed nursing and other professional journals and currently have 121 peer-reviewed journal articles (first author for more than 90), three peer-reviewed conference proceedings, 51 peer-reviewed presentations, 11 non-peer-reviewed articles, one professional book, and four book chapters. My research focuses target both research and clinical audiences.

References

Institute for Healthcare Improvement. (2014). *The IHI triple aim.* Retrieved from http://www.ihi.org/Engage/Initiatives/TripleAim/Pages/default.aspx

Karten, S. (2015). *The Uberization of healthcare.* Retrieved from http://hitconsultant.net/2015/02/17/the-uberization-of-healthcare

Thompson, B. M. (2015). *Why what works for Uber may not work for medical apps.* Retrieved from http://mobihealthnews.com/45826/why-what-works-for-uber-may-not-work-for-medical-apps

Tzeng, H. M., & Ketefian, S. (2002). The relationship between nurses' job satisfaction and inpatient satisfaction: An exploratory study in a Taiwan teaching hospital. *Journal of Nursing Care Quality, 16*(2), 39–49.

Tzeng, H. M., & Yin, C. Y. (2013). Frequently observed risk factors for fall-related injuries and effective preventive interventions: A multihospital survey of nurses' perceptions. *Journal of Nursing Care Quality, 28*(2), 130–138.

Tzeng, H. M., & Yin, C. Y. (2015). Perceived top 10 highly effective interventions to prevent adult inpatient fall injuries by specialty area: A multihospital nurse survey. *Applied Nursing Research, 28*(1), 10–17.

Tzeng, H. M., Yin, C. Y., Fitzgerald, K., & Graham, K. (2015). *iEngaging* user testing: Lessons learned from inpatients, adults 65 years or older and health care providers. *Journal of Nursing Care Quality, 30*(3), 275–283.

CHAPTER 10

Nursing Informatics at the University of Michigan School of Nursing

A View of the Past, Perspectives on the Future

Patricia A. Abbott, PhD, RN, FAAN
Marcelline Harris, PhD, RN

SHORT PAPERS SUBMITTED FOR THIS CHAPTER

Judy G. Ozbolt
Dana Tschannen
Patricia A. Abbott
Marcelline Harris
Ivo D. Dinov

Nursing informatics emerged as a specialty in the United States in 1992; at that time, the American Nurses Association (ANA) initiated the development of the first edition of *Nursing Informatics: Scope and Standards of Practice* (ANA, 2014). Subsequently, the American Nurses Credentialing Center (ANCC; a separate entity from the ANA), developed the nursing informatics certification exam. This exam, deployed in 1995, was the first to provide a board certification for early adopters who had chosen nursing informatics as their specialty. This certification exam was forward thinking in its content and innovative in its format, as it was the first computer-based testing undertaken by the ANCC. One of us (Patti) was fortunate to be at the forefront of both of these developments in the early to mid-1990s.

The University of Michigan (UM) has a long and distinguished history in advanced information technology (IT) research and nursing science. In the 1980s and early 1990s, the "fledgling Internet ran out of Ann Arbor and the University of Michigan" (University of Michigan, 2014). Professor Douglas Van Houweling's acquisition of a $39 million grant from the National Science Foundation (NSF) in the late 1980s created NSFNET, an electronic network that connected all the NSF supercomputing centers, forming the Internet as we know it today. Van Houweling's work at UM laid the foundation for an explosion of connectivity, use, and research that led to Internet II, creating a dynamism that continues to this day. Nursing faculty were quick to recognize the potentials of IT, giving rise to several well-known scientists in nursing informatics such as Drs. Judy Ozbolt and Gail

Keenan. These women, along with others, emerged as leaders in nursing informatics over the past three decades and continue to make significant impacts in the field. The phrase "made in Michigan" takes on a whole new meaning when considering the seminal contributions of UM to the science of informatics.

How has UM influenced the present, and how does the work of current faculty reflect historical trends? The influences have been significant, and the residuals from the past have created a foundation from which a new era arises. Informatics, once viewed as the odd member of the nursing family, has risen to a position of increasing relevance and power. With the passage of time, the specialty itself has mutated and expanded, taking on new dimensions and new titles. The 1990s reference to "nursing information systems" has disappeared, having been replaced and further augmented by more expansive and holistic terms such as health informatics, health care informatics, data science, consumer informatics, and bioinformatics—reflecting a movement that has led to extensive interdisciplinarity.

Various professional associations have also contributed to defining the field. For example, the current edition of *Nursing Informatics: Scope and Standards of Practice* (ANA, 2014) defines nursing informatics as "the specialty that integrates nursing science with multiple information and analytical sciences to identify, define, manage, and communicate data, information, knowledge, and wisdom in nursing practice" (p. 4). The American Medical Informatics Association, an interdisciplinary scientific and professional society with an active nursing working group, further notes:

> Informatics researchers develop, introduce, and evaluate new biomedically motivated methods in areas as diverse as data mining (deriving new knowledge from large databases), natural language or text processing, cognitive science, human interface design, decision support, databases, and algorithms for analyzing large amounts of data generated in public health, clinical research, or genomics/proteomics. . . . The informatics community typically uses the term health informatics to refer to applied research and practice of informatics across the clinical and public health domains. (American Medical Informatics Association, n.d.)

Looking forward, the rapidly growing volumes of data generated from everything around us, new types of data storage, new methods and technologies for data and information processing, expanding bandwidth, and new types of devices will continue to enable people to interact with the Internet and each other in novel ways. There is a need for nursing as a profession to embrace emerging technologies and a need for those engaged in informatics research to contribute to future developments in the promotion and management of health, health care delivery, and improved health outcomes through accessible and computable data, information, and knowledge.

As the use of health IT has become ubiquitous in the health professions and as team-based and patient-centric care increase, the path for educational expansion becomes clearer. The new programs of science in the UM School of Nursing (UMSN) that relate to these emerging dimensions are housed in the Department of Systems, Populations, and Leadership (SPL). Drs. Patricia Abbott and Marcelline Harris have worked since 2013 to develop several emphasis areas that specifically focus on health sciences informatics, including a new master's focus and an informatics specialty certificate offered in SPL. The effort expended to create these new courses and specialty areas with the prefix of "HS" (denoting health sciences) was strategic in nature, reflecting the commitment to interprofessional education and science at UMSN.

Informatics as a specialty practice area has transformed over the decades, accompanied by concomitant changes in the scientific and educational realms. The change required in nursing education and in opening the doors to the "4th paradigm" of data-driven scientific discovery (Tansley & Tolle, 2009) involves challenging nursing academic orthodoxy. New science overlaid on massive datasets requires adjustments in the way we think about analysis and research. Moving beyond traditional hypothesis-driven and verification-based methods into innovative ways of managing and analyzing massive collections of data related to health is a change that has been under way at UMSN in recent years, as evidenced by diverse interdisciplinary recruitment and curricular reform. While some express the opinion that nursing programs are continuing to implement curricula better suited to the past, not the future, of nursing science (Wyman & Henly, 2015; Henly et al., 2015), UMSN is proving to be an exception to the rule. The science of informatics and data is increasing within UMSN, mirroring the trends in major U.S. industries. The potential for funding and collaboration continues to increase.

Support for health informatics research comes from a variety of sources. The National Library of Medicine of the National Institutes of Health (NIH) has historically funded "basic" health informatics research applied across specialty areas such as translational bioinformatics, clinical research informatics, clinical informatics, consumer health informatics, and public health informatics. Other NIH institutes, including the National Institute of Nursing Research, and federal agencies such as the Agency for Healthcare Research and Quality often fund research that includes the use or development of informatics tools, although in the context of specific health care problems. The innovation that occurs in private companies and in clinical agencies offers yet another important mechanism for engaging in informatics research.

The short papers that follow present overviews of the research and scholarship of five past and current faculty members of UMSN and demonstrate the development of health informatics research over time. Dr. Ozbolt is among the earliest nurses in the country to launch a focused research program in informatics; she is further recognized as one of the early proponents of specialized informatics educational programs within schools of nursing. Dr. Dana Tschannen's work illustrates the contributions of a UMSN PhD graduate who, in her dissertation work, partnered with an informatics researcher in the school and then focused her research skills to studies of the clinical setting. Dr. Abbott's work demonstrates the shifting sands in the scope of informatics research as technologies and connectivity have advanced. Her work spans an early focus on data sets residing on a single, unconnected server to a very contemporary focus on mobile technology platforms that enable individuals to connect anywhere, anytime and interact directly with health care data, information, and knowledge resources. Like Ozbolt, Abbott is widely recognized for her commitment to informatics education. Dr. Harris's informatics research has been highly influenced by the early works of Ozbolt and Abbott and an interest in nursing health services research, operational responsibilities for clinical information systems, and most recently, informatics-informed infrastructures for research. Dr. Ivo Dinov's work demonstrates cutting-edge and forward-facing computational and statistical processing methodologies (i.e., data science) and their advanced applications in health care education and research. UMSN is fortunate to have Dinov's expertise available to help shape curriculum for our doctoral students. Jointly, the five overviews that follow demonstrate the unique and ongoing commitment of UMSN to improvements in health outcomes and care delivery systems through informatics research.

References

American Medical Informatics Association. (n.d.). The science of informatics. Retrieved from https://www.amia .org/about-amia/science-informatics

American Nurses Association. (2014). *Nursing informatics: Scope and standards of practice* (2nd ed.). Washington, DC: Author.

Henly, S. J., McCarthy, D. O., Wyman, J. F., Stone, P. W., Redeker, N. S., McCarthy, A. M., . . . Moore, S. M. (2015). Integrating emerging areas of nursing science into PhD programs. *Nursing Outlook, 63*(4), 408–416.

Tansley, S., & Tolle, K. M. (Eds.). (2009). *The fourth paradigm: Data-intensive scientific discovery* (vol. 1). Redmond, WA: Microsoft Research.

University of Michigan. (2014). *Internet pioneer honored for building the web's first backbone* [Press Release]. Retrieved from http://www.ns.umich.edu/new/releases/22109-internet-pioneer-honored-for-building-the-web -s-first-backbone

Wyman, J., & Henly, S. (2015). PhD programs in nursing in the United States: Visibility of American Association of Colleges of Nursing core curricular elements and emerging areas of science. *Nursing Outlook, 63*(4), 390–397.

Building a Foundation for Nursing Informatics Science

Judy G. Ozbolt, PhD, RN, FAAN, FACMI, FAIMBE

I began my research program in nursing informatics in 1972 while a student in the University of Michigan's master of science specialty in medical-surgical nursing. The inspiration was a lecture by Professor Samuel Schultz II describing computer programs that were being developed to formulate difficult medical diagnoses. Would it be possible, I asked, to develop a computer program that could use data from the nursing assessment to formulate nursing diagnoses? Yes, Professor Schultz responded, a prior student in the program, Suzanne Lagina, had developed a program to diagnose patients' anxiety levels (Lagina, 1971). With my research partner, fellow student Bernadine Symons Edwards, I undertook the project that would become the foundation of my research career.

The literature offered little guidance. There was no consensus that nurses were licensed to make diagnoses of any sort. A "nursing problem" was any problem a nurse might address in professional practice, a definition that could not be more circular or unenlightening. The organization that would evolve into the North American Nursing Diagnosis Association had not yet convened its first meeting. Bernadine and I had to conceptualize what constituted a nursing diagnosis and then populate that conceptual model with terms. Furthermore, we had to demonstrate the place of diagnosis in the nursing process by creating a model of the process. And we had to determine what assessment data were needed to reach each diagnosis. As the early conceptual and modeling work proceeded, I took a course in programming in Fortran IV and Bernadine acquired the keypunching skills needed to write each line of the program onto an individual paper card.

More than a year and 6,000 lines of code later, the program ran and nurses evaluated it. They concluded that the program would probably help them to make better diagnostic decisions but that it took too long to enter the assessment data and receive the diagnoses (Goodwin & Edwards, 1975; prior to 1980, I published as Judy Ozbolt Goodwin). That criticism reflected the technological constraints of the time. Because there were no computer terminals in the patient care areas of the University of Michigan Medical Center, nurses had to assess the patients, make written notes, and return to the computer laboratory in the School of Nursing to enter the data. Nurses connected with the University of Michigan's mainframe computer, an IBM 360-67, by dialing a telephone and, when the signal was established, snapping the handset into an acoustic coupler on the side of a printing terminal. (The School of Nursing had no cathode-ray terminals with screens.) Consequently, nurses had to wait while a printer slower than a skilled human typist laboriously presented each question of the assessment and each of the multiple-choice response options. The nurse would type the letter of the selected response, and the process would repeat. It took about an hour to enter the data and receive the diagnoses.

The fundamental questions explored in that master's research project continued to guide my research. What basic concepts and relationships defined each stage of the nursing process? What decisions were required at each stage, and what data were needed to reach effective decisions? How did the philosophic perspective of nursing (e.g., optimizing functional abilities vs. supporting self-care vs. promoting adaptation) affect the terms applied at each stage? How could the quality and effectiveness of nursing care be defined and measured? How could evolving information technologies help represent nursing phenomena, support nursing decisions, and document nursing assessments, diagnoses, goals, actions, and outcomes? And finally, what statistical approaches could be applied to precisely defined and measured data stored in electronic records to evaluate the effectiveness and the efficiency of care and thus promote better processes and outcomes?

My employment during graduate school on a project to develop measures of patient outcomes that would reflect nursing quality (Clinton, Denyes, Goodwin, & Koto, 1977) gave me knowledge of a variety of methods to define and measure the quality of care. When I moved to France after earning my PhD to teach in that nation's only master's program in nursing, I learned that measuring the quality of nursing or medical care was a novel idea in France. I participated on a high-level panel discussion with French nurses, physicians, health care executives, and educators exploring definitions of quality of care and methods of assessment. While in France, I published several articles on the topic in French nursing and medical journals.

I returned to the University of Michigan as an associate professor in 1980 and developed several more prototype programs to support nursing decisions. During the 1980s, I gained opportunities for leadership in promoting computer applications in nursing and medicine. I served on a study section for the National Center for Health Services Research and Technology Assessment (now the Agency for Healthcare Research and Quality) and was the first nurse elected to the board of directors of the Symposium on Computer Applications in Medical Care (now subsumed into the American Medical Informatics Association [AMIA]). In 1988, I cochaired the scientific program committee of an invitational working conference in nursing informatics sponsored by the International Medical Informatics Association (IMIA). That work, conducted in Killarney, Ireland, led to publication of a book, *Decision Support Systems for Nursing* (Ozbolt, Vandewal, & Hannah, 1990) that won a Book of the Year award from the American Nurses Association.

Beginning in 1989, I chaired an expert panel for the National Center for Nursing Research (now the National Institute of Nursing Research) to identify research priorities in nursing informatics. That report (Ozbolt, 1993) guided funding decisions for nursing informatics research for the next decade.

In the 1990s, then at the University of Virginia as associate dean of research and director of the PhD program, I served AMIA as a founding member of the board of directors and sequentially as first chair of the nursing informatics working group, secretary of the board, and chair of the scientific program committee for the annual symposium (Ozbolt, 1994), as well as serving numerous terms on the board and its executive committee. I was also elected to the American College of Medical Informatics, the honorary society associated with AMIA. During the 1990s, I continued to pursue standardized terminologies that would provide valid and reliable clinical data to investigate nursing phenomena and the effectiveness of nursing care (Ozbolt, 1996; Ozbolt, Russo, & Stultz, 1995).

In 1998, I joined the innovative team in biomedical informatics at Vanderbilt University as Independence Foundation Professor of Nursing and Professor of Biomedical Informatics. The dean of the School of Nursing, Colleen Conway-Welch, charged me with resolving the conflicting camps of clinical nursing terminology so that nursing data could be used for research and quality improvement. With support from the National Library of Medicine and from vendors of electronic health records, I convened all the American developers of nursing terminologies along with interdisciplinary experts in biomedical data, terminologies, and standards to confer about what was required for nursing terminology standards. The first Nursing Terminology Summit in 1999 achieved agreement that a concept-based nursing terminology reference model was required.

The 2000, the Nursing Terminology Summit brought in experts from Europe, Asia, Australia, and Latin America to join with North Americans in considering how to arrive at an international standard that all could support. Subsequent to the discussions at the summit, the nursing informatics group within IMIA established technical and advisory panels, and in 2001, IMIA submitted a reference terminology model to the International Standards Organization that was quickly adopted, based on the global support for the model. Other investigators used the summits (which continued for 10 years) as a springboard to establish standards for nursing terminology and data in other standards organizations, including the Systematic Nomenclature of Medicine—Clinical Terms (SNOMED-CT); the Logical Object Identifiers, Names, and Codes (LOINC); and the Committée Européen de Normalisation (the European Standards Committee) (Ozbolt, 2003). On the strength of these interdisciplinary accomplishments, I was named the 2001–2002 Joe B. Wyatt Distinguished University Professor at Vanderbilt.

In 2005, then president of the American College of Medical Informatics, I accepted the position of scholar at the Institute of Medicine, a component of the National Academies of Science. I led a planning effort to set priorities for the next 5 years for academies-wide studies in biomedical and health informatics.

In 2006, I became professor and specialty director for graduate studies in nursing informatics at the University of Maryland. With a grant from the Health Resources and Services Administration, over the next 3 years I recruited additional faculty members, tripled the enrollment in the master's specialty in informatics, and increased the diversity of the student body.

After my retirement from the University of Maryland in 2010, I accepted a request to chair a technical expert panel on the unintended consequences of electronic health records and their meaningful use, commissioned by the Office of the National Coordinator for Health Information Technology in the U.S. Department of Health and Human Services. Among the products of that effort was a report on which I was lead author, *Building Better Consumer eHealth* (Ozbolt et al., 2012).

Finally, following staff turnover in the Office of Professional Development and a consequent loss of institutional memory at the University of Maryland School of Nursing, I agreed to return to chairing the annual Summer Institute in Nursing Informatics. I served in that role for several years and relinquished it for full retirement after the 2015 symposium.

I trace the heritage of my research from Florence Nightingale, who decried the lack of "hospital records fit for any purpose of comparison" (Nightingale, 1863), and through my mentor Harriet Werley, a champion since the 1950s of standardized nursing data sets that could be used to evaluate the quality of care and improve patient outcomes. Today, thanks to interdisciplinary and international collaboration, data and terminology standards exist that, when incorporated into electronic health records, enable nurses to conduct research on clinical data "to save life and suffering and improve the care of the sick" (Nightingale, 1863).

References

Clinton, J. R., Denyes, M. J., Goodwin, J. O., & Koto, E. M. (1977). Developing criterion measures of nursing care: Case study of a process. *Journal of Nursing Administration, 7,* 41–45.

Goodwin, J. O., & Edwards, B. S. (1975). Developing a computer program to assist the nursing process: Phase I—From systems analysis to an expandable program. *Nursing Research, 24,* 299–305.

Lagina, S. M. (1971). A computer program to diagnose anxiety levels. *Nursing Research, 20*(6), 484–492.

Nightingale, F. (1863). *Notes on hospitals* (3rd ed.). London: Longman, Green, Longman, Roberts, and Green.

Ozbolt, J. G. (Chair). (1993). *Nursing informatics: Enhancing patient care.* Bethesda, MD: National Center for Nursing Research, National Institutes of Health.

Ozbolt, J. G. (Ed.). (1994). *Proceedings of the Eighteenth Annual Symposium on Computer Applications in Medical Care* [Symposium suppl.]. *Journal of the American Medical Informatics Association.* Philadelphia, PA: Hanley & Belfus.

Ozbolt, J. G. (1996). From minimum data to maximum impact: Using clinical data to strengthen patient care. *Advanced Practice Nursing Quarterly, 1*(4), 62–69.

Ozbolt, J. (2003). The Nursing Terminology Summit Conferences: A case study of successful collaboration for change. *Journal of Biomedical Informatics, 36*(4–5), 362–374.

Ozbolt, J., Sands, D. Z., Dykes, P., Pratt, W., Rosas, A. G., & Walker, J. M. (2012). *Summary report of consumer eHealth unintended consequences work group activities.* Washington, DC: Office of the National Coordinator for Health Information Technology. Retrieved from http://www.healthit.gov/sites/default/files/final_report _building_better_consumer_ehealth.pdf

Ozbolt, J. G., Russo, M., & Stultz, M. P. (1995). Validity and reliability of standard terms and codes for patient care data. In J. G. Ozbolt (Ed.), *Proceedings of the Eighteenth Annual Symposium on Computer Applications in Medical Care* [Symposium suppl.] (pp. 37–41). *Journal of the American Medical Informatics Association.* Philadelphia, PA: Hanley & Belfus.

Ozbolt, J. G., Vandewal, D., & Hannah, K. J. (Eds.). (1990). *Decision support systems in nursing.* St. Louis, MO: Mosby.

* Prior to 1980, Ozbolt published as Judy Ozbolt Goodwin.

Patient Care Quality and Safety Through Technology and Clinical Information

Dana Tschannen, PhD, RN

My scholarly work has focused on advancing the science of quality and patient safety through the application of technology and clinical information. The patient record contains a wealth of data and information that provide the health care team with the knowledge needed to plan and implement the most optimal care. The difficulty, or potential barrier, is providing the information in a way that is meaningful and actionable to members of the health care team. The purpose of my scholarship is to positively impact safe patient care at the bedside through application of technology to improve knowledge acquisition, evidence-based practice adoption, care delivery, and workflow.

My interest in nursing informatics began during my doctoral studies at the University of Michigan (UM), where I worked with Dr. Gail Keenan on the Hands-On Automated Nursing Data System (HANDS) project. HANDS, an electronic plan-of-care tool, supports care across the continuum through a standardized, streamlined process for planning and evaluating patient care. Using the North American Nursing Diagnosis Association's definitions and classifications—Nursing Intervention Classifications (NIC) and Nursing Outcome Classifications (NOC)—nurses are able to enter and update a patient's plan of care, providing a framework for information sharing at care transitions and handoffs among the interdisciplinary team. In a longitudinal, multisite study, eight units in four hospitals implemented the HANDS intervention for 12 (n = 4 units) and 24 (n = 4 units) months (Agency for Healthcare Research and Quality R01 HS015054). Findings revealed an exceptional improvement in the compliance rate of updating the plan of care (78%–92% overall compliance for updating the plan of care each shift during the study months), with evidence supporting the use of the HANDS tool as intended (e.g., stable changes in plans of care were noted over the course of a patient's stay) (Keenan et al., 2012). In addition, use of the HANDS tool created a standardized set of data elements captured at similar time points that can be used for benchmarking and identifying best practices.

As I transitioned from student to faculty, my desire to improve quality and safety for patients remained strong, with an initial focus on using technology to improve knowledge acquisition of evidence-based practices among students and staff nurses. This included studies using technology, such as a multiuser environment (e.g., Second Life [SL]) as a learning platform and video case simulations for nursing staff training. An eight-bed virtual nursing unit was developed in SL and has been used to engage students and staff in acquiring knowledge related to communication and teamwork, priority setting, diabetes self-management education, and conflict management. An initial quasiexperimental study, funded by the Center for Research on Learning and Teaching at UM, was conducted to explore the use of virtual simulations in SL to improve the knowledge transfer of senior-level nursing students. In SL, participants interact with one another in the virtual environment using an avatar (e.g., an online manifestation of self). All students (n = 115) received education on topics related to conflict management, priority setting, and patient safety, with the intervention group also participating in three virtual simulations. Knowledge transfer (e.g., the ability of students to utilize intellectual resources learned in one situation and apply them to another) was evaluated by having students complete individualized high-fidelity simulations. Scores for the intervention group were significantly higher than scores for the control group, providing support for the use of virtual simulations to improve knowledge transfer (Tschannen, Aebersold, McLaughlin, Bowen, & Fairchild, 2012).

Additional studies using SL have been completed to improve teamwork among nursing staff. Using a quasiexperimental design, 43 nursing staff participated in a series of virtual simulations in SL that focused on common teamwork problems experienced in the hospital setting. Perceptions of teamwork pre- and postparticipation were measured using the Nursing Teamwork Scale. Findings noted an improvement in mean teamwork scores, with the intervention having a significant effect on three of the teamwork subscales (e.g., trust, team orientation, and backup) (Kalisch, Aebersold, McLaughlin, Tschannen, & Lane, 2015).

An additional study was conducted using video simulation to improve knowledge acquisition among nursing staff at the UM Health System. In collaboration with nursing leaders and clinical experts, a series of simulations were developed and filmed for use in the annual nursing competency. The full intervention included prerequisite work, which included online learning modules with embedded questions and a pretest, followed by participation in two 20-minute simulation videos and a discussion. The simulation videos were based on the nursing-sensitive quality indicators that impacted 80% of nursing areas: restraint alternatives, pressure ulcer prevention, fall prevention, catheter-associated urinary tract infection (CAUTI) prevention, infection control, deep vein thrombosis (DVT) prophylaxis, and stroke recognition and intervention. Following participation in the video simulations, staff completed a posttest to ensure competency was achieved. Overall, the nursing staff (n = 1,500 nurses and 500 assistive personnel) was very positive about the intervention, with 48% of staff rating the use of video simulations as being extremely effective (e.g., 10 on a 1–10 scale) and more than 86% rating the effectiveness at an 8 or higher. Additionally, improvements in competency were noted for staff nurses (improvement in scores of 34% from pre- to posttest) and assistive personnel (improvement of 27% from pre- to posttest) (Tschannen, Aebersold, Woloskie, & DeVries, 2014).

These highlighted studies provided evidence to support the use of technology (e.g., videos, virtual learning platforms) for improving knowledge acquisition. Yet knowledge alone does not result in better outcomes, as operational processes and workflow must align for optimal provider performance. For this reason, the next phase of my work aimed at (a) understanding nursing workflow within the delivery of patient care and (b) creating tools and processes that aided nurses in implementing evidence-based interventions in a timely and meaningful way.

When health information technology does not integrate into current work patterns or standards within the organization, failure can occur despite the technology itself being appropriate. For this reason, my work has included a focus on the impact of technology on nursing workflow. The purpose of the initial study—which was done in collaboration with students and staff at the UM Health System—was to determine the impact of a computerized physician order entry system (CPOE) on nursing workflow. Specifically, an exploratory study using mixed methodology (observations and semistructured interviews) was conducted on two units, an adult intensive care unit and a pediatric general care unit. A total of 86 observations of the medication administration process (e.g., from order review to documentation of administered medication) were completed. Despite the variation in populations of study, the barriers to workflow were relatively consistent, including systems issues (e.g., medication reconciliation difficulty, long order sets) and less frequent interaction among the health care team. The modality used for communicating became primarily asynchronous (e.g., pagers), which required more time to resolve care-based issues (Tschannen, Talsma, Reinemeyer, Belt, & Schoville, 2011). Findings from this study noted a fragmented system such that information required to optimize the patient's plan of care was not easily accessible in a format that allowed for synthesis and action.

Upon understanding workflow and care delivery processes such as was noted in the CPOE workflow study, tools can be developed that aid nurses in implementing evidence-based interventions in a timely and meaningful way. The Clinical Care Daily project began with the primary purpose of reducing the presence and severity of pressure ulcers among hospitalized patients through the implementation of an automated daily report with patient risk and the current status of skin breakdown. Clinical Care Daily, an automated daily feedback tool using currently collected patient information, was developed to help nurses to identify pressure ulcer risk, changes in risk, and prevention and treatment interventions to reduce the development of hospital-acquired pressure ulcers. The study intervention. which was developed using the translating research into practice model, included the Daily

Automated Pressure Ulcer Tool ("Daily"), daily rounds conducted by a clinical champion, coaching of nursing staff, and policy revisions as needed to align with the skin assessment requirements (Tschannen, Talsma, Gombert, & Mowry, 2011). The intervention was pilot tested on one intensive care unit. The clinical nurse specialist reviewed the "Daily" each morning and made rounds on the unit, assessing the skin of patients who were noted to have pressure-related breakdown; educating staff on pressure staging, assessment, and treatment alternatives as applicable; and collaborating with other health care providers on treatment modalities. Initial success was evidenced by a 34% reduction in pressure ulcer rates and an 86% reduction in missed care in turning patients 3 months postimplementation of the "Daily" intervention in the pilot unit (Tschannen, Talsma, Gombert, et al., 2011; Talsma, Tschannen, Guo, & Kazemi, 2011). Subsequently the tool was rolled out to several other intensive care and general care units within the health system. Currently the tool is being refined to include patient risk factors associated with other nursing-sensitive adverse outcomes (e.g., CAUTIs, falls, DVT) for use in other hospital facilities.

As noted from my work, technology can be applied in a variety of ways to impact the quality and safety of health care. Technology can be (a) the platform, as noted in my studies related to knowledge acquisition; (b) the item for evaluation (e.g., CPOE workflow study); or (c) the intervention, as described in the Clinical Care Daily project. Regardless, it is important to maximize the utilization of technology in a manner that will ensure a knowledgeable workforce, optimize workflows, and improve the quality and safety of care to our patients and families.

References

Kalisch, B., Aebersold, M., McLaughlin, P., Tschannen, D., & Lane, S. (2015). Using virtual simulation to improve nursing teamwork: A feasibility study. *Western Journal of Nursing, 37*(2), 164–179.

Keenan, G., Yakel, E., Yao, Y., Xu, D., Szalacha, L., Tschannen, D., . . . Wilkie, D. (2012). Maintaining a consistent big picture: Meaningful use of a web-based POC EHR system. *International Journal of Nursing Knowledge, 23*(3), 199–133.

Tschannen, D., Aebersold, M., McLaughlin, E., Bowen, J., & Fairchild, J. (2012). Use of virtual simulations for improving knowledge transfer among baccalaureate nursing students. *Journal of Nursing Education and Practice, 2*(3), 15–24.

Tschannen, D., Aebersold, M., Woloskie, S., & DeVries, L. (2014, October). *Use of online modules and video simulation in annual nursing staff competency blitz.* Paper presented at the 20th Annual Online Learning Consortium International Conference, Orlando, FL.

Tschannen, D., Talsma, A. N., Gombert, J., & Mowry, J. (2011). Using the TRIP model to disseminate an IT-based pressure ulcer intervention. *Western Journal of Nursing Research, 33*(2), 427–442.

Tschannen, D., Talsma, A. N., Reinemeyer, N., Belt, C., & Schoville, R. (2011). Nursing medication administration and workflow using computerized physician order entry. *CIN: Computers, Informatics, Nursing, 29*(7), 401–410.

Talsma, A. N., Tschannen, D., Guo, Y., & Kazemi, J. (2011). Evaluation of the pressure ulcer prevention clinical decision report for bedside nurses in acute care hospitals. *Applied Clinical Informatics, 2*(4), 508–521.

Informatics

The Road Less Taken

Patricia A. Abbott, PhD, RN, FAAN, FACMI

Informatics is an evolving and dynamic discipline, and my career has mirrored these characteristics of the field. In the late eighties, the concept of a nurse focusing her attention in informatics was almost unheard of. Educational and research opportunities were concomitantly scarce. In 1992, I was only the seventh nurse in the United States to receive a master's degree in nursing informatics. Prior to 1992, nursing informatics was not a recognized nursing specialty in the United States or abroad and job positions and doctoral educational programs did not exist for a nurse with informatics interests. Continuing my education; growing my research portfolio; and finding a position that aligned with my education, background and interests during this era was very challenging and highly rewarding. It required creativity, perseverance, and a willingness to span boundaries.

Entering the field when I did gave me the rare opportunity to define a nursing specialty from its inception. I coauthored the original American Nurses Association *Nursing Informatics: Scope and Standards of Practice*; directed the first graduate program in nursing informatics for 5 years during a period of rapid growth and transition that included initialization of the PhD in nursing informatics; coauthored the American Nurses Credentialing Center Nursing Informatics Board Certification exam; and developed new avenues of research for myself and my students. Many roles with national and international informatics boards, National Institutes of Health (NIH) study sections, and expert panels both within nursing and medicine have arisen over the years. Currently, I am the first (and only) woman elected to serve on the board of directors for the Open Source Electronic Health Records Alliance, an organization funded by the U.S. Department of Veterans Affairs to build a vendor-neutral community for the creation, evolution, promotion, and support of open-source electronic health records (EHR).

Remaining in academia, I have continued to study and develop new dimensions of informatics science and pedagogy. A prominent and recent example of activity in this regard was the award of a $1.8 million grant from the NIH/Department of Health and Human Services (DHHS), Curriculum Development Center for Healthcare Information Technology Workforce (1U24OC000013-01; Abbott, PI), in which I led the development of informatics courses and advanced educational simulators for deployment across 10,000 academic institutions in the United States and Puerto Rico. As part of the American Recovery and Reinvestment Act of 2009, this funding enabled not only the development of a simulated

EHR system for workforce scale-up and health professional education but also the development of four 3-credit fully online and 508-compliant courses, all of which are open source and in the public domain via DHHS. The use of this educational EHR system (based on the U.S. Department of Veterans Affairs electronic health record and called "VistA for Education" [VFE]) has been extended for use at UM in the School of Information, the UM Medical School, and most recently, the UM School of Nursing (UMSN). The integration of VFE into the UMSN pediatric nurse practitioner program in March 2016 was designed to educate and emphasize the safe and effective use of EHRs in patient encounters. Additionally, the use of EHRs, while required in clinical care, can be very disruptive to the clinician-patient relationship; therefore, additional interventions to study (and then alter) how our students communicate while utilizing EHRs are part of this integration project.

In regard to educational innovation with informatics at the UMSN, a collaborative project with the U.S. Air Force Academy and the UM Comprehensive Cancer Center has just begun. I and my colleagues are prototyping immersive environments, based on virtual reality, for advanced simulation research in techniques for communicating bad news to patients regarding breast cancer diagnoses. Interestingly, increasing public access to online resources for health has resulted in something nicknamed the "Jolie effect," which is producing challenging clinical communication environments, particularly with newly diagnosed breast cancer patients. Immersive simulation experiences in virtual worlds similar to Second Life, with interactive "artificially intelligent" simulated patients (including voice recognition and response, similar to iPhone's "Siri"), gives providers the opportunity to interact with challenging patients and difficult conversations. The design and development process itself opens new avenues for informatics inquiry, while the impact of the approach in the simulation environment provides additional areas for study.

The two decades spent in nursing informatics, has resulted in the identification of several other themes that drove (and still drive) my curiosity. Branching from my master's thesis in 1992, understanding how humans interact with computing technology, primarily in relation to health and health care, remains very intriguing to me. In 2006, I competed for a midcareer postdoc via NIH and won. This launched a 2-year fellowship in computer science at the Human-Computer Interaction Lab at the University of Maryland, College Park, where I studied not only human computer interaction but also visualization techniques and usability.

Why choose visualization? My dissertation research in 1999 was in a relatively new field at the time called knowledge discovery in large datasets (KDD). Demonstrating that which was old can be new again, KDD has now morphed into big data analytics, which (in distinct contrast to 1999, when my research was disparaged by the nursing profession in general) is now a major field in informatics and related sciences. The result of the KDD dissertation experiment was the generation of patterns in the data that were uninterpretable by the average human cognitive engine. What good were results if they could not be visualized and interpreted? Visualization techniques and human-computer interaction are foundational underpinnings to nearly all applications of informatics science. How can the clinical EHR interface be developed to match the user's cognitive model of the task being undertaken? How can we translate complex results into a display on a cell phone that an 87-year-old woman can understand and interpret? How can we tap into (and interpret) the very large streams of data originating from Open.gov efforts, social media, and sensor-based health technologies? How can we use cellular telephony displays in low-resource settings to relay vital health information that could save a woman dying from postpartum hemorrhage? How can we design devices that ease the access to critical information at the bedside, in the home, in a rural community, or for vulnerable populations who live in the highlands of Western Guatemala? Understanding the usability and the comprehension of health data requires not only the use of information science and visualization but also an understanding of cognition, behavior change, global health, engineering, cultural context, and design. In the quest to answer one question, a million more are spawned.

These questions, and others like them, drove a decade of inquiry, from studying the usability of handheld clinical information appliances (Abbott, 2012); to the study of health IT-enabled care management in rural, frontier, and other underserved populations (Effken & Abbott, 2009); to global telehealth (Abbott & Liu, 2013); and work with the U.S. Department of Commerce/National Institute of Standards and Technology in developing usability guidelines (Lowry et al., 2012; Schumacher et al., 2012) in 2012 and 2013. Interwoven with these studies came an increasing interest in global electronic health (eHealth) and the complexity of its implementation across various types of users (Abbott, Foster, Marin, & Dykes, 2013). As cellular connectivity increasingly spanned the globe, disconnected populations were suddenly able to access and utilize digital networks, opening thousands of new areas for application and inquiry.

An initial foray into the global aspect of informatics arose when I assumed directorship of the Johns Hopkins School of Nursing's World Health Organization (WHO) Collaborating Center. The first of its kind, this center was designed specifically to address the clamor for nursing and health-related communications across the globe and was named the Center for Nursing Knowledge and Information Management (KIMS). A major product that emerged from KIMS Center was the development of the Global Alliance for Nursing and Midwifery electronic community of practice (eCoP) that was managed for nearly a decade from the KIMS Center. This eCoP quickly became a major global communication platform for information and knowledge exchange among nurses, midwives, and community health workers. It served as a model for additional efforts and continues to operate successfully from the Johns Hopkins University School of Nursing to this day. Several publications arose from this work, but its true impact is being the first of its kind to provide a sustainable mechanism for knowledge exchange among formerly disconnected nurses and midwives all over the world (Lori, Ortiz, Oyarzo, Abbott, & Land, 2010).

An additional effect from the confluence of informatics and nursing in the global context is the publication of several works regarding workforce scale-up using information and communication technologies (Abbott & Coenen, 2008). A Center for Research on Learning and Teaching grant (UM) obtained in 2014 (Abbott, PI), titled Extending the Global Reach of Nursing Education in Haiti, enabled the purchase, installation, development, and deployment of advanced fiber optic infrastructure into the Faculté des Sciences at Infirmières de l'Université d'Haïti (FSIL) School of Nursing. Based on this work, FSIL and UMSN embarked on, and still maintain, cross-school classes in community health. This infrastructure and deployment work has resulted in further expansion and successful subsequent funding for other members of the faculty for educational outreach. Most recently, a WHO-commissioned analysis, titled "An Exploration of National Policies and Effective Practices for Electronic and Mobile Learning for Nursing and Midwifery Education" (Abbott et al., 2016), was conducted at the UM under my direction. I was also honored to be invited to serve as a member of the eHealth Technical Advisory Group for the WHO, which is an indicator of my reputation and impact in the unique space of informatics, global health, and usability. In closing, serving as director of the Hillman Program in Nursing Innovation at UMSN has allowed me to witness the innovation and creativity that the UM has become known for. New approaches, new discoveries, and new ways of thinking and doing at the UM continue to drive the advancement of nursing science.

References

Abbott, P. (2012). Effectiveness and clinical usability of a handheld information appliance. *Nursing Research and Practice, 2012*. doi:10.1155/2012/307258

Abbott, P., & Coenen, A. (2008). Globalization and advances in information and communication technologies: The impact on nursing and health. *Nursing Outlook, 56*(5), 238–246.

Abbott, P., Foster, J., Marin, H., & Dykes, P. (2014). Complexity and the science of implementation in health IT-knowledge gaps and future visions. *International Journal of Medical Informatics, 83*(7), e12–22. doi:10.1016/j.ijmedinf.2013.10.009

Abbott, P., & Liu, Y. (2013). Scoping review of the Telehealth literature. *International Medical Informatics Association Yearbook, 8*(1), 51–88.

Abbott, P., Omollo, K., Hammond, N., Mwenesi, R., Bell, S., Mutumba, M., . . . Jiang, Y. (2016, Embargoed Release). *An exploration of national policies and effective practices for electronic and mobile learning for nursing and midwifery education*. Geneva: World Health Organization.

Effken, J., & Abbott, P. (2009). *The nursing role in health IT-enabled care management in rural, frontier, and other underserved populations* (Commissioned white paper). Agency for Healthcare Quality and Research. *Journal of the American Medical Informatics Association*. doi:10.1197/jamia.M2971

Lori, J., Ortiz, D., Oyarzo, S., Abbott, P., & Land, S. (2010). Developing nursing and midwifery communities of practice for making pregnancy safer. *Journal of Knowledge Management & E-Learning, 2*(2), 122–133.

Lowry, S. Z., Quinn, M. T., Ramaiah, M., Brick, D., Patterson, E. S., Zhang, J., . . . Gibbons, M. C. (2012). *A human factors guide to enhance EHR usability of critical user interactions when supporting pediatric patient care* (NIST Interagency/Internal Report 7865). National Institute of Standards and Technology, U.S. Department of Commerce. Retrieved from http://www.nist.gov/manuscript-publication-search.cfm?pub_id=911520

Schumacher, R., Patterson, E., North, R., Zhang, J., Lowry, S., Quinn, M., . . . Gibbons, M. (2012). *Technical evaluation, testing and validation of the usability of electronic health records* (NIST Interagency/Internal Report 7804). National Institute of Standards and Technology, U.S. Department of Commerce. Retrieved from http://www.nist.gov/manuscript-publication-search.cfm?pub_id=909701

Clinical and Research Informatics

Joint Contributions to Research Infrastructure

Marcelline Harris, PhD, RN

My interests in informatics arose while I was a PhD student at the University of Nebraska Medical Center, College of Nursing. After nearly 15 years in clinical practice, I pursued a research doctorate, focusing on then-emerging methods of outcomes research. Near the end of my program, I attended a preconference at the Midwest Nursing Research Society on informatics for research. One of the panelists, Dr. Christopher Chute, was codirector of a National Institute of Health/National Library of Medicine postdoctoral training program in medical informatics, jointly run by the University of Minnesota and the Mayo Clinic. Beginning in 1997, I spent 3 years in that postdoctoral program, working with Dr. Chute and focusing on the role of terminology systems in what was then the emerging development of computer-based patient records. Just 15 years later, it is hard to imagine a patient record system that is not computer based! During that postdoc, I was fortunate to participate in early vocabulary summits hosted by Dr. Judy Ozbolt at Vanderbilt University. There were rarely more than 30 invitees at these summits; it is interesting to note now that Drs. Ozbolt, Patricia Abbott, Gail Keenan (dissertation chair for Dr. Dana Tschannen), and Marcelline Harris, participants in those summits, have all been drawn to the University of Michigan School of Nursing at various points in their careers.

Two complementary research foci, semantic approaches to system infrastructures and nursing health services research, have merged here at the University of Michigan, where I am is currently leading a data and infrastructure group that is laying the foundation for an extensive Clinical Data Research Network (CDRN), funded by the national Patient-Centered Clinical Research Network. When completed, this national network will greatly expand the capacity to conduct both randomized trials and observational comparative effectiveness studies in new and novel ways, fully engaging a range of stakeholders (patients, providers, payers, health systems) in the design and implementation of research studies. This major effort assures that the opportunities presented by "big data" are brought to research that aims to improve health care outcomes.

Bridging domain-specific knowledge representations and data integration based on current operational and legacy systems while planning for forward-facing technologies and systems is a challenge facing the many informaticists who span research and operational roles. Not surprisingly, the careers of nurse scientists who pursue a research path in informatics are characterized by working with interdisciplinary teams, particularly those with deep technical and information science expertise. My research on semantic-based approaches to systems was launched at the Mayo Clinic, where I held a position as a career scientist and later served as nurse administrator for nursing research and then for informatics (the equivalent of what is now commonly called a chief nursing information officer). Similar to the career pathway described by Ozbolt, my work has been supported by the National Library of Medicine, the Agency for Healthcare Research and Quality, and the Robert Wood Johnson Foundation. I have served as a member and chair of study sections focused on the use of technology in health care delivery systems. I also served as chair or cochair of the World Health Organization (WHO) terminology reference group, where I played a key role in ensuring that the International Classification of Nursing Practice was included in the WHO listing of International Classifications. A few of my research studies are summarized below.

As a discipline, nursing has long placed tremendous effort into the development and use of standardized terminology systems. Yet harmonizing those systems into common representations that can be processed by computer systems has long eluded us. A study I led examined the underlying structures of our published knowledge of patient conditions that are known to be sensitive and responsive to the effects of nursing interventions (e.g., pressure ulcers, pain, etc.). Among the findings was that the implicit structures of these knowledge bases could be expressed in explicit information and terminology models (Harris, Graves, Solbrig, & Chute, 2000). Collaborating with colleagues from the terminology summits, a study examining documentation systems from multiple agencies demonstrated that nursing interventions could be expressed in an international standard for information systems such as Health Level 7 (HL7; http://www.hl7.org) with extensions to that system (Danko et al., 2003). Those recommendations were worked through the HL7 standards development organization and became fully integrated into reference information models that underlie many of today's electronic health records. This work was brought full circle in another study of multivendor, multisite nursing documentation systems and the binding of computable terminology systems (also called ontologies) to the standard reference information model. The output of this work resulted in a challenge sponsored by the Office of the National Coordinator of Health Information Technologies, with prize money awarded to three vendors who successfully implemented these fully harmonized approaches to nursing knowledge in an actual point of care system (Harris et al., 2015).

Nursing health services research has long focused on demonstrating the effects of nursing practice on patient outcomes. Among the challenges in this research have been the cross-sectional nature of studies and the absence of data that could link patient's exposure to nurse staffing levels to patient outcomes. Because of my joint roles as a career scientist and a nurse executive with an overview of the nursing information systems at Mayo, I was able to see that the data resources at Mayo could address this challenge and perhaps move along the discussion of whether nurse staffing makes a difference. Partnering with

Jack Needleman and Peter Buerhaus, authors of seminal research on the effects of nurse staffing, these investigators demonstrated in a longitudinal, linked data study that not only gaps in nurse staffing but also high rates of patient turnover independently and jointly contributed to higher risk of mortality. Because of the nature of the data, our team was able to apply advanced biostatistical approaches that for the first time demonstrated a direct effect of nurse staffing variability on inpatient mortality. The study was published in the *New England Journal of Medicine* and remains one of the few studies to demonstrate such a direct effect (Needleman et al., 2011). In follow-up work, my colleagues and I exploited new coding systems, such as the present-on-admission codes associated with International Classification of Diseases billing codes, to improve the sensitivity and specificity of nurse-sensitive measures, such as failure-to-rescue, that are constructed using administrative data sets (Needleman, Buerhaus, Vanderboom, & Harris, 2013).

In summary, these studies demonstrate novel advances to assuring nursing data, information, and knowledge are embedded in information systems and that those data are usable for research. It is exciting to think about what nursing informatics research can contribute when platforms such as the CDRN's described above are fully functional.

References

Danko, A., Kennedy, R., Haskell, R., Androwich, I., Button, P., Correia, C., . . . Russler, D. (2003). Modeling nursing interventions in the Act Class of HL7 RIM Version 3. *Journal of Biomedical Informatics, 36*(4–5), 294–303.

Harris, M. R., Graves, J. R., Solbrig, H. R., & Chute, C. G. (2000). Embedded structures and representations of nursing knowledge. *Journal of the American Medical Informatics Association, 7*(6), 539–549.

Harris, M. R., Langford, L. L., Miller, H., Hook, M., Dykes, P. C., & Matney, S. A. (2015). Harmonizing and extending standards from a domain-specific and bottom-up approach: An example from development through use in clinical applications. *Journal of the American Medical Informatics Association, 22*(3), 545–552.

Needleman, J., Buerhaus, P. I., Pankratz, V. S., Leibson, C. L., Stevens, S. R., & Harris, M. R. (2011). Nurse staffing and inpatient hospital mortality. *New England Journal of Medicine, 364*, 1037–1045.

Needleman, J., Buerhaus, P. I., Vanderboom, C. E., & Harris, M. R. (2013). Using present-on-admission coding to improve exclusion rules for quality metrics: The case of failure-to-rescue. *Medical Care, 51*(8), 722–730.

Health Science Analytics

Data- and Technology-Driven Approaches for Addressing Health Care Challenges, Advancing Well-Being, and Enhancing Nursing Education

Ivo D. Dinov, PhD

There are many health care challenges that currently inhibit our ability to respond quickly, effectively, and decisively in addressing acute and chronic, urgent and ambulatory, and short- and long-term care. At the same time, there are enormous opportunities for change, improvement in health practice and scientific advances that are driven by rapid scientific progress, national health care policies, accelerated IT developments, and tremendous training and curricular improvements.

Challenges

Globally, there is a significant push to improve short-term and long-term self-management care; reduce individual, institutional or government costs associated with a multitude of acute and chronic conditions; and develop effective evidence-based decision-support systems. The Patient Protection and Affordable Care Act (2010) promotes health care coverage for low- and middle-income families and businesses; however, it may be years before its impact on individuals and the entire health system is fully understood (e.g., compliance, benefits, costs, detriments, potential to advance our knowledge, and ability to deliver and track care). Addressing these challenges requires a broad range of expertise, a commitment to transdisciplinary science, the development of new training curricula, continued scientific advances, reliable, and scalable infrastructure for data management and analytics. Other critical factors include efficient and sustained funding support and effective regulatory and policy frameworks that maximize returns on investment, protect personal information, and secure sensitive materials (e.g., biohazards) (Toga & Dinov, 2015). There are also substantial IT challenges that demand considerable attention and tangible progress. For instance, transitioning to the 10th revision of the World Health Organization's International Statistical Classification of Diseases and Related Health Problems (ICD-10; http://www.CMS.gov/Medicare/Coding/icd10) required care providers to allocate time, resources, and staff for its effective implementation and emersion in clinical practice to meet the regulatory October 2015 deadline. Figure 10-a shows the new alphanumeric labeling nomenclature for annotating and cataloging human health conditions, diseases, symptoms, abnormal findings, and injuries.

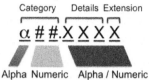

Figure 10-a. Format of the newest version of the World Health Organization's International Statistical Classification of Diseases and Related Health Problems (ICD-10), which uses an alphanumeric labeling nomenclature for classifying health conditions.

Big Data Science

The following are some of the very distinctive characteristics that make big data unique and very different from traditional (small) data: (a) size—the volume of data often exceeds standard storage, memory and, computational capabilities; (b) incongruency—big data samples, cases, and observations may be highly nonhomologous, which requires special treatment; (c) incompleteness—big data might be sparse, with (random and nonrandom causes of) missing values due to the en masse nature of its generation and assembly; (d) complexity—as the dimension of the data increases, distance metrics between observations become degenerate (curse of dimensionality), leading to considerable computational and interpretation challenges, (e) multiscale—big data frequently includes observations from micro to macro scales spanning time, space, and frequency spectra; and (f) multisource—numerous digital, analogous, and mixed data are produced by devices and instruments, which demand special protocols for the integration (fusion) of relevant data within and beyond the scope of any specific research study. The model, algorithm, and tool development necessary to cope with these specific challenges make "standard scientific methods" impractical for understanding big data. Cleveland (2001) introduced the notion of *data science* as an independent discipline, extending the field of statistics to incorporate six technical areas: multidisciplinary investigations, models and methods for data, computing with data, pedagogy, tool evaluation, and theory. Data science is an applied scientific field crossing many discipline boundaries to derive valuable insights and actionable knowledge from complex observable phenomena. Data science practitioners require a versatile and unique set of skills to manage, process, interrogate, and extract information from complex systems.

Opportunities

Significant health care opportunities derive from three complementary sources: ubiquitous big health care datasets, enormous methodological and technological advances, and the emergence of data science analytics. Figure 10-b shows two examples of the very rapid increase of the volume and complexity of data acquired to support a wide spectrum of biomedical, clinical, and health care needs. This data avalanche presents generous opportunities to examine, model, treat, and track normal and pathological conditions (Dinov et al., 2014).

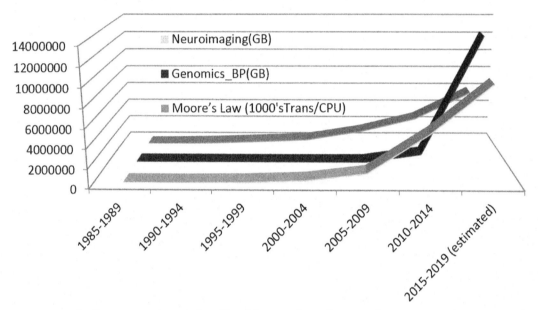

Figure 10-b. Exponential growth of health care data illustrated using neuroimaging and genomics. The misalignment between the rapid rate of increase of the volume of data and the increase of computational power necessary for the information processing is the result of enormous technological advances and improvements in data resolution, streaming efficiency, and censoring equipment. By 2015, more than 10^6 whole human genomes will be sequenced, totaling more than 100 petabytes of data.

The impressive methodological and technological advances in health care introduced since 2010 include scientific discoveries, methodological improvements, and technological products that collectively alleviate suffering, cure diseases, improve quality of life, and provide the foundation for bigger breakthroughs in the near future. Examples of such innovative developments include smart clinical trials; protocols for deep understanding of the phenology, genetics, and environmental effects on neurodegeneration (e.g., Alzheimer's and Parkinson's); rapid and effective blood tests using microsamples; high-frequency wireless wearable technologies (Figure 10-c), and powerful data analytic approaches (work by Dinov under review).

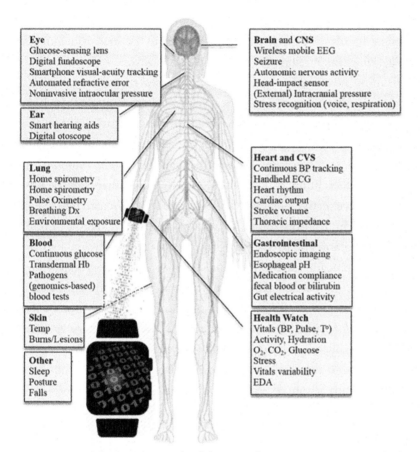

Figure 10-c. The innovative health care advances since 2010 include continuous monitoring using wearable technologies. This provides big health care data associated with location, time, and metabolic and biological characteristics that can be harvested, streamed, modeled, analyzed, visualized, and interpreted in real time.

The emergence of data science analytics coincides with a wave of innovative scientific discoveries that enable predictive modeling and high-throughput analytics that are critical for interrogating big health care data and gaining insights about patterns, trends, connections, and associations in the data. The unique characteristics of such datasets trade off the importance of traditional hypothesis-driven inference and statistical-significance with computational-efficiency, protocol-complexity, and methods-validity (Dinov, Siegrist, Pearl, Kalinin, & Christou, 2015; Husain, Kalinin, Truong, & Dinov, 2015).

Nursing and Health Science Research and Education

Effective management and efficient health care delivery depend on rapid evidence-based, big-data driven, vibrant, robust decision making. Effective management requires unique skill sets; broad knowledge; hands-on experience; teamwork; and the successful integration of human knowledge, machine intelligence, and powerful hardware resources. Many communities and organizations involved in nursing and health research, training, funding, and practice advocate for a significant overhaul in health science training. This includes approaches, techniques, and the implementation of basic and advanced statistical and analytical methods in the undergraduate and graduate health science curriculum, at the PhD level (Wyman & Henly, 2015), and at earlier levels of education as well. Prior recommendations (Bednash, Breslin, Kirschling, & Rosseter, 2014) include enhancing the links between rigorous education and effective practice, modernization of the curriculum (e.g., advanced methods, IT integration, transdisciplinary training), ongoing valuation of training effectiveness, apprentice programs and partnerships for innovative data-driven discoveries, placements in appropriate clinical residency programs, active methodological learning, the blending of domain-specific knowledge, clinical abilities and data analytic skills, and pairing rigorous scientific training with clinical reasoning and quantitative literacy. For instance, the report *The Research-Focused Doctoral Program in Nursing: Pathways to Excellence* (American Association of Colleges of Nursing, 2010) recommends that PhD nursing students be exposed to formal and informal learning experiences; build scientific depth in an identified area of study; learn advanced research design and statistical methods; and develop skills for data, information, and knowledge management, efficient processing, and hands-on analysis.

The adoption of innovative scientific methods in advanced nursing education, health care research, and clinical practice could be improved. Many factors may inhibit the adoption of advanced analytical methods into the training curriculum, for example, care demands on practicing health care providers, demographics of learners and instructors, the DNP/PhD dichotomy, and the powerful inertia of the status quo (Smeltzer et al., 2015). There may not be one unique solution for improving the analytical and scientific skills of nursing professionals. We should enhance the quality and increase the robustness of nursing research while we simultaneously refine the baccalaureate, master's, and doctoral programs. The community needs to review the broad spectrum of modern scientific methods for health sciences and identify key statistical and analytic concepts critical for students' growth as skilled health care professionals, scholars, and practitioners. Some statistics techniques are already an integral part of nursing practice and research.

The faculty of the University of Michigan School of Nursing designed and implemented a novel core statistical and analytics training program for nursing professionals that includes a blend of courses emphasizing the theoretical foundations, model assumptions, computational tools, and applied research practice involving contemporary qualitative and quantitative methods. Table 10-a illustrates this series of four graduate courses (4 credits each) that provide the foundation for a new graduate-level nursing methods and analytics curriculum.

Table 10-a. Example of a Four-Course Series on Analytical Methods for Health Sciences

Foundation courses		Advanced courses	
Fundamentals	**Applied Inference**	**Linear Modeling**	**Special Topics**
Objectives	*Objectives*	*Objectives*	*Objectives*
Apply data management strategies to sample data files	Understand the commonly used statistical methods of published scientific papers	Compare and contrast advanced statistical concepts, grasp model assumptions/limitations, and apply them to quantitative analyses in health care research	Research, employ, and report on recent advanced health sciences analytical methods
Carry out statistical tests to answer common health care research questions using appropriate methods and software tools	Conduct statistical calculations/analyses on available data	Apply multivariate statistical modeling, enabling consistency between research questions and selected advanced statistical analyses	Read, comprehend, and present recent reports of innovative scientific methods applicable to a broad range of health problems
Understand the core analytical data-modeling techniques and their appropriate uses	Use software tools to analyze specific case-study data	Critique and select appropriate advanced statistical linear models.	Experiment with real Big Data
	Communicate advanced statistical concepts/techniques	Conduct multivariate statistical analyses	
	Determine, explain, and interpret assumptions and limitations		

Table 10-a. Example of a Four-Course Series on Analytical Methods for Health Sciences *(continued)*

Foundation courses		Advanced courses	
Fundamentals	**Applied Inference**	**Linear Modeling**	**Special Topics**
Topics	*Topics*	*Topics*	*Topics*
Exploratory data analytics	Epidemiology	Multiple regression	Scientific visualization
	Correlation/regression	General linear model	PCOR/CER methods
Parametric inference	ρ and slope inference, 1–2 samples	ANOVA	HTE
Probability theory		ANCOVA	Big Data / Big Science
Odds ratio/relative risk	ROC curve	MANOVA	Missing data
Distributions	ANOVA	MANCOVA	GWAS
Exploratory data analysis	Nonparametric inference	Repeated measures ANOVA	Medical imaging
			Data networks
Resampling/simulation	Cronbach's α	Partial correlation	Adaptive clinical trials
Design of experiments	Measurement reliability/validity	Time-series analysis	Databases/registries
Intro to epidemiology		Fixed, randomized, and mixed models	Meta-analyses
Estimation	Survival analysis		Causality/causal inference
Hypothesis testing	Decision theory	Hierarchical linear models	
Experiments vs. observational studies	Central limit theorem		SEM
	Association tests	Mixture modeling	Classification methods
Data management	Bayesian inference	Surveys	Time-series analysis
Power, sample-size, effect-size, sensitivity, and specificity	PCA/ICA/factor analysis	Longitudinal data	GIS
	Point/interval estimation (CI)	Generalized estimating equations (GEE) models	Rasch measurement model
Association vs. causality	Study/research critiques	Model fitting and model quality (KS-test)	MCMC Bayesian inference
Clinical vs. statistical significance	Common misconceptions		Network analysis
Statistical independence Bayesian rule			

The value of this new nursing/health science curricular redesign is threefold. First, it will build the trainees' core skills for dealing with an avalanche of health care data, which will promote swift data-driven decision making, smart reactions, and competent responses to varying health care observations. Second, it will enable and galvanize transdisciplinary collaborations among basic scientists, clinical investigators, and health care practitioners to solve complex biomedical problems. Third, the new curriculum aims to enhance the processes of patient diagnosis, treatment, prevention of human disease or injury, and management of other physical and mental impairments. These benefits might be realized by utilizing modern scientific techniques, embedding data-driven inference in the decision-making discoveries, and avoiding common mistakes in various health care settings.

Past, Present, and Future

Much of the foundation of modern health and nursing science is deeply rooted in the development and utilization of innovative scientific methods for data modeling, statistical analysis, and evidence-based practice. For instance, Florence Nightingale (1820–1910), the founder of modern nursing science, established the first professional nursing school at St. Thomas' Hospital in London (King's College London). She recognized early on the importance of broad-based scientific training, including mathematics and statistics, to aggregate, analyze, and demonstrate evidence-based health care practice. Nightingale was a pioneer in the graphical presentation of information and developed the widely used polar area plot for radial display of frequency patterns, which she used to depict the observed cyclical trends of soldier mortality (Figure 10-d). More of these core data analytic contributions, statistical methodological developments and fundamental scientific discoveries are necessary to attract and train skilled nursing and health care scientists, advance the biomedical and health care research, bridge across transdisciplinary boundaries, and ultimately improve human health.

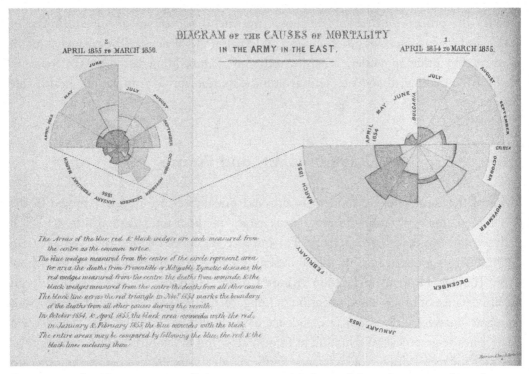

Figure 10-d. Nursing scientific innovation—Nightingale's polar area plot showing observed cyclical trends of soldier mortality.

In the past year, we have developed a mechanism to integrate dispersed multisource data; service the mashed information via human and machine interfaces in a secure, scalable manner; and enable joint data analytics (Husain et al., 2015). This new platform includes a device agnostic tool (Dashboard web app: http://socr.umich.edu/HTML5/ Dashboard) for graphical querying and navigating and exploring the multivariate associations in complex heterogeneous datasets (Figure 10-e).

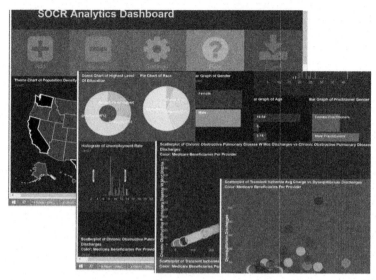

Figure 10-e. Interactive data assembly, management, and visual analytics.

References

American Association of Colleges of Nursing. (2010). The research-focused doctoral program in nursing: Pathways to excellence. Washington, DC: Author.

Bednash, G., Breslin, E. T., Kirschling, J. M., & Rosseter, R. J. (2014). PhD or DNP planning for doctoral nursing education. *Nursing Science Quarterly, 27*(4), 296–301.

Cleveland, W. S. (2001). Data science: An action plan for expanding the technical areas of the field of statistics. *International Statistical Review, 69*(1), 21–26. doi:10.1111/j.1751-5823.2001.tb00477.x

Dinov, I. D., Petrosyan, P., Liu, Z., Eggert, P., Zamanyan, A., Torri, F., . . . Toga, A. W. (2014). The perfect neuroimaging-genetics-computation storm: Collision of petabytes of data, millions of hardware devices and thousands of software tools. *Brain Imaging and Behavior, 8*(2), 311–322.

Dinov, I. D., Siegrist, K., Pearl, D. K., Kalinin, A., & Christou, N. (2015). Probability distributome: A web computational infrastructure for exploring the properties, interrelations, and applications of probability distributions. *Computational Statistics, 594,* 1–19. doi:10.1007/s00180-015-0594-6

Husain, S. S., Kalinin, A., Truong, A., & Dinov, I. D. (2015). SOCR Data dashboard: An integrated big data archive mashing Medicare, labor, census and econometric information. *Journal of Big Data, 2*(13), 1–18. doi:10.1186/s40537-015-0018-z

Patient Protection and Affordable Care Act, 42 U.S.C. § 18001 (2010).

Smeltzer, S. C., Sharts-Hopko, N. C., Cantrell, M. A., Heverly, M. A., Nthenge, S., & Jenkinson, A. (2015). A profile of U.S. nursing faculty in research- and practice-focused doctoral education. *Journal of Nursing Scholarship, 47*(2), 178–185.

Toga, A. W., & Dinov, I. D. (2015). Sharing big biomedical data. *Journal of Big Data, 2*(1), 7.

Wyman, J. F., & Henly, S. J. (2015). PhD programs in nursing in the United States: Visibility of AACN core curricular elements and emerging areas of science. *Nursing Outlook, 63*(4), 390–397.

Nursing Leadership

CHAPTER 11

Innovation Leadership

Daniel J. Pesut, PhD, RN, PMHCNS-BC, FAAN

Introduction

Dr. Pamela Hinds and colleagues (2015) have proposed legacy mapping as a means to plan for and document meaningful work in nursing. Legacy mapping begins with two questions: (a) What do you want to improve in nursing through your efforts, and (b) What would you like to be best known for? The purpose of this chapter is to describe and discuss the highlights of my professional contributions through time and to answer the two questions related to my professional legacy, innovation leadership, and attention to the value of personal and professional renewal.

My education and development in the PhD program at the University of Michigan School of Nursing (1981–1984) instilled a spirit of inquiry and innovation in me that has resulted in a program of scholarship and a significant number of publications (Google Scholar Profile) that document the impact and influence of my work in the areas of nursing practice, education, and research. Over time, my scholarship has evolved from clinical research interests in volitional psychosomatic self-regulation to educational interests in the area of metacognition and the self-regulation of creative thought in nursing. My interest in metacognition and creative thinking evolved into a deep commitment to and development of innovations associated with teaching, learning, and educational research focused on the acquisition, mastery, and evaluation of clinical reasoning skills in nursing. Along the way, I developed a keen interest in the role futures thinking plays in visionary, resilient leadership (Pesut, 1997, 2000, 2015; Pesut & Thompson, 2015; Allison-Napalitano & Pesut, 2015). Innovation leadership best describes my professional contributions over time.

Early Inspiration: Clinical Nursing Research Interests

During my doctoral program at the University of Michigan, I had the good fortune to be mentored by and work with Dr. Jean Wood. We had a mutual interest in mind-body interactions and the phenomena of volitional psychosomatic self-regulation. Starting with patient interviews and qualitative methods, Jean and I described the mental phenomena people use to manage their recovery from episodes of illness (Wood & Pesut, 1981, 1982). From these interviews, we developed categories of self-regulation strategies and eventually created the Carolina Self-Regulation Inventory (CSRI) and instrument to measure these self-regulation strategies (Massey & Pesut, 1991; Pesut & Massey, 1992). The CSRI has been used by a number of studies examining the role of self-regulation with a variety of acute and chronic health conditions such as chronic pain and weight management. We were early pioneers in scoping out patient awareness of self-regulatory phenomena. Jean moved on to an administrative position at the University of Illinois and continued with various aspects of the clinical self-regulation research. With the loss of my mentor and grounding in the concepts of self-regulation, I began to consider other strategic areas of research that would impact and positively influence the profession.

As my doctoral studies progressed, it became increasingly clear to me that if nursing was to strategically advance its scientific agenda, then nurses needed to develop a creative and innovative mind-set. Simply put, I reasoned that science presupposes creativity. And if creativity is a prerequisite to scientific thinking, then one strategy and tactic to enhance scientific activity would be to enhance and develop the creative thinking skill set of nurses. A focus on creativity and innovation seemed to be the most strategic way forward to advance the nursing science and research agenda. I believed it was essential to help nurses develop their own creativity and innovation leadership skill. Creative nurses were more likely to develop innovative solutions to complex patient care challenges. I reasoned that nurses with a more innovative leadership skill set were more likely to develop creative questions and hypotheses that could be put forth to advance nursing science, knowledge development, and research. Helping nurses self-regulate creative thought became the focus of my dissertation and laid the foundation for my enduring interest in creative thinking, clinical reasoning, and innovation leadership. Throughout my professional career, I have been interested in how the creative process supports personal and professional development, enhances reasoning, and stimulates future thinking and supports innovation leadership and professional renewal.

Thinking About Thinking: The Self-Regulation of Creative Thought in Nursing

My PhD dissertation, *Metacognition: The Self-Regulation of Creative Thought in Nursing* (Pesut, 1984), set the stage for research, development, and testing of innovative educational practices and models that support teaching and learning of creative and clinical reasoning skills. It made sense to me that most creative thinking strategies, tactics, and techniques were heuristic devices or tools that helped people think about their own thinking and develop their creative thinking abilities. As an educator, I realized that one of the most important things I did was to help people self-regulate and manage their own creativity and thinking processes. I assisted students and nurses in practice to make tacit assumptions, values, and beliefs explicit. I challenged nurses and students to "think about their thinking" and then created scaffolding, strategies, and structures for them to build on their knowledge, skills, and abilities. My dissertation provided a new definition of creativity (Pesut, 1985) and a conceptual model that framed creative thinking as a self-regulatory metacognitive process (Pesut, 1990). As it turns out, there are important distinctions to be made between cognitive and metacognitive skills in the development of clinical reasoning (Kuiper & Pesut, 2004) and mastery of innovative leadership agility (Pesut & Thompson, 2015).

Acting on my vision and logic, I created and evaluated a creativity training program for practicing registered nurses using concepts, theories, and principles from the literature on creative thinking, self-instructional cognitive behavior modification training, and research in the area of metacognition. Through focused attention to self-regulation (self-monitoring, self-evaluation, and self-reinforcement), the research revealed that nurses are able to self-regulate creative thought. Intentionally helping nurses master specific strategies, tools, and techniques that support the development of self-perceived creativity resulted in significant differences on tests of creative thinking. My doctoral research served as the foundation of my scholarship. I continue to develop ideas about the relationship of metacognition to critical and creative thinking that support clinical reasoning in nursing and the thinking and actions that foster innovation (Pesut, 2013; Moody, Horton-Deutsch, & Pesut, 2007). Throughout the course of my career, I have worked with more than 50 doctoral students to advance innovations in nursing education research. As associate dean for graduate programs and director of the PhD program at Indiana University (2005–2012), I taught all incoming PhD students and helped them articulate their research interests through the use of mind maps and integral theory perspective taking. Working with PhD students at the University of South Carolina, Indiana University, and the University of Minnesota, I continue to help students articulate and clarify their research interests through the use of creative and innovative teaching and learning methods.

Innovation Leadership and the Transformation of the Nursing Process: The Outcome Present State Test Model of Clinical Reasoning

My work in creative thinking and metacognition provided insights into clinical reasoning thinking strategies that support the development of clinical reasoning skills (Pesut & Herman, 1992). The clinical thinking of nurses evolves over time. In fact, one can discern transformations of the nursing process approximately every 20 years. Noting this distinction resulted in identification of three generations of nursing process (Pesut & Herman, 1998) and provided the impetus to create an innovative model of clinical reasoning, the

Outcome Present State Test (OPT) Model of Reflective Clinical Reasoning (Pesut & Herman, 1998, 1999). Changing the paradigm of the nursing process and how nurses reason about complex patient care challenges (Pesut, 2008) is a significant example of innovation leadership. The OPT model provides a structure and process for evolving nursing content and standardized nursing terminologies and focuses on outcome specification and makes explicit the nature and dynamics associated with clinical judgment. While refining and developing the OPT model, there was a concurrent evolution and development of nursing knowledge classification systems such as the North American Nursing Diagnosis Association (NANDA), Nursing Intervention Classification (NIC), and Nursing Outcome Classification (NOC). The OPT model provided a structure for the use of these nursing classification systems. Research documented significant differences in clinical reasoning skill acquisition of students through the use of reflection and self-regulated learning and adoption and use of standardized terminologies in nursing (Kautz, Kuiper, Pesut, & Williams, 2006). The OPT model has been adopted in many national and international clinical and educational contexts. Nurse educators in the United States, Spain, Italy, Iceland, Brazil, Mexico, Taiwan, Thailand, and China are using and conducting research with the OPT model. The original work by Pesut and Herman (1999) was translated into Mandarin in 2007. Research teams continue to evaluate the teaching and learning strategies associated with the model and its impact on student thinking and reasoning (Kuiper, Pesut, & Kautz, 2009; Kautz, Kuiper, Pesut, Knight-Brown, & Daneker, 2005). As of this writing, a team is working on the development of a care coordination clinical reasoning model based on the original OPT structure, strategies, and techniques. The model supports and emphasizes the critical, creative, systems, complexity thinking involved in care coordination from several perspectives (Kuiper, Pesut, & Arms, 2016).

Leaders Create the Future: Inspiration and Renewal

In 1993, I received the Edith Moore Copeland Founder's Award for Excellence in Creativity. This award is one of the highest honors bestowed by the Honor Society of Nursing and served as recognition of my professional contributions and innovation leadership skills (McBride, 2004). In 1995, I was inducted into the American Academy of Nursing. With an eye toward stimulating innovation leadership with a futures orientation, I agreed to author "Future Think," a feature that appeared in *Nursing Outlook*, the official journal of the American Academy of Nursing. These 36 editorial thought pieces (over a 5-year period) challenged members of the nursing profession to think about the future and reflect on how nursing could respond to the cross impact of health care and educational trends and issues (Pesut, 1997). Additionally, I provided feedback and evaluation and served on the editorial board for the journal *Nurse Educator* from 1984 to 2004. I also contributed time and talent as the assistant editor for the education column of the *Journal of Professional Nursing* from 2002 to 2004. I continue to prompt reflections through the *Meta-Reflections* blog sponsored by Sigma Theta Tau International.

It was an honor to serve on the board of directors of the Honor Society of Nursing, Sigma Theta Tau International, for 8 years (1997–2005). The highlight of my professional service contributions through the years was serving as president of the Honor Society of Nursing, Sigma Theta Tau International (2003–2005). Innovation leadership themes surfaced as I developed my presidential call to action: "Create the Future Through Renewal" (Pesut, 2004). I believe professional renewal is crucial for creating and sustaining an innovation mind-set. In recognition of my innovation leadership, a generous nurse philanthropist instigated the creation of the Daniel J. Pesut Spirit of Renewal Award. This international award is bestowed at the biennial convention of the Honor Society of Nursing on an individual who best meets the following criteria for the award: service to others through civic, professional, and/or community engagement; scholarly habits that stimulate reflective practice in self and others; commitment to the development of knowledge, learning, and service; organizational contributions that foster professional growth, development, and renewal in others; mentoring and coaching that foster renewal; and the ability to raise the spirit of colleagues, self, and other associates. The award represents what I would like to be known for by others—the second of the legacy map questions— fostering a spirit of renewal and inspiration in others (Allison-Napolitano & Pesut, 2015).

Working with fellow doctoral students at the University of Michigan; faculty in the Department of Psychology, the Institute for Social Research (ISR), and the School of Nursing; and colleagues at the Neuropsychiatric Institute (NPI) and University Hospital, I was well educated to develop an innovative leadership mind-set. Grounded in principles and practices of innovation leadership, I continue to advance the creative knowledge, skills, and abilities of students, colleagues, doctoral students, and nurses in practice. I am committed to facilitating the innovation leadership skill development of the next generation of leaders because innovation leadership will be required to create a desired 21st-century health care system.

References

Allison-Napolitano, E., & Pesut, D. (2015). *Bounce forward: The extraordinary resilience of nursing leadership.* Silver Springs, MD: American Nurses Association.

Hinds, P. S., Britton, D. R., Coleman, L., Engh, E., Humbel, T. K., Keller, S., & Walczak, D. (2015). Creating a career legacy map to help assure meaningful work in nursing. *Nursing Outlook, 63*(2), 211–218.

Kautz, D. D., Kuiper, R., Pesut, D. J., Knight-Brown, P., & Daneker, D. (2005). Promoting clinical reasoning in undergraduate nursing students: Application and evaluation of the Outcome Present State Test (OPT) model of clinical reasoning. *International Journal of Nursing Education Scholarship, 2*(1), 1–21.

Kautz, D., Kuiper, R., Pesut, D., & Williams, R. (2006). Using NANDA, NIC and NOC language for clinical reasoning with the Outcome–Present State Test Model. *International Journal of Nursing Terminologies and Classification, 17*(3–4), 129–138.

Kuiper, R. A., & Pesut, D. J. (2004). Promoting cognitive and metacognitive reflective reasoning skills in nursing practice: Self-regulated learning theory. *Journal of Advanced Nursing, 45*(4), 381–391.

Kuiper, R. A., Pesut, D. J., Arms, T. (2016). *Clinical reasoning and care coordination for the advanced practice nursing.* New York, NY: Springer.

Kuiper, R. A., Pesut, D. J., & Kautz, D. (2009). Promoting the self-regulation of clinical reasoning skills in nursing students. *Open Nursing Journal, 3*, 76–85.

Massey, J., & Pesut, D. (1991). Self-regulation strategies of adults, *Western Journal of Nursing Research, 13*(5), 640–647.

McBride, A. (2004). Daniel J. Pesut gentleman, creative leader. *Reflections on Nursing Leadership, 30* (1), 16–23.

Moody, R., Horton-Deutsch, S., & Pesut, D. J. (2007). Appreciative inquiry for leading in complex systems: Supporting the transformation of academic nursing culture. *Journal of Nursing Education, 46*(7), 319–324.

Pesut, D. J. (1984). Metacognition: The self-regulation of creative thought in nursing. Doctoral dissertation, University of Michigan. *Dissertation Abstracts International, 45*, 515.

Pesut, D. J. (1985). Toward a new definition of creativity. *Nurse educator, 10*(1), 5.

Pesut, D. J. (1990). Creative thinking as a self-regulatory metacognitive process—A model for education, training and further research. *Journal of Creative Behavior, 24*(2), 105–110.

Pesut, D. J. (1997). Future think. *Nursing Outlook, 45*(3), 107.

Pesut, D. J. (2000). Looking forward: Being and becoming a futurist. In F. Bower (Ed.), *Nurses taking the lead: Personal qualities of effective leadership* (pp. 39–65). Philadelphia, PA: W. B. Saunders.

Pesut, D. J. (2004). Create the future through renewal. *Reflections on nursing leadership/Sigma Theta Tau International, Honor Society of Nursing, 30*(1), 24.

Pesut, D. J. (2008). Thoughts on thinking with complexity in mind. In C. Lindberg, S. Nash, & C. Lindberg (Eds.), *On the edge: Nursing in the age of complexity* (pp. 211–238). Bordentown, NJ: Plexus Press.

Pesut, D. J. (2013). Creativity and innovation: Thought and action. *Creative nursing, 19*(3), 113–121.

Pesut, D. J. (2015). Avoiding derailment: Leadership strategies for identity, reputation and legacy management. In J. Daly, S. Speedy, & D. Jackson (Eds.), *Leadership & nursing contemporary perspectives* (2nd ed., pp. 251–261). Sydney: Churchill Livingstone, Elsevier.

Pesut, D. J., & Herman, J. (1992). Metacognitive skills in diagnostic reasoning: Making the implicit explicit. *International Journal of Nursing Terminologies and Classifications, 3*(4), 148–154.

Pesut, D. J., & Herman, J. (1998). OPT: Transformation of nursing process for contemporary practice. *Nursing Outlook, 46*(1), 29–36.

Pesut, D. J., & Herman, J. (1999). *Clinical reasoning: The art and science of critical and creative thinking.* New York, NY: Delmar.

Pesut, D. J., & Massey, J. (1992). Self-management of recovery: Implications for nursing practice. *Journal of the American Academy of Nurse Practitioners, 4*(2), 58–62.

Pesut, D. J., & Thompson, S. (2015). Leadership and reflective practice: Leadership agility designed to create the future. In G. D. Sherwood & S. Horton-Deutsch (Eds.), *Reflective organizations: On the frontlines of QSEN and reflective practice implementation* (pp. 339–359). Indianapolis, IN: Sigma Theta Tau International.

Wood, D. J., & Pesut, D. J. (1981). Self-regulatory mental processes and patient recovery. *Western journal of nursing research, 3*(3), 262–267.

Wood, D. J., & Pesut, D. J. (1982). Psychosomatic self-regulation and recovery from surgery. *Nursing Research, 31*(3), 189–190.

CHAPTER 12

Leadership as Scholarship

Joanne Disch, PhD, RN, FAAN
Linda R. Cronenwett, PhD, RN, FAAN
Jane Barnsteiner, PhD, RN, FAAN

An Expanding View of Scholarship

In 1992, Margaret Wheatley called for a new science with a "movement toward holism, toward understanding the system as a system and giving primary value to the relationships that exist among seemingly discrete parts" (p. 9). She challenged the conventional wisdom that was based on a Newtonian image of the universe, where the world is expected to be predictable and scholars search for better ways of perceiving and explaining it. What would be necessary would be better understandings of change and chaos, of key patterns and principles, of organizational design, and of leadership that was more relational rather than autocratic.

At about the same time, Boyer (1990) proposed what he believed to be a necessary expansion in the academy's definition and expressions of scholarship. Rather than focusing on only research and teaching in the traditional style, he encouraged us to "enlarge the perspective" and to rethink what it means to be a scholar. He proposed that we consider the scholarship of discovery, integration, application, and teaching.

Several years later, the Carnegie Foundation for the Advancement of Teaching launched its Carnegie Initiative on the Doctorate (CID) (Walker, Golde, Jones, Bueschel, & Hutchings, 2008). Devoting 5 years to the study of the PhD, the initiative's goal was to rethink doctoral education and make recommendations for "moving it into the future." Several themes emerged that expanded our thinking of doctoral education as a complex process of ongoing formation applicable in many situations: (a) *scholarly integration*, which supports the idea that teaching and research are synergistic and that both require intellectual effort; (b) *intellectual community*, which describes the importance of the culture and environment in which scholarship occurs; and (c) *stewardship*, which refers to fostering renewal and creativity in assuring the continuing health of the discipline. The authors noted that the PhD is a route to many destinations and different careers, yet all who pursue it can be considered scholars, since scholarship is a function not of setting but of purpose and commitment:

A fully formed scholar should be capable of generating and critically evaluating new knowledge; of conserving the most important ideas and findings that are a legacy of the past and current work; and of understanding how knowledge is transforming the world in which we live, and engaging in the transformational work of communicating their knowledge responsibly to others. (Walker et al., 2008, p. 12)

Leadership as Scholarship

Leadership is a form of scholarship that helps us "move into the future." Leaders usually influence others through relationships; they advance the collective work of the group (Porter-O'Grady & Malloch, 2016). They apply evidence and expertise to situations, when available, and generate evidence when necessary. They are unsatisfied with the status quo and seek continuously to improve systems and processes. They create environments within which people can do their very best work (Disch, 2009). They inspire others to pursue a particular path and help give meaning to chaos, change, and uncertainty. Recognizing that the whole is greater than the sum of the parts, they collaborate broadly to set direction and craft solutions. On the other hand, Max DePree (1989, p. 12) reminds us that success is less about the leader and more about the followers: "The measure of leadership is not the quality of the head, but the tone of the body."

As members of the doctoral student community at the University of Michigan School of Nursing in the early 1980s, the three of us were privileged to draw from the resources of outstanding faculty at the school and across the campus. We were challenged to learn to think differently, to draw from diverse bodies of knowledge, to formulate and address questions of importance to society, to lead boldly, and to contribute to the professional literature. We developed connections among ourselves, other nurses, and colleagues from other disciplines that continue today and form strong networks for current and future work. In the following sections, each of us describes the leadership journey she has taken and its impact on her life as a scholar.

Joanne Disch, PhD, RN, FAAN

Definition of Leadership

My leadership journey began in eighth grade when a classmate and I were nominated by our school for the city-wide Boy and Girl leadership contest. I don't recall any specific leadership competencies that I had, but I do recall the coaching by the mother of another classmate in getting our applications ready. I regularly use her strategies today when applying for, or nominating someone else for, an award: (a) consider all the activities you've engaged in and find a link to the requirements of the award; (b) use powerful verbs to indicate leadership and action; and (c) don't leave any questions or boxes blank. Move something from another category if you have to so that you demonstrate achievement in each area. Her advice worked: Both my classmate and I won our respective awards.

Filling out an application to receive a leadership award isn't the same thing as being a leader. But over the years, I have come to appreciate the subtle lessons on leadership that Mrs. Pfeiffer also imparted: First impressions are crucial; you have to believe that you have something to offer; you have to be willing to put yourself forward; impact can be demonstrated in a number of ways; and leaders need followers and partners to succeed. Actually, Mrs. Pfeiffer's words came back to me when I applied for the board of AARP. I faced a significant blank section when filling out the application: prior service with AARP. I had had none. There was nothing to move from another category. So I framed my answer to make an advantage out of a deficit, along the lines of "All organizations need individuals with long histories with the organization—and one or two people who bring fresh eyes and experiences. I would be that person." I also spoke about my nursing lens and my experiences as a leader and colleague in interprofessional activities, helping the selection committee understand what a nurse could bring to a board. I was pleased to be invited to join the board and, eventually, become its chair.

My definition of leadership has evolved over the years through the diverse leadership roles I have held, such as chief nurse executive at two major medical centers; president of the American Association of Critical-Care Nurses and the American Academy of Nursing; interim dean of the University of Minnesota School of Nursing; board member of Allina Health and Aurora Health Care; board member and chair of AARP; and currently chair of the board of trustees of Chamberlain College of Nursing. Interestingly, my definition of leadership finally gelled when teaching leadership to undergraduate nursing students and explaining why they needed to develop leadership skills: *to work with and through others to improve something.* While the phrase is simple, the competencies that are needed are challenging. Improving something requires an awareness of what's working and what's not, what the alternative options are, how things could be done better, and how to intentionally apply quality improvement and change principles. Improving something is different from getting the work done, although both are often done concurrently. Working with and through others is equally challenging. This requires engaging people, getting their ideas, offering inspiration and assistance, knowing when and how to give feedback or support, and sharing good news when available and bad news when necessary. Fortunately, there are many approaches to leadership.

Personal Journey as Leader

Several common threads have characterized my particular leadership journey.

Having concurrent roles in practice and education. All my clinical leadership positions were part of a joint or dual role with a research-intensive school of nursing. Thus I have extensive experience in the clinical side of health care, so I understand the challenges and pressures of a 24/7/365 operation where lives truly are at stake. Alternatively, I have held academic positions ranging from teaching assistant to division chair, so I understand the challenges faced by faculty and the need to shift toward establishing environments for student-centered learning amid growing resource constraints.

Spanning boundaries. Similar to integrating practice and education, much of my leadership journey has been focused on bringing together groups and individuals who have distinct roles and responsibilities, or differing backgrounds and views, to work on issues of common concern. One example is the work I led as president of American Association of Critical Care Nurses. At that time in the early 1980s, there was antagonism between the American Nurses Association (ANA) and the specialty nursing organizations. A primary goal of my presidency was to create better relationships between the two groups. I realized that for nursing to be a strong force, we needed to come together. The executive director of the American Association of Critical Care Nurses and I invited the president and executive director of ANA to dinner—which launched a strong personal and professional relationship that enabled us to jointly work together and model collaboration to other leaders.

A second example is the work that was required when integrating two very distinct nursing staffs into one after the purchase of the University of Minnesota Hospital and Clinic by Fairview Health Services in 1997. The staffs were physically separated by the Mississippi River, half were from an academic health center and the others from a community hospital, and half of the nurses were covered by a union contract that the other half had voted against a few years earlier. As before, for nursing to be a strong force and for patient and family care to be safely delivered, we needed to work together. A third example is the research I have done over the past several years on nurse and physician coleadership of patient care areas.

Embracing paradox. Within health care today are many paradoxes: for example, do more with less, improve quality and reduce cost, strengthen nursing and create strong interprofessional teams, and be competitive yet collegial. Within health care education, paradoxes also exist, such as (a) incorporate new content (e.g., genomics, informatics, social determinants) while keeping programs of reasonable length; (b) be an expert educator, researcher, clinician, and nursing leader; (c) expand student enrollment in the face of decreasing resources. I have come to appreciate that we must find ways to successfully manage these polarities, which usually requires keeping an eye on new trends, seeing why both realities are important for the collective, and learning to think differently. Also, pursuing "both/and" approaches gives better solutions, as opposed to "right/wrong," "good/bad," or "your way/my way." Asking, for example, "Under what conditions could we improve quality and reduce cost?" is a very effective strategy for helping people identify points of commonality.

In a related fashion, *seeking ambiguity* has also characterized my work. Definitive black-and-white strategies rarely work in today's dynamic environment. I have learned that reframing a potential problem into a broader issue can often bring new options. For example, rather than working to hire more nurses, could we explore options for expanding the capacity of an organization to provide nursing care? The latter question allows for a wide range of options, such as allowing part-time nurses to work full-time, bringing back retired nurses, or hiring nursing assistants to do tasks that do not require nurses' expertise.

Core Values

In addition to the characteristics listed above, mentors in my leadership journey have instilled in me some core values that have influenced my career and personal life. Here are a few:

- **Information is power, but relationships are the key.** Historically touted sources of power, such as positional, expert, and referent, are helpful to a point. But at the end of the day, one's relationships and interdependence with others are what enhance a leader's effectiveness the most.
- **Focus and make an impact.** Rather than doing many things at a time, select a handful that are priorities and target your energy, attention, and resources to these few. That's not to say that leaders don't have to advance several priorities at the same time, but keeping a laser-like focus on those most important ensures movement in these key areas.
- **Work hard, play hard, rest hard.** Many years ago, a valued colleague pointed out that the traditional balance of working hard and playing hard isn't adequate for today's fast-paced environment. Leaders need to build in periods where they can rest hard, rejuvenate, and reestablish balance in their work and personal lives.

Neuman, Newman, and Holder (2000, p. 62) stated, "Leadership and scholarship should be viewed as requisite to each other." Effective leaders offer an evidence-based course of action and identify goals and relevant activities that constitute a form of scholarship. I have certainly engaged in traditional methods of creation and dissemination, such as through publications, presentations, scholarly papers, and research. Of greatest impact, however, might be the role modeling that I have been privileged to provide through formal leadership positions in a variety of organizations, as well as one-to-one mentoring, coaching, and collaborating. This has occurred at the local, organizational, and international levels and with nursing students, nurses, colleagues from other disciplines, and consumers. Most importantly, the focus has remained on strengthening relationships and creating environments in which individuals can flourish.

Linda R. Cronenwett, PhD, RN, FAAN

Definition of Leadership

For most of my career, I thought about leadership as the process of influencing others—mostly followers—toward shared goals. As an incoming freshman to the University of Michigan in 1962, I participated in a leadership-development program during my first weekend on campus. I had been a leader of clubs and student government in high school, decided to attend the University of Michigan after participating in Girls' State in Ann Arbor, and assumed I would continue to be a "leader" among the university's "leaders and best." I can't remember what I learned that first weekend, but I was *not* drawn to leadership activities or politics on my new campus. I was (and still am) not someone who waved my hand to say, "I want to lead," but someone who stepped up after being chosen to lead.

Since 2009, I have partnered with the executives, faculty, and staff of the Center for Creative Leadership (CCL) (the third largest leadership development firm in the world) in Greensboro, North Carolina, to lead the Robert Wood Johnson Foundation (RWJF) Executive Nurse Fellows (ENF) program. I have come to deeply appreciate CCL's view of leadership as the processes of setting direction, creating alignment, and maintaining commitment (DAC) in collectives (Velsor, McCauley, & Ruderman, 2010), a definition that reflects a broader understanding of who produces leadership from "leadership as being produced solely by individuals who are recognized as leaders" to "leadership as being produced by the entire collective" (p. 21). The focus of the CCL definition is on the *outcomes* of leadership. Asymmetrical power vested in leaders within a hierarchy can accomplish effective leadership outcomes (such as my days as a young U.S. Navy Nurse Corps Officer leading 10–15 corpsmen to deliver nursing care to a ward full of sailors and marines wounded in Vietnam). But the CCL definition recognizes that collectives can use other processes as well, including lateral influence among peers (the nursing shared governance models we nurtured at Dartmouth-Hitchcock Medical Center); the emergence of ideas and shared leadership practices that arise as people with a collective of talents work together over time (e.g., scientific teams or the shared leadership of the Quality and Safety Education for Nurses [QSEN] initiative; Cronenwett, 2012a); and forms of leadership that can be derived from boundary-spanning efforts among interdependent groups, such as the multiple initiatives to improve quality and safety education and practice that emerged from an interprofessional group of nurse, physician, and hospital administrator educational leaders known as the Dartmouth Summer Symposium, for which I served as the nursing member of Paul Batalden's "Kitchen Cabinet" (Batalden & Gordon, 2012).

The DAC definition of leadership also recognizes that people in organizations can and do lead from "top," "middle," and "bottom" positions, sometimes compensating for weaknesses at another level but achieving the best outcomes when leadership is nurtured, rewarded, and developed at each level of the collective. Looking back, I was clearly leading (with various levels of effectiveness) from the day I became a navy officer upon graduation from my bachelor's degree in nursing program, but leader development was spotty and informal, as it is for most nurses, even today.

Personal Journey as Leader

Since 2009, I have had the pleasure of reading more than 400 applications for the RWJF ENF program and can attest to the fact that people who become executive nurse leaders in academic and practice settings report having been selected to lead early in their careers. I, too, found that others expected me to lead early on, probably because I learned quickly, trusted others, built and maintained relationships fairly easily, and modeled my family of origin's commitments to integrity and service. These gifts to me were nurtured at home and in school many years ago, as they were for many young women with strong personal initiative and drive who became nurses. But the path onward was a series of learning by trial and error (too little reflection and leader development) as I struggled with the downsides of overusing my strengths (e.g., my ability to assert a clear and compelling message could too easily veer into being perceived as strident or "know it all"), avoiding conflict and roles in conflict resolution, and relying too heavily on my preferred modes of exerting influence (asserting/inspiring/rationalizing vs. bridging and negotiating).

Because I happened (for personal life reasons, not good planning) to receive my baccalaureate, master's, and doctoral education at two great schools of nursing (University of Michigan and University of Washington) along with a semester at the University of California, San Francisco (where I had courses from Shirley Chater and Rheba de Tornyay), I was exposed to nursing leaders at each stage of professional development. My dean at the University of Michigan, Carolyne Davis, who went on to lead the Health Care Financing Administration, housed me in Washington when we lobbied for the National Center for Nursing Research (the predecessor of the National Institute of Nursing Research at NIH). These individuals were my role models for making a difference in nursing and the world at large.

In my master's program, it became clear that I was expected to write for publication, and the hard work of learning to craft a well-written manuscript was nurtured by the early editors of *Nursing Research* and *Research in Nursing and Health*, Florence Downs and Harriet Werley. They gave clear (and copious amounts of) constructive feedback, and I learned both how to improve my writing and how to pick myself up from negative feedback, learn something, and not take it personally. Given that one of my strengths as leader has been an ability to influence through publications and presentations, these early lessons served me well.

My professional socialization also included an emphasis on contributing to the improvement of the profession and health care through professional organization and policy work.

I was socialized to consider it mandatory to belong and pay dues to professional organizations, but my role models were also *leaders* of these organizations. Over my career, I contributed to leadership efforts in areas of science (as a member of the ANA Council of Nurse Researchers Executive Committee, the chair of the committee that founded the Eastern Nursing Research Society, and a member of the National Advisory Council for Nursing Research); practice (as president of the New Hampshire Nurses Association and chair of the ANA Congress of Nursing Practice); education (as president of the North Carolina Nursing Deans and Directors and on the board of directors of the Josiah Macy Jr. Foundation); and policy (on the board of directors of the Institute for Healthcare Improvement, the North Carolina Institute of Medicine, and the North Carolina Quality Center). I also held formal leadership roles in both practice (as director of professional practice at Dartmouth-Hitchcock Medical Center) and academic settings (as dean for 10 years at University of North Carolina–Chapel Hill). As a result, I understood and valued all domains of professional commitment (Batalden & Gordon, 2012)—namely, improving patient care, improving system performance, and improving professional development—and this breadth helped me develop important leadership abilities to think and act strategically across boundaries of settings, professions, and roles.

To analyze the attributes that helped me lead, I will describe two areas of impact (in addition to QSEN, which follows this section as an example of these authors' shared leadership). As one of the early nurse researchers in a practice setting, I pioneered efforts to integrate research and practice. In the 1980s, practicing nurses were rarely exposed to science. From 1985 to 1990, I edited a newsletter, *Research Review: Studies for Nursing Practice*, specifically for nurses in practice. The publication was picked up by Williams & Wilkins in its last 3 years and marketed throughout the country. I was simultaneously leading 10 years of "Research Days for Clinicians" conferences, where nurses presented summaries of areas of science and results of research utilization projects. I wrote editorials on leading research and research utilization in practice settings for the *Journal of Nursing Administration* from 1985 to 1987 and spoke at numerous hospital and research conferences. Along with a peer network of other researchers in practice settings, we set direction and created alignment toward the goal of integrating research and nursing practice. Decades later, almost all nursing journals and professional organization publications and conferences maintain a commitment to this integration.

A second example of leadership impact relates to my contributions to creating alignment among licensure, education, and certification of advanced practice. As chair of the ANA Congress of Nursing Practice from 1990 to 1994, I led the revision of ANA's *Nursing's Social Policy Statement* (Cronenwett et al., 1995) as we bridged efforts with multiple nursing organizations to move the descriptors of levels of nursing practice from generalist/specialist to basic/advanced. I had to develop new methods of influencing others and hone my listening, communication, and conflict-resolution skills for this politically challenging activity. When it was over, I gave numerous presentations and wrote an article for *Nursing*

Outlook that was reprinted (Cronenwett, 2012b) so that all nurses could ponder the dilemmas we faced and the rationale for the results. I co-led a Josiah Macy Jr. Foundation Conference on primary care (Cronenwett & Dzau, 2010) and coauthored the 2010 *Health Affairs* article that advocated for updating of state licensure laws for APRNs (Pohl, Hanson, Newland, & Cronenwett, 2010). I was dean during the period when nursing organizations decided that the doctorate of nursing practice (DNP) degree should be required for entry into advanced practice. Again, I used publications and presentations to stimulate debate, and an article by six deans has been one of *Nursing Outlook*'s most downloaded since its publication (Cronenwett, Dracup, Grey, et al., 2011). Regrettably (to me), nursing faces a difficult path ahead if we are to ever again meet workforce needs while achieving alignment among licensure, education, and certification of advanced practice.

Outside of running for the ANA Congress of Nursing Practice, where I did have to wave my hand and say, "Pick me," I have usually led at the request of communities and groups I serve. I benefit from extensive networks of leaders upon whom I can call for insight, support, and assistance with strategic thinking. When others value my leadership, they say it is because I show up, prepare well, follow through, discern cutting-edge issues, inspire others to action in person and through publications, and care deeply about nursing and its contributions to better health and health care for all.

Jane H. Barnsteiner, PhD, RN, FAAN

Definition of Leadership

The foundation for my career was set during my first year of nursing practice, when, as a staff nurse in the neonatal intensive-care unit (NICU) at the Children's Hospital of Philadelphia (CHOP), I cared for the first human to receive total parenteral nutrition. While this therapy is commonplace today, in 1967 it was groundbreaking. Working closely together, a finely honed team of physicians and nurses at CHOP, with bench scientists from the University of Pennsylvania, kept a child with very little bowel function alive for 18 months.

What I learned during that experience infused me with an unwavering commitment to two principles: (a) a team working well together can overcome any obstacle; and (b) professional practice has to be evidence based if it is to guide sound decision making, just as research has to have some association with real-life situations if it is to be relevant and helpful. Thus my philosophy can be summed up in two words—*relationships* and *relevance*—which have served as the basis of my definition of leadership.

My definition of leadership evolved over my career to most closely fit the situational leadership model, which calls for using different styles of leadership—directive, coaching, supporting, or delegating—according to the situation. Initially developed by Paul

Hersey (1985) and then popularized by Ken Blanchard, the flexible model calls for assessing people on their competency and commitment and then using one of the four leadership approaches as the situation indicates. An example of using the model was when I was charged by the chief executive officer at CHOP to lead an interdisciplinary quality improvement project on decreasing adverse chemotherapy events. Team members were chosen by top leadership, and none of the team members was enthused about the project or my leadership, as I was not an oncology expert. Initially, my leadership style was directive as the group learned the quality improvement process and I gained the commitment of members to the potential life-saving outcomes of the project. As the team became more knowledgeable and participants began to trust me and to appreciate the benefits of the project, I was able to change my approach to coaching through the process, supporting team members as we conducted tests of change and then delegating the continuation of the initiative to the subject matter experts. An example of our success was the group's enthusiasm for publishing the project work, which has been cited multiple times (Womer et al., 2002).

From 1984, when I completed my PhD in clinical nursing research, through 2011, I was a clinician educator on the standing faculty in the School of Nursing at the University of Pennsylvania (Penn). I was always in a dual role, and from 1984 to 1995, I was the director of nursing practice and research at CHOP, and from 1995 to July 2008, I was the director of nursing translational research at the Hospital of the University of Pennsylvania (HUP). My focus as a clinician educator was grounded in the duality of relationships and relevance, bringing the realities of clinical practice to the learning environment and the scholarship of the academy to the clinical setting. My leadership drew on my expertise as a pediatric nurse, an international expert on patient safety and quality improvement in health care, and an effective champion for translating evidence into practice.

My journey as a leader in education and practice was greatly influenced by Claire Fagin, dean emerita of Penn School of Nursing and former interim president of the university, and by educational theorist Parker Palmer. According to Fagin, nursing is a practice discipline centered on relationship-based care. The relationship between the nurse and the recipient of care—whether it be a patient, family, or community—is the foundation on which healing can occur or change can be accepted. Similarly, the relationship between faculty member and student is an important foundation that is needed if learning is to occur. Having been on the faculty during Fagin's deanship, I learned how the integration of education, research, and clinical care advances the science of nursing, shapes the structure and quality of health care, and provides continuity in patient care and student teaching. From Palmer's writings, I gained appreciation for life as a journey, which if openly taken can lead us to a place where our deep sense of purpose meets society's needs. The matching of my abilities and interests with student, clinician, and societal needs has evolved into a career-long journey that has benefited others while providing me with a tremendously rewarding experience.

Personal Journey as a Leader

My strength as a leader lay in generating new applications and ways of thinking, often creating ripples of change that transformed others' thinking and actions. Several examples are listed below.

On the education of students. I returned to Penn Nursing after completing my doctorate in 1984 as the field of advanced practice nursing was evolving. I identified the need for pediatric nurses to have advanced education in caring for the sickest of the sick newborns and children, and with an award of more than $500,000 from the Division of Nursing, Department of Health and Human Services, I developed the first Pediatric Critical Care Advanced Practice Nursing Program in the world, preparing clinical nurse specialists (CNSs) and nurse practitioners. During the 20 years I directed the program, it grew in stature, attracting students from across the United States and throughout the world. I consulted with many schools of nursing that developed a similar specialty focus, and our graduates went on to work in major children's hospitals across the United States, Thailand, Taiwan, England, Singapore, and Canada.

On quality improvement and patient safety. A major focus of my work on the clinical side related to the quality of patient care and patient safety. In 2004, I instituted a National Patient Safety Conference cosponsored by the School of Nursing and HUP. This annual conference, continuing today, brings cutting-edge knowledge on quality and safety to faculty, students, and clinicians.

In 2005, I developed an interprofessional course, Foundations of Patient Safety, open to undergraduate and graduate students across the university. Reviewing the content covered in our curriculum and that of other schools of nursing on this topic, I realized the content was not diffusing into the curricula of schools of nursing. Thus was born my participation in the QSEN project described at the end of this chapter.

To disseminate the QSEN competencies, RWJF funded me, Joanne Disch, and a core group of others to design a standard curriculum and to hold regional train-the-trainer workshops for faculty from schools of nursing across the country. This work led to multiple publications (Barnsteiner, 2011; Barnsteiner et al., 2013; Disch, Barnsteiner, & McGuinn, 2013) and visiting professorships (a) at Saginaw Valley State University to bring together faculty and leaders in clinical agencies to develop patient safety and quality improvement initiatives and (b) at the University of Hong Kong Department of Nursing, assisting the faculty in developing a pediatric acute care graduate program and integrating evidence-based practice into their pedagogies.

On interprofessional education and collaboration. My teaching and collaborative work at the national level extended beyond the discipline of nursing. I served as a nurse consultant with the American Board of Internal Medicine on the development of competencies and milestones for resident physician education related to quality, safety, and professionalism. I coauthored articles with physician colleagues on chemotherapy safety with

Dr. Rick Womer and colleagues (2002) at CHOP; on instituting a disruptive conduct policy for medical staff with Dr. Thomas Spray and colleagues (Barnsteiner, Madigan, & Spray, 2001) at CHOP; and on both quality improvement and interprofessional education with Dr. Leslie Hall (Barnsteiner, Disch, Hall, Mayer, & Moore, 2007; Hall, Moore, & Barnsteiner, 2008).

On the Professional Practice of Nursing

My leadership extended beyond the university to professional associations, schools of nursing, and clinical settings nationwide. In addition to being a frequently invited keynote speaker and presenter, I was a founding member of the Society of Pediatric Nurses, the only professional nursing organization addressing the health care needs of children and their families. As the editor for translational research and quality assurance for the *American Journal of Nursing*, I ensure publication of sound integrative literature reviews, quality improvement projects, and clinical research results that influence frontline clinicians (Kennedy, Barnsteiner, & Daly, 2014).

On the Professional Practice Environment

A health care culture focused on excellence and world-class patient care requires that nursing research and evidence-based practice are integrated into professional practice models and nursing care delivery. My goal is to fuel a love of knowledge, an enthusiasm for questioning the status quo, and an interest in exploring new approaches to practice based on emerging science and national standards. My work at CHOP and HUP, and consulting with numerous health care executives nationally and internationally, has provided entrée to influence the practice setting and learning environment for clinical nurses.

In summary, the value I placed on relationships and relevance enabled my efforts to improve all aspects of professional commitment—the education of students, the professional practice of nursing, and the quality of the professional practice environment.

Quality and Safety Education for Nurses

A Collective Journey

The leadership skills of the three of us came together in a national initiative to improve the quality and safety competencies of all nurses (and health professionals generally). With the support of 7 years of funding from the Robert Wood Johnson Foundation (2005–2012), QSEN made it possible for leaders to describe quality and safety competencies and specific curricular learning objectives for each competency related to the knowledge, skills, and attitudes needed for both basic and advanced practice. Faculty members in QSEN pilot schools from all types of programs generated teaching strategies, and QSEN faculty and others across the country contributed content for a compendium of faculty resources to support faculty development. Regional train-the-trainer institutes; annual QSEN National Forums where faculty could showcase their innovations; and partnerships involving key regulatory stakeholders, textbook authors and publishers, and interprofessional quality and safety organizations enhanced the spread and penetration of the work (Cronenwett, 2012a). Ten years later, QSEN competencies have been incorporated into curricular frameworks, accreditation criteria, nursing education textbooks, models for new graduate residency programs, and nursing job descriptions and performance appraisals. As QSEN leaders, we have frequently advised leaders of other initiatives on how to make this happen.

Shared Leadership

Many leaders became involved in QSEN over time, but QSEN originated in the Dartmouth Summer Symposiums, where we three were part of a group of 10 nurses regularly invited to participate on topics related to improving the quality of health care through better professional development. Medicine had begun its work to require evidence of quality and safety system competencies, and each summer, we nurses pledged to support each other if anyone could successfully find funding for an initiative in nursing. Not surprisingly, if you read our stories above, the three of us brought our common and individual strengths to these efforts and played central leading roles in this effort that was shared with the profession at large.

We shared a commitment to improving patient care, improving system performance, and improving professional development. Jane consistently led across these domains, while Joanne and Linda led in each domain, though not always at the same time. We also shared a history of professional organizational leadership throughout our careers and thus had deep networks on which to draw when it came to linking QSEN work to nursing licensure, accreditation, and certification. Whenever we asked the "leaders and best" in nursing to take part in QSEN in some way, they always said yes. Finally, we were all nurse leaders who spanned boundaries across professions to contribute to quality and safety initiatives. Thus we were linked into the larger health care quality improvement initiatives of which QSEN was a part. We benefited from the thinking of other disciplines—and vice versa, as QSEN objectives for knowledge, skills, and attitudes were adopted by interprofessional groups.

In terms of the individual strengths we brought to QSEN, Jane was the pioneer in developing a course on the foundations of patient safety and could provide firsthand inspiration with stories from what she learned. She inspired QSEN pilot school faculties and their clinical partners by being an exemplar from both worlds and co-led the curricular development portion of the regional train-the-trainer institutes with Joanne and the American Association of Colleges of Nursing. During QSEN's last phase, Jane coedited the first major textbook, *Quality and Safety Education in Nursing* (Sherwood & Barnsteiner, 2012). Her *relationships and relevance* core values were embedded in her work.

Linda was the leader who successfully developed the program officer relationships and grant proposals that led to RWJF funding for QSEN. Concurrently with QSEN, Linda was serving on the Institute for Healthcare Improvement's (IHI) board of directors and benefited from IHI's experiences in finding that effective leaders of large-scale change understood the difference between simply raising awareness and ensuring broad-scale implementation of a change. IHI recommended, and QSEN was built to attend to, three major streams: build will, generate a supply of ideas for change, and attend to the skills needed for a day-to-day execution of change (McCannon, Berwick, & Massoud, 2007). Linda enhanced our use of theories of large-scale change in planning, implementing, and disseminating QSEN work. She edited the two special issues of *Nursing Outlook* in 2007 and 2009 that laid out the rationale and framework for the work to be done. She also set the tone as principal investigator for sharing leadership and credit for QSEN accomplishments among QSEN leaders, the leaders of nursing's professional regulatory bodies, and nurse-educator innovators nationwide.

During the QSEN years, Joanne was leading in the Dartmouth Summer Symposium, the AARP board, and as president-elect and president of the American Academy of Nursing (AAN). She was the thought leader for the work on the QSEN competency on teamwork and collaboration, in keeping with her leadership and lived values of boundary spanning and interprofessional activities, and contributed to numerous publications and presentations. The collaboration with AACN during the broad-scale faculty development phase was enhanced by her relationships across leading professional organizations, and she used her presidency of AAN to write editorials related to QSEN (Disch, 2012). Joanne's special ability to inspire and mentor attracted faculty members to be "QSENistas"—a label that has lasted now through seven QSEN National Forums. Her motto to "work hard, play hard, rest hard" was embraced by QSEN Faculty and Advisory Board members, resulting in a special camaraderie that made our work fun as well as meaningful.

Conclusion

As three alumnae from the University of Michigan's doctoral program, we forged personal relationships as we studied together for our doctorates in the early years of the School of Nursing's doctoral program. What we learned about leadership and scholarship led to numerous contributions to the profession and society at large. Thirty years later, we collaborated in the leadership of a national initiative, Quality and Safety Education for

Nurses. The impact of this QSEN initiative on improving care, health care system performance, and professional development is one of the many proud legacies of the University of Michigan alumni.

References

Barnsteiner, J., Madigan, C., & Spray, T. (2001). Instituting a disruptive conduct policy for medical staff. *AACN Clinical Issues, 12*(3), 378–382.

Barnsteiner, J., Disch, J., Hall, H., Mayer, D., & Moore, S. (2007). Interprofessional education: It can't be left to chance. *Nursing Outlook, 55,* 144–150.

Barnsteiner, J. (2011). Teaching the culture of safety. *Online Journal of Issues in Nursing, 16*(3), 1.

Barnsteiner, J., Disch, J., Johnson, J., McGuinn, K., Chapell, K., & Swartout, E. (2013). Diffusing QSEN competencies across schools of nursing: The AACN/RWJF Faculty Development Institutes. *Journal of Professional Nursing, 29*(2), 68–74.

Batalden, P., & Gordon, T. (Eds.). (2012). *Sustainably improving health care: Creatively linking care outcomes, system performance, and professional development.* London: Radcliffe Publishing.

Boyer, E. L. (1990). *Scholarship reconsidered: Priorities of the professoriate.* Stanford, CA: Carnegie Foundation for the Advancement of Teaching.

Cronenwett, L. (2012a). A national initiative: Quality and safety education for nurses (QSEN). In G. Sherwood & J. Barnsteiner (Eds.), *Quality and safety in nursing: A competency approach to improving outcomes* (pp. 49–64). Hoboken, NJ: Wiley-Blackwell.

Cronenwett, L. R. (2012b). Molding the future of advanced practice nursing [Originally published in 1995; Reprinted in Nursing Outlook's Special 60th Anniversary Issue with commentary]. *Nursing Outlook, 60*(5), 241–249.

Cronenwett, L., Dracup, K., Grey, M., McCauley, L., Meleis, M., & Salmon, M. (2011). The doctor of nursing practice: A national workforce perspective. *Nursing Outlook, 59*(1), 9–17.

Cronenwett, L., & Dzau, V. (2010). In B. Culliton & S. Russell (Eds.), *Who will provide primary care and how will they be trained?* Proceedings of a Conference Sponsored by the Josiah Macy, Jr. Foundation. New York, NY: Josiah Macy, Jr. Foundation. Retrieved from http://www.macyfoundation.org/docs/macy_pubs/JMF_PrimaryCare_Monograph.pdf

Cronenwett, L. R., Pokorny, B. E., Barnard, K., Doughty, S. E., Hall, B., Harkness, G. A., . . . Walker, M. K. (1995). *Nursing's social policy statement.* Washington, DC: American Nurses Publishing.

DePree, M. (1989). *Leadership is an art.* New York, NY: Dell Publishing.

Disch, J. (2009). Generative leadership. *Creative Nursing, 15*(4), 172–177.

Disch, J. (2012). QSEN? What's QSEN? *Nursing Outlook, 60*(2), 58–59.

Disch, J., Barnsteiner, J., & McGuinn, K. (2013). Taking a "Deep Dive" on integrating QSEN content in San Francisco Bay Area schools of nursing. *Journal of Professional Nursing, 29*(2), 75–81.

Hall, L., Moore, S., & Barnsteiner, J. (2008). Quality and nursing: Moving from a concept to a core competency. *Urologic Nursing, 28*(6), 417–430.

Hersey, P. (1985). *The situational leader.* New York, NY: Warner Books.

Kennedy, M. S., Barnsteiner, J., & Daly, J. (2014). Honorary and ghost authorship in nursing publications. *Journal of Nursing Scholarship, 46*(6), 416–422.

McCannon, C. J., Berwick, D. M., & Massoud, M. R. (2007). The science of large-scale change in global health. *JAMA, 298*(16), 937–1939. doi:10.1001/jama.298.16.1937

Neuman, B., Newman, D. M. L., & Holder, P. (2000). Leadership-scholarship integration: Using the Neuman Systems Model for 21st-century professional nursing practice. *Nursing Science Quarterly, 13*(1), 60–63.

Pohl, J. M., Hanson, C., Newland, J. A., & Cronenwett, L. (2010). Unleashing nurse practitioners' potential to deliver primary care and lead teams. *Health Affairs, 29*(5), 900–905.

Porter-O'Grady, T., & Malloch, K. (2016). *Leadership in nursing practice: Changing the landscape of health care* (2nd ed.). Burlington, MA: Jones & Bartlett Learning.

Sherwood, G., & Barnsteiner, J. (Eds.). (2012). *Quality and safety in nursing: A competency-based approach to improving outcomes.* Hoboken, NJ: Wiley-Blackwell.

Velsor, E. V., McCauley, C. D., & Ruderman, M. N. (Eds.). (2010). *The Center for Creative Leadership handbook of leadership development* (3rd. ed.). San Francisco, CA: Jossey-Bass.

Walker, G. E., Golde, C. M., Jones, L., Bueschel, A. C., & Hutchings, P. (2008). *The formation of scholars: Rethinking doctoral education for the twenty-first century.* Stanford, CA: Carnegie Foundation for the Advancement of Teaching.

Wheatley, M. (1992). *Leadership and the new science.* San Francisco, CA: Berrett-Koehler Publishers.

Womer, R. B., Tracy, E., Soo-Hoo, W., Bickert, B., DiTaronto, S., & Barnsteiner, J. H. (2002). Multidisciplinary systems approach to chemotherapy safety: Rebuilding processes and holding the gains. *Journal of Clinical Oncology, 20*(24), 4705–4712.

CHAPTER 13

Commentary on Leadership Papers

Kathleen Potempa, PhD, RN, FAAN

In 2017, the University of Michigan, founded in 1817, will enter its third century. Now housing 19 colleges and research units at the Ann Arbor campus, the university most often characterizes itself as having both breadth and depth of academic strength. Among other factors that set Michigan apart is its interdisciplinarity stemming from this breadth and depth. In review of the two chapters by four University of Michigan School of Nursing doctor of philosophy (PhD) alumni ("Innovation Leadership" by Pesut and "Leadership as Scholarship" by Disch, Cronenwett, and Barnsteiner), the academic context of Michigan—the "Michigan Difference"—is apparent in their development as leaders and scholars.

Pesut describes working with Jean Wood as his early mentor, but he also worked with colleagues and faculty from psychology, the Institute for Social Research, and the Neuropsychiatric Institute at Michigan. The theoretical framework he developed and used in later work drew from nursing, psychology, psychiatry, and other social sciences, including related research methodologies. Similarly, Disch, Cronenwett, and Barnsteiner talk about working with fellow doctoral students in nursing and other departments in the development of their ideas and research. The interdisciplinary context of Michigan as the backdrop and foundation of doctoral education is evident in the descriptions these authors offer of their early scholarly development. The hallmark of the Michigan PhD is that it brings about collaboration and creative endeavors among a diverse group of disciplines and schools of thought.

Another characteristic of the School of Nursing at Michigan is that it encourages independent thinking in the creation of models, frameworks, and approaches to discovery, knowledge, and research. Never describing itself as ascribing to a particular school of thought, it has produced scholars with a range of interests and paradigms. The diversity of perspectives is reflected in Pesut, who conceived of a cognitive/reflective model of leadership as a "thought process" that influences behavior and action (e.g., nursing practice). The impact of his work is seen in the volume of writing and in the education of many doctoral students in the framework of discovery and innovation.

Disch, influenced by the work of Wheatley and others, describes leadership as "relational" in terms of enhancing others and the work group rather than being autocratic.

Disch is and has been a leader of action. Serving in many leadership capacities in universities, institutes, boards, and associations, she has lived the scholarship of relational leadership through her actions. Through the years, Disch has demonstrated the basic principle that "leadership is a form of scholarship that helps us 'move into the future'" (see Chapter 12). Her participation in the development and leadership of Quality and Safety Education for Nurses (QSEN) illustrates the futuristic view as one of the first recognized efforts to focus on the quality and safety of nursing practice.

Cronenwett, who is also action oriented, focuses on the outcomes of leadership. Through her early leadership experiences as a navy officer and her years of experience at Dartmouth as a leader of a large health care organization, Cronenwett uses the framework of setting direction, alignment, and maintaining commitment in influencing organizations. Also a major leader of QSEN, Cronenwett has used her writing, her organizational leadership experience, and her commitment to sustaining progress to "turn the head of the field" toward patient outcomes.

Finally, Barnsteiner describes one of her early influences, the situational leadership model, which emphasizes *relationship* and *relevance* as key factors in leadership. Barnsteiner has demonstrated the impact of her scholarship through the advancement of pediatric advanced practice and education based on these principles. Her leadership was visionary in that she developed a program for the future based on her understanding of the relevance of advanced practice in the evolving health care needs of children and systems. Also a QSEN leader, Barnsteiner made the work relevant to the care of children in the evolving context of knowledge and health care.

"Leaders and best" are words synonymous with Michigan and its School of Nursing. The pathways described in these manuscripts by Pesut and Disch, Cronenwett, and Barnsteiner reflect a grounding in the breadth and depth of multiple disciplinary influences and relationships developed during their PhD education at Michigan. The pathways chosen also illustrate that relationships so constructed in the Michigan context of learning create lifelong synergies that enhance creativity, innovation, and leadership enactment. Whether through writing, organizational leadership, or educating future generations of leaders, the authors have continued to expand and grow networks of leaders. These Michigan PhDs have refocused nursing, which is historically process oriented, on creating better patient outcomes.

Going Forward

The papers presented herein provide a small glimpse of the contributions to leadership, theory, and practice by a sample of the School of Nursing's esteemed PhD alumni. As is true of history, we should build upon and learn from our past as we remain poised for the future. The challenges of today and tomorrow are inevitably different from the challenges and contexts that influenced our alumni. Today, significant national driving influences include the call for health care reform, a need to provide more with fewer financial resources in both higher education and health care, sociopolitical tensions that are polarizing rather than uniting, and a global context that poses both opportunities and significant challenges.

In terms of health care reform, nursing was front and center in the landmark Institute of Medicine report *The Future of Nursing* (IOM, 2010). The results of the first 5 years of activity to meet the goals proposed in the report were documented and evaluated in the 2015 follow-up report (IOM, 2015). While some goals have been met and many are on the way toward significant improvement, there remain many gaps in achieving the Institute of Medicine's vision. For example, the doctor of nursing practice degree student population is expanding, while the production of research doctoral trainees has had only modest increases since 2004 (Redman, Pressler, Furspan, & Potempa, 2015). A future challenge is not only to expand the educational preparation of nurses but to utilize the graduates in ways that enhance health care quality, accelerate research, and drive innovation.

Competition among health professionals to "seize the day" in leading health care reform and expanding professional services provides challenges and opportunities to consider. While nursing has been in the vanguard of health promotion and prevention, advanced practice nurses continue to focus on practice expansion around diagnosis and pharmaceutical interventions. That focus has been and will remain a valuable tool to expand access to quality health care, yet there is vast unmet need in developing healthy behaviors among individuals and communities that do not require medically ordained services and interventions. Nursing leadership in these areas will require a much stronger voice and a willingness to develop evidence-based and sustainable models of prevention services. There is much that nurses can do in communities, and entrepreneurial approaches might provide avenues for new service delivery.

Innovation in care, educational models, and research will also require a sense of cost-conscious practicality. Solutions to emerging issues will need to be affordable, accessible to a broad public, and adaptable in the context of rapidly changing technology. How are we helping our students to develop in an era ripe for innovation, entrepreneurship, and rapid change? Perhaps one of our most compelling challenges is preparing nurses at all levels of education for this era, already upon us, of rapid change.

We can find the wisdom and courage to make change from the leaders of our Michigan history who drove innovations, created change despite resistance, and led the way with clarity and purpose. The salient message from the examples of leadership provided is that "we can and we must." The Michigan heritage is that we step up: We find new pathways, find new solutions, and take up the challenges that confront us.

References

Institute of Medicine. (2010). *The future of nursing: Leading change, advancing health.* Washington, DC: National Academies Press.

Institute of Medicine. (2015). *Assessing progress on the Institute of Medicine Report: The future of nursing.* Washington, DC: National Academies Press.

Redman, R. W., Pressler, S., Furspan, P., & Potempa, K. (2015). Nurses in the U.S. with a practice doctorate: Implications for leading in the current context of health care. *Nursing Outlook, 63*(2), 124–129.

Short Papers Submitted for Chapters 1–6

SHORT PAPERS SUBMITTED FOR CHAPTER 1

Hala Darwish
Donna McCarthy
Brenda K. (Smith) Richards

Cognitive and Behavioral Neuroscience Research

Hala Darwish, PhD, RN

Study and understanding of cognitive function—such as learning and memory and the biological, social, behavioral, and environmental factors that may lead to its impairment or enhancement—are the focus of my nursing research program. This area of study falls under biobehavioral nursing. Nursing care is holistic; thus the different interactions among all factors and influences that impact a complex mechanism such as cognitive function ought to be thoroughly studied, understood, and controlled for the effective delivery of full nursing care.

During my doctoral education at the University of Michigan School of Nursing (UMSN), I have utilized neuroscience knowledge and basic science research skills to answer my dissertation questions that emanated from my nursing clinical observations.

In my dissertation, I conducted series of experiments using a rat model of head injury and examined the effect of traumatic brain injury of mild to moderate intensity on different memory functions, such as recognition and spatial learning. Two different treatment modalities were tested: environmental enrichment and simvastatin. The results showed that traumatic brain injury of mild to moderate intensity leads to persistent cognitive deficit up to 35 days postinjury in the rat. These spatial learning and object recognition memory deficits are associated with impairment at the synaptic level as well. In addition, these deficits benefited from both pharmacological and behavioral interventions (Darwish, Mahmood, Schallert, Chopp, & Therrien, 2012; Darwish, Mahmood, Schallert, Chopp, & Therrien, 2014). This concurs with patients' self-reported memory deficits that persist up to 1 year or more postinjury. Moreover, it puts emphasis on the role of nurses in coordinating both physical and cognitive rehabilitation after traumatic brain injury.

Later, during my postdoctoral training, my mentor and I explored the effect of vitamin D supplementation on cognitive function and inflammatory responses in aged animals; the results suggested that vitamin D supplementation lessened age-related memory impairment and led to a decrease in proinflammatory levels and amyloid burden in the brains of the aged animals. This indicated that vitamin D might be a useful therapeutic option to alleviate the effects of aging on cognitive function (Briones & Darwish, 2012). Therefore, when I joined the American University of Beirut (AUB) as an assistant professor, my interest in vitamin D deficiency as a contributing factor to cognitive impairment continued, and I pursued it using clinical research methods, especially when I realized that vitamin D deficiency is surprisingly prevalent among the Lebanese. I continued the same line of research, and I conducted a study about the vitamin D levels and cognitive performance in adults and older adults. Just as in rats, lower serum 25 hydroxyvitamin D was associated with impaired cognitive performance in adults and older adults (Darwish et al., 2015). Given the increased prevalence of vitamin D insufficiency in Lebanon, this has an impact on clinical practice; the need to correct and supplement vitamin D early on as a measure to strengthen cognitive performance was recommended.

The biobehavioral nursing approach is interdisciplinary by nature and requires collaborations with different fields of medicine, basic science, and health sciences for successful clinical outcomes. In 2011, I was appointed as managing director of the Abu Haidar Neuroscience Institute and the Nehme and Therese Tohme Multiple Sclerosis (MS) Center at the AUB Medical Center. Interestingly, the evidence was mounting showing that MS is affected by vitamin D levels and also has cognitive impairment sequelae. At the MS center, I was involved in research looking at risk factors associated with MS, such as age, smoking and low vitamin D, and the Epstein-Barr virus, in addition to facilitating and supervising the research of graduate students from various faculties at AUB and other universities in Lebanon—for instance, in the Departments of Public Health and Psychology (Mouhieddine et al., 2015; Fawaz et al., 2015; Farran, Ammar, & Darwish, 2016). I also have partaken in a clinical trial to collect cognitive data on a group of MS patients before and after vitamin D supplementation. The results of this study showed that vitamin D predicts cognitive performance in patients with MS and that vitamin D supplementation improves cognitive performance (research in progress). The results of this clinical trial were recently presented at the European Committee for Treatment and Research in Multiple Sclerosis and Society for Neuroscience annual meetings, and the results of this clinical trial were recently presented at the European Committee for Treatment and Research in Multiple Sclerosis and Society for Neuroscience annual meetings; the results were featured online on *Medpagetoday* (http://www.medpagetoday.com/MeetingCoverage/SFN/54172).

Studying cognitive performance in Lebanon is necessary. With my collaborators from the Faculty of Health Sciences and the Faculty of Medicine (Gerontology), we have recently been awarded a grant to conduct a systematic cohort study of dementia among older adults who will be recruited and assessed for a more accurate detection and prevalence measure of dementia in the Lebanese community. Our long-term goal is to establish the first community-based cohort study to improve our understanding of dementia risk and etiology and provide knowledge of caregivers' burden and health status.

Since my return to Lebanon from the United States, validating the cognitive assessment tools in Arabic has been a priority. I am currently working on a project that aims to validate the Brief International Cognitive Assessment for MS (BICAMS) in Arabic. The tool's reliability and validity will be measured, and the normative values for each test will be determined for use in screening and follow-up. This will allow more accurate clinical practice and research utilizations of these measures in the Arab world.

Along the same line, more experiments focusing on therapeutic interventions—such as environmental enrichment, vitamin D, and possible drug trials to improve learning and memory following traumatic brain injury in small animals—are under way.

In my role as managing director of the Neuroscience Institute and the MS center, I am involved in managing the MS center's staff and supervising daily operations, as well as coordinating the neuroscience outpatient center patient care and training of nurses in the area of multiple sclerosis and outpatient neuroscience nursing. In this role, I serve as a resource to the nurses and patients to eliminate barriers to operative work performance. I have coordinated the training of Lebanese and Iraqi physicians and nurses in the area of multiple sclerosis nursing and have emphasized the role of nurses in caring for patients with MS. Moreover, I oversee and guide the neuroscience unit clinical educators to ensure they are all trained to provide the best, evidence-based nursing care.

Before completing my PhD, I finished my master's degree as an acute care nurse practitioner at UMSN, which has given me the needed clinical skills to perform as an advanced nurse and supervise the clinical nursing performance at the MS center and the neuroscience outpatient center. I am also involved in the teaching, clinical training, and supervision of graduate students in the adult track at the AUB School of Nursing, especially those interested in neuroscience nursing.

In the early course of my graduate studies, I was introduced to cognitive neuroscience and was familiarized with several types of research methods, clinical and basic science. As a graduate research assistant at UMSN, I learned how to conduct clinical research trials. Though the research trial I was part of was not directly related to my field of study, it was an opportunity to advance my knowledge of the methods of conducting nursing clinical research and to later utilize the information in developing my current research program. The work then involved many tasks necessary for successfully conducting clinical trials, which ranged from subject recruitment, to retention techniques, to data collection and communication with the institutional review board.

My nursing doctorate study of neuroscience was my introduction to basic science research. I trained in two different laboratories at the University of Michigan and learned new laboratory techniques. These techniques ranged from handling animals, such as mice and rats, to immunohistochemistry and in-situ hybridization. Moreover, I did behavioral testing to measure different cognitive and affective functions in animals, such as spatial memory (Morris water maze) and anxiety (elevated plus maze). Because of this intensive training and mentorship by several principal investigators, I was able to adopt novel techniques of behavioral tests and introduce them in the clinical and laboratory settings where I conducted my dissertation experiments, postdoctoral research, and academic research.

The mastery of several research techniques and methods allowed me to examine the factors leading to impairment and improvement of learning and memory over time at a behavioral and molecular level and build my ongoing research program.

References

Briones, T. L., & Darwish, H. (2012). Vitamin D mitigates age-related cognitive decline through the modulation of pro-inflammatory state and decrease in amyloid burden. *Journal of Neuroinflammation, 9*(1), 244–257.

Darwish, H., Mahmood, A., Schallert, T., Chopp, M., & Therrien, B. (2012). Mild traumatic brain injury (MTBI) leads to spatial learning deficits. *Brain Injury, 26*(2), 151–165.

Darwish, H., Mahmood, A., Schallert, T., Chopp, M., & Therrien, B. (2014). Simvastatin and environmental enrichment effect on recognition and temporal order memory after mild-to-moderate traumatic brain injury. *Brain Injury, 28*(2), 211–226.

Darwish, H., Zeinoun, P., Ghusn, P., Khoury, B., Tamim, H., & Khoury, S. J. (2015). Serum 25-hydroxyvitamin D predicts cognitive performance in adults. *Journal of Neuropsychiatric Disease and Treatment, 11*, 2217–2223.

Farran, N., Ammar, D., & Darwish, H. (2016). Quality of life and coping strategies in Lebanese multiple sclerosis patients: A pilot study. *Multiple Sclerosis and Related Disorders, 6*, 21–27.

Fawaz, C., Makki, S., Kazan, J., Gebara, N., Andary, F., Itani, M., . . . Mondello, S. (2015). Neuroproteomics and miRNAS in multiple sclerosis: Transforming research and clinical knowledge. *Expert Review in Proteomics, 12*(6), 637–650.

Mouhieddine, T. H., Darwish, H., Fawaz, L., Yamout, B., Tamim, H., & Khoury, S. J. (2015). Risk factors for multiple sclerosis and associations with anti-EBV antibody titers. *Clinical Immunology, 158*(1), 59–66.

Untangling the Biology of Sickness Symptoms

Donna McCarthy, PhD, RN, FAAN

My program of research seeks to understand the pathobiology of sickness symptoms. My doctoral work at the University of Michigan (1981–1985) was directed by Dr. Charlotte Mistretta (Nursing) and Dr. Matthew Kluger (Physiology). My dissertation research used an animal model to study the association between fever and anorexia during infection and was funded by the Rackham Graduate School, the National Institutes of Health (NIH) (F31), and the American Nurses Foundation. Findings suggested that fever did not contribute to the loss of appetite, and both were mediated by a small protein produced by activated leukocytes, later identified by Dr. Kluger and others as interleukin-1 (IL-1). These findings suggested that anorexia was part of the acute phase response to infection. (Sample publication[s] are presented for each section of this brief. The list is intended as illustrative only.)

- McCarthy, D. O., Kluger, J. J., & Vander, A. J. (1984). The role of fever in appetite suppression following endotoxin administration. *American Journal of Clinical Nutrition, 40*, 310–316.

My postdoctoral study at the University of Rochester, New York (1985–1987), was supervised by Dr. Norbert Roberts (Medicine) and Dr. Jean Johnson (Nursing) and funded by an award from the Robert Wood Johnson Clinical Nurse Scholars Program. My project focused on understanding why influenza infection conferred immunity to the virus, while infection with respiratory syncytial virus (RSV) did not. We found that leukocytes exposed to RSV produced an inhibitor of IL-1, which prevents activation of the immune response to the virus. There are now two known inhibitors of IL-1 activity—namely, IL-1 receptor antagonist and IL-1 soluble receptors.

- Salkind, A. R., McCarthy, D. O., Nichols, J. E., Domurat, F. M., Walsh, E. E., & Roberts, Jr., N. J. (1991). Interleukin-1 inhibitor activity induced by respiratory syncytial virus: Abrogation of virus-specific and alternative human lymphocyte responses. *Journal of Infectious Disease, 163*, 71–77.

In 1987, I took a position at the University of Wisconsin–Madison, where I used an animal model to study symptoms of cancer and cancer treatment, focusing first on anorexia and weight loss. Early work demonstrated that appetite reduction after injection with IL-1 was associated with gastroparesis and increased plasma levels of cholecystokinin, a hormone that affects gastric emptying after meals. We also demonstrated that weight loss occurred in association with increased expression of IL-1 in animals with various tumors that did or did not induce weight loss. However, we found that it was not possible to increase food intake or total caloric intake of tumor-bearing rats. This work was funded by the American Institute for Cancer Research and the National Institute of Nursing Research (NINR) (R29, R03). In another study, funded by Sigma Theta Tau, we demonstrated that nutritional supplements only marginally improved food intake, but did not prevent weight loss, during radiotherapy for cancer. These experiments demonstrated that anorexia is a regulated or defended response to tumor growth, not due solely to the effects of cancer treatment.

- McCarthy, D. O., & Daun, J. M. (1992). The role of gastric stasis in tumor-induced anorexia in rats. *Cancer, 70*, 1601–1604.

- McCarthy, D., & Weihofen, D. (1999). The effect of nutritional supplements on the food intake of radiotherapy patients. *Oncology Nursing Forum, 26,* 897–900.

Similarly, my doctoral student, Terry Lennie, who is presently a professor and associate dean for PhD studies at the University of Kentucky, demonstrated that weight loss after traumatic injury is also a regulated response that is affected by preinjury body mass. His work was funded by an NIH predoctoral fellowship (F31).

- Lennie, T. A., McCarthy, D. O., & Keesey, R. E. (1995). Relationship of body energy status and the metabolic response to injury. *American Journal of Physiology, 269,* R1024–R1031.

In 2000, I began to study muscle wasting in a mouse model of cancer-related fatigue. My doctoral student, Sadeeka Al-Majid, who is presently a professor at California State University–Fullerton, demonstrated that loss of muscle mass could be prevented with resistance exercise. Her work was funded by the Oncology Nurses Foundation. We went on to show that anti-inflammatory drugs could reduce muscle wasting in tumor-bearing mice. I continued this research as a visiting scientist in the intramural program of the National Institute of Nursing Research.

- Al-Majid, S., & McCarthy, D. O. (2001). Resistance exercise training attenuates wasting of the EDL muscle in mice bearing the Colon-26 adenocarcinoma. *Biological Research for Nursing, 2,* 155–166.
- Hitt, A., Graves, E., & McCarthy, D. O. (2005). Indomethacin preserves muscle mass and reduces levels of E3 ligases and TNF receptor type 1 in the gastrocnemius muscle of tumor-bearing mice. *Research in Nursing & Health, 28,* 56–66.

In 2007, I became the associate dean for research at the Ohio State University College of Nursing. I continued to study the pathobiology of cancer-related fatigue and found that myocardial muscle was also affected by tumor growth, producing a decline in systolic function that was associated with reduced exercise tolerance of the tumor-bearing mice. We went on to show that treatment with a drug commonly used to treat heart failure would improve myocardial function and preserve muscle mass in the tumor-bearing mice, but it did not improve voluntary exercise of the tumor-bearing mice.

- Stevens, S. C., Velten, M., Clark, Y., Jing, R., Reiser, P. J., Bicer, S., Devine, R. D., McCarthy, D. O., & Wold, L. E. (2015). Losartan treatment attenuates tumor-induced myocardial dysfunction. *Journal of Molecular and Cellular Cardiology, 85,* 37–47.

We thus began to explore the occurrence of depression in our mouse model of cancer-related fatigue. This work was funded by the Oncology Nurses Foundation and the NINR (R15, R01). We found that depression-like behaviors precede fatigue-like behaviors; a drug that blocked cytokine production reduced depression-like behaviors but did not improve muscle mass or fatigue behaviors. Treatment with an antidepressant drug also reduced depression-like behavior without affecting cytokine production. Lastly, treatment with an anti-inflammatory drug improved both depression and fatigue-like behaviors and reduced cytokine production. We are currently conducting experiments to determine if aerobic exercise will reduce muscle wasting and depression-like behaviors in our mouse model of cancer-related fatigue.

- Norden, D. M., Bicer, S., Clark, Y., Jing, R., Henry, C. J., Wold, L. E., Reiser, P. J., Godbout, J. P., & McCarthy, D. O. (2014). Tumor growth increases neuroinflammation, fatigue and depressive-like behavior prior to alterations in muscle function, *Brain, Behavior & Immunity, 43*, 76–85.

During my postdoctoral study in New York, I came to know the work of Drs. Robert Ader and Nicholas Cohen, two pioneers in the area of psychoneuroendocrinology—the effects of the stress response on immune cell function. At the University of Wisconsin–Madison, I continued to look at stress and immune function with graduate students, particularly with Duck-Hee Kang, who went on to become the Lee and Joseph D. Jamail Distinguished Professor at the University of Texas Health Science Center at Houston. This work was funded by Sigma Theta Tau International, the American Lung Association of Wisconsin, and an NINR predoctoral fellowship (F31).

- Kang, D-H., Coe, C. L., McCarthy, D. O. (1996). Academic examinations significantly impact immune responses, but not lung function, in healthy and well-managed asthmatic adolescents. *Brain, Behavior, and Immunity, 10*, 164–181.
- Sribanditmongkol, S., Neal, J. L., Szalacha, L. A., & McCarthy, D. O. (2015). Effect of perceived stress on cytokine production in healthy college students. *Western Journal of Nursing Research, 37*, 481–493.

Discovering the Genetics of Diet Preference

Carbohydrates Versus Fats

Brenda K. (Smith) Richards, PhD

The aim of my research program is to identify genetic determinants of macronutrient selection and total energy intake, eating behaviors that are fundamental to the development of obesity phenotypes. Eating behaviors involving appetites for fat-, carbohydrate-, or protein-rich foods are influenced by an array of molecular signals throughout the body, including those involved in neural and metabolic processes. Despite growing evidence for a strong genetic influence on food choices in both children and adults, the specific genes that encode these molecular signals and contribute to macronutrient-specific appetites are virtually unknown. Using molecular genetic methods, it is possible to identify specific genes that contribute to individual differences in food preferences. Understanding the biological processes that bring about macronutrient selection and ensuring that those choices are healthy are critical for addressing the epidemics of obesity, diabetes, and cardiovascular disease.

Our early work discovered key evidence that macronutrient selection is a quantitative or complex genetic trait—that is, it is measurable in nature and continuous in distribution, reflecting the actions of numerous genes and the environment. First, we developed an experimental model system for measuring macronutrient selection in mice, in which animals compose their own diet while choosing among individual sources of fat, carbohydrate, and protein. Next, we evaluated a dozen mouse inbred strains and discovered that proportional fat intake was continuously distributed, ranging widely from 26% to 83% of total energy (Smith, Andrews, & West, 2000; see Figure 1-a), suggesting a quantitative trait. Complementary studies showed that this macronutrient selection phenotype in selected mouse inbred strains generalized across a variety of experimental diet paradigms, indicating a robust model for investigation. These findings established that macronutrient selection is a complex trait, amenable to genetic analysis, and enabled us to identify a suitable model: two inbred strains that exhibit markedly different preferences for eating fat- versus carbohydrate-rich diets.

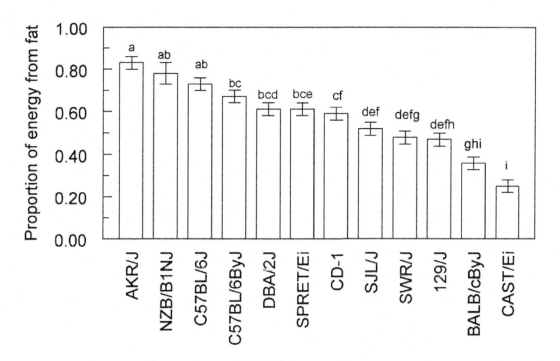

Proportional fat intake (mean ± SE) of 12 mouse strains self-selecting from separate macro-nutrient sources of fat, carbohydrate, and protein. Values were derived based on total calorie intake from day 12 to the end of the 4-week study. Values without common letters are significantly different at $p < 0.05$.

Figure 1-a. Natural variation in self-selected fat intake across 12 mouse strains.
Smith, B. K. et al. (2000). *American Journal of Physiology—Regulatory, Integrative and Comparative Physiology, 278*(4), R797–R805. © 2000 by American Physiological Society.

Continuing the work described above, we intercrossed two inbred strains of fat-preferring (C57BL/6J) and carbohydrate-preferring (CAST/EiJ) mice and evaluated their second-generation offspring (F2 animals) for macronutrient selection. A genome-wide scan conducted in the F2 population found nine quantitative trait loci (QTL) where a section of DNA (the locus or genotype) was highly significantly correlated with variation in the quantitative trait or phenotype (Smith Richards et al., 2002). We discovered QTL for the preferential intake of fat kcal on chromosomes 8, 18, and X; the preferential intake of carbohydrate kcal on chromosomes 6, 17, and X; and total kcal intake (adjusted for body weight) on chromosomes 17 and 18. An additional locus for total kcal intake was identified on chromosome 2, which was body weight dependent. These results constitute strong evidence for multiple genetic controls on total energy and macronutrient-specific intakes. Subsequent work focused on the region encompassing chromosome 17 QTL *Mnic1* (macronutrient intake-carbohydrate) and *Kcal2* (kilocalorie intake). First, we validated that the *Mnic1/Kcal2* QTL specified the original linked traits using a congenic strain generated in our laboratory through breeding and genotyping strategies. This congenic strain (B6.CAST-17.1) possesses a differential DNA segment (encompassing the *Mnic1/Kcal2* QTL region) of the carbohydrate-preferring CAST/EiJ strain, introgressed on the genetic background of the second, fat-preferring strain (C67BL/6J). This new congenic strain ate 30% more carbohydrate and 10% more total calories per body weight, yet similar amounts of fat, compared to the genetic background control (Kumar, DiCarlo, Volaufova, Zuberi, & Smith Richards, 2010). Thus, by transferring a small region of chromosome 17 DNA from CAST mice, we changed the fat-preferring C57BL/6J strain into a carbohydrate-preferring strain and confirmed that the differential chromosome 17 segment contains a gene(s) responsible for the genetic determination of these traits. Recently, we narrowed and precisely localized the causative interval to a 19.0 Mb region using high-resolution genetic fine-mapping techniques in a subcongenic-derived F2 mapping population (Gularte-Mérida et al., 2014). Notably, no genetic linkage for fat intake was detected for this region, clearly emphasizing the carbohydrate-specific effects of this locus. By combining sequence analyses, gene ontologies, comprehensive expression profiling, and functional studies, we have identified several highly plausible candidate genes, located within the fine-mapped QTL region, that are expressed in trait-relevant tissues such as the hypothalamus and stomach (e.g., see Gularte-Mérida et al., 2014, and Kumar et al., 2008). By determining the causative DNA variation underlying preferential carbohydrate and total calorie intake in this animal model, we will improve our understanding of the genetic factors influencing food preferences in humans.

My laboratory is also investigating the role of fat oxidation in the metabolic control of fat intake and fat preference. Overall, our work addresses the novel proposition that loss of a specific enzyme in the mitochondrial beta oxidation of fatty acids alters macronutrient selection/intake. This is based on our finding that mice with a complete genetic inactivation of *Acads*, encoding short-chain acyl-CoA dehydrogenase (SCAD), shift food consumption away from fat and toward carbohydrate when offered a choice between macronutrient-rich diets, while maintaining total energy intake that is equivalent to that of wild-type controls (Smith Richards, Belton, York, & Volaufova, 2004). These results suggest a mechanism for metering small changes in available energy from the diet. To our knowledge, this is the first report of an alteration in eating behavior associated with deficiencies in the acyl-CoA dehydrogenases. Our further results suggest hypothalamic AMP-kinase as the cellular energy sensor linking impaired fat oxidation to feeding behavior in this model (Kruger, Kumar, Mynatt, Volaufova, & Richards, 2012). How the basic neural circuitry responsible for the homeostatic regulation of total energy intake is used to control consumption of specific macronutrients remains unanswered. In addition to a general appetitive drive, specific nutrient appetites are likely encoded by unique molecular changes in the hypothalamus that occur via largely unknown variations in interoceptive signaling (Berthoud, Munzberg, Richards, & Morrison, 2012). Gratification of these particular appetites then will involve engaging the brain's motivational system.

References

Berthoud, H.-R., Munzberg, H., Richards, B. K., & Morrison, C. (2012). Neural and metabolic regulation of macronutrient intake and selection. *Proceedings of the Nutrition Society*, *71*(3), 390–400.

Gularte-Mérida, R., DiCarlo, L. M., Robertson, G., Simon, J., Johnson, W. D., Kappen, C., . . . Richards, B. K. (2014). High-resolution mapping of a genetic locus regulating preferential carbohydrate intake, total kilocalories, and food volume on mouse chromosome 17. *PLOS ONE, 9*(10), e11042.

Kruger, C., Kumar, K. G., Mynatt, R. L., Volaufova, J., & Richards, B. K. (2012). Brain transcriptional responses to high-fat diet in *Acads*-deficient mice reveal energy sensing pathways. *PLOS ONE, 7*(8), e41709.

Kumar, K. G., Byerley, L., Volaufova, J., Drucker, D. J., Churchill, G. A., Li, R., . . . Smith Richards, B. K. (2008). Genetic variation in *Glp1r* expression influences the rate of gastric emptying in mice. *American Journal of Physiology Regulatory Integrative and Comparative Physiology, 294*(2), R362–R371.

Kumar, K. G., DiCarlo, L. M., Volaufova, J., Zuberi, A. R., & Smith Richards, B. K. (2010). Increased physical activity co-segregates with higher intake of carbohydrate and total calories in subcongenic mice. *Mammalian Genome, 21*(1–2), 52–63.

Smith, B. K., Andrews, P. K., & West, D. B. (2000). Macronutrient self-selection in thirteen mouse strains. *American Journal of Physiology Regulatory Integrative and Comparative Physiology, 278*(4), R797–R805.

Smith Richards, B. K., Belton, B. N., Poole, A. C., Mancuso, J. J., Churchill, G. A., Li, R., . . . York, B. (2002). QTL analysis of self-selected macronutrient diet intake: Fat, carbohydrate, and total kilocalories. *Physiological Genomics, 11*(3), 205–217.

Smith Richards, B. K., Belton, B. N., York, B., & Volaufova, J. (2004). Mice bearing *Acads* mutation display altered postingestive but not 5s orosensory response to dietary fat. *American Journal of Physiology Regulatory Integrative and Comparative Physiology, 286*(2), R311–R319.

SHORT PAPERS SUBMITTED FOR CHAPTER 2

Cynthia Arslanian-Engoren
Margaret L. Campbell
Jesus M. Casida
Nancy Kline Leidy
Samar Noureddine
Susan Pressler
Terri Voepel-Lewis

Decision Making and Coronary Heart Disease

Cynthia Arslanian-Engoren, PhD, RN, FAAN

As a nurse scientist with decision-making expertise, my program of research focuses on the cardiac triage decisions of emergency department triage nurses and the self-care decisions of women to reduce their risk of coronary heart disease. As part of this work, I developed and tested an intervention that included a decision aid to improve emergency department nurses' cardiac triage decisions for women who present with symptoms of an acute myocardial infarction (Arslanian-Engoren, Hagerty, & Eagle, 2010) and also developed an instrument to measure emergency department nurses' cardiac triage decisions (Arslanian-Engoren & Hagerty, 2013). As part of my work examining self-care decisions, I qualitatively and quantitatively examined women's knowledge and risk perceptions for coronary heart disease.

I recently expanded my work to include both the examination of cognitive dysfunction in older adults hospitalized for acute heart failure (Arslanian-Engoren et al., 2014) and sleep-related factors (e.g., fatigue, sleep loss) that might influence decision regret among critical care nurses (Scott, Arslanian-Engoren, & Engoren, 2014; Arslanian-Engoren & Scott, 2014). These areas represent a logical extension of my decision-making work. As more adults are living with coronary heart disease and surviving acute myocardial infarction, an increasing number are developing heart failure and are being hospitalized for acute decompensated heart failure. Cognitive dysfunction in older adults with heart failure affects self-care management decisions necessary to engage in behaviors that reduce illness burden and hospital readmission and improve health-related quality of life. Inadequate sleep and fatigue in nurses affect cognitive performance in the domains of executive function and decision making.

Emergency Department Nurses' Cardiac Triage Decisions

My emergency department nurse triage research has revealed (a) age and gender differences in nurses' cardiac triage decisions, (b) the inability of nurses' triage decisions to predict admission diagnosis for acute coronary syndromes, (c) a mismatch between symptoms experienced by women who have a myocardial infarction and those used by nurses to triage women for suspected acute coronary syndromes, and (d) that goals of practice for nurses do not always align with acute myocardial infarction guidelines (Arslanian-Engoren, Eagle, Hagerty, & Reits, 2011). As part of this work, I constructed genetic algorithms to examine the prediction rules of emergency department nurses for persons with suspected acute coronary syndromes and showed that nurses use different prediction rules for triaging male and female vignette patients with acute coronary syndromes. I was one of the first to show that female patients presenting with possible cardiac symptoms face gender inequities in nurses' triage decisions, placing these patients at risk for life-threatening delays in acute cardiac treatment.

To improve nurses' cardiac triage decisions, I lead an interdisciplinary research team that developed and tested the effectiveness of a multifocused intervention (education, vignettes, decision aid). Improvements were seen in nurses' knowledge of women's myocardial infarction presentation, adherence to American College of Cardiology/American Heart Association myocardial infarction practice guidelines, and patient outcomes (likelihood of obtaining a timely electrocardiogram). Results were sustained 3 months postintervention and resulted in practice changes (Arslanian-Engoren et al., 2010). The importance of my research was highlighted in a 20-year literature review of factors affecting nurses' triage decisions for acute coronary syndromes (Kuhn, Page, Davidson, & Worrall-Carter, 2011).

I continue to lead this area of science and research with the development and testing of an instrument to measure emergency department nurses' cardiac triage decisions (Arslanian-Engoren & Hagerty, 2013). This is the first published instrument to quantify the decision-making processes of emergency nurses who triage men and women who enter the emergency department for complaints suggestive of myocardial infarction. Factor analysis of the theoretically derived, empirically based, 30-item instrument revealed three factors (patient presentation, unbiased nurse reasoning process, and nurse action) with good internal consistency and sample adequacy. This instrument has the potential to improve patient safety and outcomes related to early identification and treatment of myocardial infarction. Further evaluation is planned.

Self-Care Decisions to Reduce the Risk of Coronary Heart Disease

Because the overall goal of my program of research is to reduce coronary heart disease in women, I also examine women's coronary heart disease risk perceptions. Building on my earlier studies, which include rural and urban women's knowledge and risk perceptions for coronary heart disease, treatment-seeking decisions of women with myocardial infarction, and gender and age differences in acute coronary syndromes symptoms, I have examined women's coronary heart disease risk factors and screening, physiological and anatomical bases for sex differences in acute coronary syndromes, and acute coronary syndromes in older adults. My work recently found that social support helped women engage in heart-healthy behaviors to reduce their risk for coronary heart disease and stroke (Arslanian-Engoren, Eastwood, DeJong, & Berra, 2015).

Cognitive Dysfunction in Older Adults With Acute Heart Failure

This groundbreaking work was one of the first to show cognitive dysfunction in older adults hospitalized for acute decompensated heart failure (Arslanian-Engoren et al., 2014). It showed that more and worse acute heart failure symptoms were associated with cognitive dysfunction. I coauthored the original American Heart Association scientific statement on the presentation of acute heart failure syndromes in the emergency department, treatment, and disposition and have coauthored other papers examining the sequela of living with heart failure, including cognitive dysfunction, mortality, health-related quality of life, and exercise self-concepts.

Fatigue and Nurses' Clinical Decisions

I recently expanded my program of research to include sleep-related factors (e.g., fatigue, sleep loss) that might influence clinical decision regret among critical care nurses. Critical care nurses often make decisions under conditions of uncertainly that are time limited and complex. Inadequate sleep adversely affects cognitive function (e.g., decision making, working memory), impairs decision making, and jeopardizes patient safety. Decision regret, reported by 29% of critical care nurses, was more likely among nurses who reported more acute fatigue, daytime sleepiness, and poorer intershift recovery and sleep quality (Scott, Arslanian-Engoren & Engoren, 2014). This paper was one of the key references included in the 2014 American Nurses Association Position Statement addressing nurse fatigue to promote safety and health. Qualitative analysis of critical care nurses' descriptions of clinical decisions when sleepy revealed six themes: (a) failure to adhere to standards of practice, (b) failure to ensure patient safety, (c) failure to be a patient advocate, (d) failure to communicate in a professional manner, (e) impaired cognition, and (f) negative affective responses. Results provide compelling insight into the decisions of sleep-deprived nurses and the negative affect experienced by nurses who fail to meet their professional and societal obligations to make decisions that support the delivery of high-quality, safe patient care (Arslanian-Engoren & Scott, 2014).

My work has been widely disseminated in high-impact journals (e.g., *American Journal of Cardiology*, *Circulation*, *Journal of Cardiovascular Nursing*, *Journal of Cardiac Failure*) and has informed practice guidelines and clinical practice. My research has advanced the frontier of knowledge in decision making and coronary heart disease. My reputation as a scholar has been recognized by several notable awards (e.g., Midwest Nursing Research Society Decision Making Research Section Senior Nurse Researcher, Acute Care Distinguished Scientist) and by colleagues and peers in cardiovascular nursing. In 2008, I was inducted as a fellow of the American Heart Association. In 2012, I was inducted as a fellow of the American Academy of Nursing in recognition of my measurable, outstanding, and sustained impact on nursing and health care.

References

Arslanian-Engoren, C., Eagle, K. A., Hagerty, B. M., & Reits, S. (2011). Emergency department triage nurses' self-reported adherence with American College of Cardiology/American Heart Association myocardial infarction guidelines. *Journal of Cardiovascular Nursing, 26*(5), 408–413. doi:10.1097/JCN.0b013e3182076a98

Arslanian-Engoren, C., Eastwood, J.-A., DeJong, M. J., & Berra, K. (2015). Participation in heart-healthy behaviors: A secondary analysis of the American Heart Association Go Red Heart Match data. *Journal of Cardiovascular Nursing, 30*(6), 479–483.

Arslanian-Engoren, C., Giordani, B. J., Algase, D., Schuh, A., Lee, C., & Moser, D. K. (2014). Cognitive dysfunction in older adults hospitalized for acute heart failure. *Journal of Cardiac Failure, 20*(9), 669–678. doi:10.1016/j.cardfail.2014.06.003

Arslanian-Engoren, C., & Hagerty, B. M. (2013). The development and testing of the nurses' cardiac triage instrument. *Research and Theory for Nursing Practice: An International Journal, 27*(1), 9–18.

Arslanian-Engoren, C., Hagerty, B. M., & Eagle, K. A. (2010). Evaluation of the ACT intervention to improve nurses' cardiac triage decisions. *Western Journal of Nursing Research, 32*(6), 713–729. doi:10.1177/0193945909359410

Arslanian-Engoren, C., & Scott, L. D. (2014). Clinical decision regret among critical care nurses: A qualitative analysis. *Heart & Lung, 43*(5), 416–419. doi:10.1016/j.hrtlng.2014.02.006

Kuhn, L., Page, K., Davidson, P. M., & Worrall-Carter, L. (2011). Triaging women with acute coronary syndrome: A review of the literature. *Journal of Cardiovascular Nursing, 26*(5), 395–407. doi:10.1097/JCN.0b013e31820598f6

Scott, L. D., Arslanian-Engoren, C., & Engoren, M. (2014). The association of sleep and fatigue with decision regret among critical care nurses. *American Journal of Critical Care, 23*, 13–23. doi:10.4037/ajcc2014191

Dyspnea Assessment and Treatment at the End of Life

Margaret L. Campbell, PhD, RN, FPCN

I completed my studies and dissertation at the University of Michigan School of Nursing (UMSN) in 2006. I studied in the biobehavior track and did cognate work in neurophysiology, the science of emotions, and neurological mechanisms for fear activation and behaviors. I was advised through the completion of my dissertation by Drs. Therrien (chair), Metzger, Algase, and Maren (psychology). I was stimulated to pursue doctoral study through my clinical work as a palliative care nurse practitioner. The field of palliative care lacks the evidence base of other more established fields of clinical care. My aim with my doctoral completion was to increase the evidence base for assessing and treating dyspnea among patients at the end of life. I am proud to report that in the nearly 10 years since I completed studies at UMSN, I have achieved this aim and continue to contribute translatable evidence for clinical practice. Details about my program of research follow.

Dyspnea, also known as breathlessness, is a subjective experience of breathing discomfort that consists of qualitatively distinct sensations that vary in intensity. Dyspnea can only be known from a person's self-report. Eliciting a patient's dyspnea self-report is the gold standard for assessment, yet decreased consciousness typifies the last phase of a terminal illness, leaving many patients unable to provide a dyspnea self-report. Thus I established a biobehavioral theoretical model that *respiratory distress* is the observed corollary to dyspnea based on the person's display of physical behaviors (Campbell, 2008b).

Respiratory distress is the suffering that arises from an asphyxial threat, such as hypercarbia, hypoxemia, and inspiratory effort (Campbell, 2008b). The human respiratory system automatically produces pulmonary stress behaviors in reaction to an asphyxial threat. In addition, the amygdala is activated. Subcortical activation of the amygdala leads to a fear affective response with characteristic behaviors (see Figure 2-a).

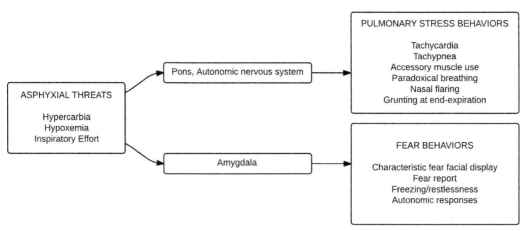

Figure 2-a. Respiratory distress model.

In my dissertation study, I undertook testing of this biobehavioral model. I observed 12 adult men and women experiencing naturally occurring dyspnea during a mechanical ventilator weaning trial in a medical intensive care unit. I videotaped the participants framed from the waist up and obtained continuous data from a capnograph/oximeter, including heart and respiratory rates, peripheral oxygen saturation, and end-tidal carbon dioxide. When the participants had been restored to comfortable ventilator-assisted breathing, I sought their reports about the emotions they experienced when short of breath through a display of pictures depicting strong emotions, one of which was fear. From these data, I established the behaviors associated with respiratory distress across cognitive states (Campbell, 2007).

Using the behaviors displayed in the previous study, I developed a Respiratory Distress Observation Scale (RDOS) and began a series of studies to establish RDOS reliability and validity. Our first RDOS psychometric study enrolled 210 participants in three groups: (a) patients with chronic obstructive pulmonary disease (COPD) undergoing pulmonary rehabilitation; (b) orthopedic surgery patients in the first 24 hours after surgery before analgesia administration; and (c) healthy volunteers. We established convergent validity with COPD patient self-reported dyspnea, discriminant validity with patients experiencing pain, and healthy volunteers. Scale reliability (α) was also established (Campbell, 2008a).

In our second psychometric study, we tested the RDOS with the intended population of terminally ill patients at risk for dyspnea and unable to provide a symptom self-report. We established construct validity; the RDOS is correlated with hypoxemia. We also established perfect interrater reliability with RDOS measurement by registered nurses (Campbell, Templin, & Walch, 2010). In that study, we also established the high frequency of inability to self-report dyspnea among this sample of patients who were near death (Campbell, Templin, & Walch, 2009).

Since its publication, the RDOS has been embraced by palliative care providers for clinical use to standardize patient assessment. Further, the RDOS has been translated into Dutch, French, and Chinese by investigators around the world for research purposes.

With a reliable, valid, objective measure of patient respiratory distress, I was able to begin a program of intervention studies. Oxygen is a routine intervention applied to patients with respiratory distress. From my clinical work, I hypothesized that patients near death, who often have decreased consciousness, could have oxygen withdrawn. I conducted a double-blind, repeated-measures observation of 32 terminally ill patients using the patients as their own control. We randomly provided oxygen, medical air, and no flow via nasal cannula in 10-minute intervals; we measured the RDOS at the end of each interval. We ascertained that most patients do not need oxygen when near death (Campbell, Yarandi, & Dove-Medows, 2013). Clinical practice changes are suggested from these findings.

Patients near death often have small amounts of retained pharyngeal secretions that resonate and make noise, sometimes referred to as "death rattle." A number of studies have been done previously to determine whether there is distress among patients with death rattle. Also, studies have been performed to determine which antisecretory medication is most effective at reducing death rattle. No one had previously established whether the patient experiences distress from death rattle. I conducted the first study to establish that there is no patient respiratory distress when patients with and without death rattle were compared. This study supports that death rattle is a normal sound, and antisecretory agents that might produce adverse effects are not indicated (Campbell & Yarandi, 2013).

Meanwhile, clinical users of the RDOS have requested distress cut-point identification. Therefore, we conducted a receiver operating characteristic curve analysis of RDOS scores among a sample of self-reporting dyspneic patients stratified at none, mild, moderate, or severe levels of dyspnea (Campbell & Templin, 2015). We have a study under way with terminally ill patients to substantiate the cut point identified by self-reporting patients.

Critically ill patients undergoing terminal ventilator withdrawal are often unable to self-report dyspnea but are at high risk for experiencing respiratory distress if the withdrawal is not well conducted. I have developed a nurse-led, RDOS-guided, algorithmic approach to this common palliative care process in intensive care units. We completed a pilot study and established feasibility and acceptability and proof of concept that the algorithm is superior to usual care in ensuring patient comfort (Campbell, Yarandi, & Mendez, 2015). An R01 application was submitted in June 2015 for a stepped wedge cluster randomized controlled effectiveness trial; a very good score was obtained from the reviewing special emphasis panel, and funding is anticipated.

Other projects are under consideration for funding. We have opened a study to determine the incidence, prevalence, and trajectory of respiratory distress among patients referred for hospice care. Previous studies of dyspnea prevalence drop patients when they can no longer self-report, so we do not know whether respiratory distress accelerates, remains unchanged, or abates as death nears. I hypothesize that it abates, but no one has rigorously followed patients' experiences until death.

Lastly, we have prepared a layperson's version of the RDOS for use in the home hospice setting. We opened a pilot study in the summer of 2015 to test whether the RDOS-family and a bundle of distress interventions taught by the hospice nurse yields positive patient and family outcomes.

In summary, the foundation in biobehavioral science I received at UMSN has enabled me to launch a program of clinical research that is changing palliative care practice here and abroad.

References

Campbell, M. L. (2007). Fear and pulmonary stress behaviors to an asphyxial threat across cognitive states. *Research in Nursing and Health, 30*(6), 572–583. doi:10.1002/nur.20212

Campbell, M. L. (2008a). Psychometric testing of a respiratory distress observation scale. *Journal of Palliative Medicine, 11*(1), 44–50. doi:10.1089/jpm.2007.0090

Campbell, M. L. (2008b). Respiratory distress: A model of responses and behaviors to an asphyxial threat for patients who are unable to self-report. *Heart & Lung, 37*(1), 54–60. doi:10.1016/j.hrtlng.2007.05.007

Campbell, M. L., Templin, T., & Walch, J. (2009). Patients who are near death are frequently unable to self-report dyspnea. *Journal of Palliative Medicine, 12*(10), 881–884. doi:10.1089/jpm.2009.0082

Campbell, M. L., Templin, T., & Walch, J. (2010). A Respiratory Distress Observation Scale for patients unable to self-report dyspnea. *Journal of Palliative Medicine, 13*(3), 285–290. doi:10.1089/jpm.2009.0229

Campbell, M. L., & Templin, T. N. (2015). Intensity cut-points for the Respiratory Distress Observation Scale. *Palliative Medicine, 29*(5), 436–442. doi:10.1177/0269216314564238

Campbell, M. L., Yarandi, H., & Dove-Medows, E. (2013). Oxygen is nonbeneficial for most patients who are near death. *Journal of Pain and Symptom Management, 45*(3), 517–523. doi:10.1016/j.jpainsymman.2012.02.012

Campbell, M. L., & Yarandi, H. N. (2013). Death rattle is not associated with patient respiratory distress: Is pharmacologic treatment indicated? *Journal of Palliative Medicine, 16*(10), 1255–1259. doi:10.1089/jpm.2013.0122

Campbell, M. L., Yarandi, H. N., & Mendez, M. (2015). A two-group trial of a terminal ventilator withdrawal algorithm: Pilot testing. *Journal of Palliative Medicine, 18*(9), 781–785. doi:10.1089/jpm.2015.0111

Innovative Therapies for Heart Failure and Circulatory Support

Jesus M. Casida, PhD, RN, APN-C

The objective of my research program is to develop and advance the science that underpins the management of critically ill patients, specifically those requiring cardiac surgery and advanced heart failure therapies by implantation of a left-ventricular assist device (LVAD)—a type of a mechanical heart. Since 2008 the majority of my research and scholarship have been centered on understanding patients' experiences with and responses to the invasive nature of cardiac surgery and LVAD implantation from biological, physiological, physical, and psychological/behavioral perspectives. My work will serve as a platform for creating a roadmap for developing and testing empirically based interventions tailored to improving care delivery processes, health, and quality-of-life outcomes among cardiac surgery and mechanical heart populations.

My research to date has had, and continues to have, an impact on advancing nursing/health sciences, research, practice, and future policy formation and can be categorized into two broad and overlapping areas: symptom management and self-management. In cardiac surgery, my research team addressed the role of sleep pattern disturbances and inflammatory response from cardiopulmonary bypass machines (i.e., heart-lung machines used during cardiac surgery). In this line of inquiry, our goal is to understand the mechanism of sleep pattern disturbances and inflammatory response and their impact on surgical (clinical), health, and quality-of-life outcomes. We found significant relationships among the domains of sleep pattern disturbances (e.g., sleep fragmentation), stress (cortisol), and inflammatory markers (C-reactive protein [C-RP] and white blood cell counts); correlation coefficients ranged from r values of .50 to 0.82, all p values < .05 (Casida, Davis, Shpakoff, & Yarandi, 2014). In conjunction with this work, we conducted an evidence-based review on the use of guided imagery in cardiac surgery with the assumption that this type of integrative mind-body therapy could be used as a sleep-promoting intervention for patients in the intensive care and step-down units. Based on our review and appraisal of seven randomized controlled trials, we found strong evidence supporting the use of guided imagery for postoperative management of pain and anxiety. Moreover, there was a consensus among authors that the pain- and anxiety-reducing effects of guided imagery may promote patients' sleep in the intensive care and step-down units (Casida & Lemanski, 2010; Casida & Nowak, 2011). Based on this sleep-promoting mechanism, we pilot tested, using a randomized controlled trial (RCT), the integration of a self-administered (or nurse-assisted) guided imagery program in busy intensive care and step-down units. We found that this intervention is feasible for and acceptable to patients; nursing staff (RNs) demonstrated by study protocol a compliance rate of 85% to 100% during postoperative nights 1 through 4. Notable findings included a significant reduction in pain and anxiety levels and narcotic analgesic consumption among guided imagery users (n = 20) versus nonusers (n = 20), $p < .05$. Although the between-group differences were not significant, we found a significant improvement in the guided imagery users' sleep patterns (i.e., lower sleep onset latency) and sleep quality and a reduction in stress (cortisol) and inflammation (C-RP) over time (postoperative nights/days 1 through 4), $p < .05$ (Casida et al., 2013). Based on these promising results, we are currently developing a larger RCT to expand this pilot work to further investigate the effects of guided imagery on sleep patterns and cardiac surgical outcomes (physical function, complications, hospitalization days, health status, and mortality).

Since sleep pattern disturbance is highly prevalent in heart failure, our research team was the first to expand this knowledge to patients with *advanced/end-stage* heart failure requiring LVADs. We found that patients' sleep was severely disrupted (e.g., high sleep fragmentation index) before LVAD, and this pattern continued up to 6 months after LVAD implantation. This finding was accompanied by patterns of excessive daytime sleepiness before and after LVAD (Casida, Davis, Brewer, Smith, & Yarandi, 2011). The severity of the sleep pattern disturbances, poor sleep quality, and associated daytime sleepiness among LVAD patients were associated with poor quality of life; correlation coefficients ranged from $r = .66$ to .84, all p values $< .05$ (Casida, Brewer, Smith, & Davis, 2012). In addition to sleep disturbances, patients also experienced high levels of fatigue, anxiety, and depression within 1 month before and up to 6 months after LVAD implantation (Casida & Parker, 2012). Recently, we completed a longitudinal study on cognition and self-care capabilities in patients with LVADs. Preliminary analysis showed significant relationships between executive function (a domain of cognition) and LVAD pump flow ($r = .72$, $p < .05$), and the patients' ability to care for themselves has shown significant upward improvement from baseline (preimplant) up to 6 months post–LVAD implant, $p < .05$ (Casida et al., ongoing analysis).

Clearly, the symptom (e.g., sleep pattern disturbances, anxiety, depression) and self-management science in LVAD is in its formative stage of development. Extensive research in this area is needed to come to a definitive conclusion about the impact of distressing symptoms on patients' self-efficacy for and adherence to the LVAD home care regimen (Casida, Wu, Harden, Chern, & Carie, 2015). Nonetheless, my work on sleep promotion and inflammation reduction in cardiac surgery, symptoms (sleep, anxiety, depression, cognition, etc.), and the emerging self-management science in patients with LVADs (Casida, Peters, & Magnan, 2009; Casida et al., 2015) has laid the groundwork for researchers to advance the science of symptom and self-management in patients who are tethered to a life-sustaining technology or an implantable artificial organ.

References

Casida, J. M., Brewer, R., Smith, C., & Davis, J. E. (2012). Sleep, daytime function, and quality of life of patients with mechanical circulatory support. *International Journal of Artificial Organs, 35*(7), 531–537.

Casida, J. M., Davis, J. E., Brewer, R., Smith, C., & Yarandi, H. (2011). Sleep and daytime sleepiness of patients with left ventricular assist devices. *Progress in Transplantation, 21,* 131–136.

Casida, J. M., Davis, J. E., Shpakoff, L., & Yarandi, H. (2014). An exploratory study of the patients' sleep patterns and inflammatory response following cardio-pulmonary bypass (CPB). *Journal of Clinical Nursing, 23*(15–16), 2332–2342.

Casida, J. M., & Lemanski, S. (2010). An evidence-based review on guided imagery utilization in adult cardiac surgery. *Clinical Scholars Review, 3*(1), 23–31.

Casida, J. M., & Nowak, L. (2011). Integrative therapies to promote sleep in the ICU. In Chlan, L., & Hertz, M. (Eds.), *Integrated Therapies in Lung Health & Sleep.* New York, NY: Springer.

Casida, J. M., & Parker, J. (2012). A preliminary investigation of symptom pattern and prevalence before and up to 6 months after implantation of a left ventricular assist device. *Journal of Artificial Organs, 15*(2), 211–214.

Casida, J. M., Peters, R., & Magnan, M. (2009). Self-care needs of patients with implantable left ventricular assist devices. *Nursing Research, Theory, & Practice: An International Journal, 23*(4), 279–293.

Casida, J. M., Wu, H. S., Harden, J., Chern, J., & Carie, A. P. (2015). Development and initial evaluation of the psychometric properties of self-efficacy and adherence scales for patients with a left ventricular assist device. *Progress in Transplantation, 25*(2), 110–115.

Casida, J. M., Yaremchuck, K., Sphakoff, L., Marrocco, A., Babicz, G., & Yarandi, H. (2013). The effects of guided imagery on sleep and inflammatory response in cardiac surgery: A pilot randomized controlled trial. *Journal of Cardiovascular Surgery, 54*(2), 269–279.

Improving Health Outcomes for People With COPD

Nancy Kline Leidy, PhD, RN

Chronic obstructive pulmonary disease (COPD) refers to a cluster of diseases, including chronic bronchitis and emphysema, characterized by a progressive reduction in expiratory airflow. It is one of the most common lung conditions seen in clinical practice and the fourth leading cause of death worldwide. As patients become more symptomatic over time, functional status declines, and acute exacerbations further the downward trajectory of obstruction, symptoms, disability, and reduced quality of life. This program of research addressed the need to understand and operationalize COPD from the perspective of the patients themselves, with the goal of furthering research to improve functional and symptomatic outcomes in this population.

Functional Status

As one of the first intramural fellows at the National Institute of Nursing Research (NINR), I immersed myself in research to understand and operationalize functional outcomes in patients with COPD, including a comprehensive review of the literature, secondary analyses of existing data, and the development of a new analytical framework for understanding functional status (Leidy, 1994). This framework outlined four key dimensions: (a) functional capacity, (b) performance, (c) reserve, and (d) capacity utilization. Functional performance can be assessed through activity monitoring or patient self-reporting, each offering a different yet complementary perspective. One of the first uses of actigraphy for evaluating functional outcomes was a controlled laboratory-based test of activity counts during physical activity (Leidy, Abbott, & Fedenko, 1997), creating a foundation for further work in this area. Qualitative research further clarified this complex area, offering a perspective on the importance of personal integrity, including "being with" and "being able." This insight also informed the development of the Functional Performance Inventory (FPI), a patient-reported outcome (PRO) measure (Leidy, 1999). The analytical framework, qualitative insight, and the FPI and FPI Short Form (SF) have been used internationally to better understand functional performance in people with COPD, including validation of a new physical activity measurement approach involving monitoring and patient self-reporting developed by the European Medicines Initiative (EMI) PRO-ACTIVE program.

Acute Exacerbations

Acute exacerbations of COPD (AECOPD) are defined as acute, sustained worsening of the patient's underlying condition beyond normal day-to-day variability leading to a change in treatment. They are disabling events for patients, that result in reduced lung function, poorer quality of life, and mortality; they also represent a significant burden to health care systems worldwide. Empirically, an AECOPD has been measured using health care resource utilization (HCRU)—that is, clinic or emergency visits with oral steroid or antibiotic treatment (moderate) or hospitalization (severe). There are a number of limitations to this definition. Clinic visits are initiated by patients and triggered by various factors, including their assessment of the episode, provider relationship, family influences, and cost. With no standardized method for clinical diagnosis and treatment, decisions are based on clinician training, treatment preferences, experiences with the patient, and health care setting, among others. Finally, as many as 50% to 70% of exacerbations are believed to be unreported, suggesting that resource-based definitions seriously underestimate exacerbation frequency.

A symptom-based method of prospectively assessing exacerbations would address many of these limitations. The **EXA**cerbations of **C**hronic Pulmonary Disease **T**ool (EXACT®) is a 14-item daily diary designed to count and characterize symptom-defined exacerbations (frequency, severity, duration) and quantify the symptomatic experiences that accompany HCRU events (Leidy et al., 2011; Leidy, Murray, Jones, Jones, & Sethi, 2014). It was developed and validated using rigorous qualitative and quantitative methods consistent with the requirements of the U.S. Food and Drug Administration (FDA) and European Medicines Agency (EMA), with the participation of a panel of experts in COPD, measurement, and drug development regulatory issues. The EXACT has been translated into more than 50 languages, used in more than 25 clinical trials (clinicaltrials.gov), and licensed to more than 50 academic investigators for clinical research. The EXACT was also the first PRO measure qualified by the FDA, an important milestone for patient-centered research and it has been reviewed by the EMA under their novel methodologies qualification program. Results of studies to date offer insight into the natural history of exacerbations and the effects of treatment.

I was pleased to initiate and lead the EXACT-PRO Initiative, the first multisponsor consortium convened to develop a standardized outcome measure for use in drug development trials and clinical research, paving the way for the C-Path PRO Consortium, the COPD Foundation Biomarker Qualification Consortium (CBQC) and other public-private partnerships to advance health outcomes research. It was a pleasure to be part of the CBQC team that successfully completed an evidence package and FDA qualification for the use of fibrinogen as a prognostic biomarker for selecting COPD patients at high risk for exacerbations or all-cause mortality for inclusion in clinical trials, the fifth of only six biomarkers qualified by the FDA to date and another first for COPD.

Respiratory Symptoms in Stable Disease

Patients with COPD experience respiratory symptoms, particularly dyspnea, when they are not exacerbating. These symptoms are not only distressing, but they are a primary cause of functional limitations. Accurate assessment is important to clinical practice and research. The Breathlessness, Cough, and Sputum Scale (BCSS), a simple three-question diary I validated in 2003, predated the FDA PRO guidance but offered an initial foray into the measurement of this important endpoint in clinical trials. The EXACT offered an opportunity to build on insight provided by the BCSS. Extending the EXACT-PRO Initiative, we developed the Evaluating Respiratory Symptoms (E-RS) diary, using 11 items from the EXACT (Leidy, Sexton, et al., 2014). The E-RS has been reviewed by the EMA and is in the final stages of PRO qualification review by the FDA. Like the EXACT, it is being used in a number of international studies.

Assessing Symptoms and Impact in Clinical Practice

Assessing symptoms in clinical practice requires effective clinician-patient interaction to ensure the right information is gathered to inform treatment decision making. The COPD Assessment Test (CAT) offers clinicians a validated, standardized clinical tool for this purpose (Jones et al., 2009). The brief 8-item measure is patient self-administered, with the information presented to the clinician in a format that allows the practitioner to quickly detect areas of greatest difficulty in need of further evaluation. The instrument is used in practices worldwide and often serves as a health outcome measure in clinical research, with more than 200 related publications to date.

Finding Patients With Undiagnosed, Clinically Significant COPD in Primary Care

Evidence suggests that a significant portion of patients with COPD are undiagnosed. Many of these patients have substantial loss of lung function or are at risk for exacerbation. Identifying individuals with undiagnosed clinically significant COPD ($FEV_1 < 60\%$ predicted or exacerbation risk) should set in motion interventions to improve short- and long-term health outcomes. A 2008 National Institutes of Health (NIH)-COPD Foundation workshop suggested a three-stage approach for identifying these patients: a questionnaire to eliminate those unlikely to have severe disease; a simple measure of expiratory airflow to exclude those with normal or near normal pulmonary function; and diagnostic evaluation, including clinical assessment and spirometry.

Dr. Fernando Martinez, David Mannino, and I are serving as coinvestigators of an NIH-funded grant (the National Heart, Lung, and Blood Institute [NHLBI]: R01 HL 114055, 2012–2015) to develop a simple yet precise screening strategy for identifying undiagnosed patients with clinically significant COPD. The project involved pulmonologists, primary care physicians, and nurses from across the United States and participation of the COPD Foundation. The multimethod empirical approach included a comprehensive literature review and qualitative focus groups (Leidy et al., 2015), the latter designed to understand how patients themselves describe risk factors and manifestations of COPD.

Random forests analyses were performed on three existing databases for additional insight into the key attributes that characterize COPD and the categories and types of variables that might be useful in case identification. Results were used in conjunction with the literature review and qualitative research to develop a pool of 44 candidate items covering 6 categories of information ready for empirical testing. A prospective, case-control multisite study was conducted with 186 cases of clinically significant COPD and 160 controls, including those with no COPD and those with mild COPD. A systematic item-reduction process uncovered a set of five simple questions capable of differentiating cases and controls. A threshold for peak expiratory flow (PEF) was also determined. Results suggest that asking patients a set of five simple questions with selective use of PEF might be an effective and efficient approach for identifying patients needing diagnostic evaluation for clinically significant COPD. The study was presented as a featured late-breaking podium presentation at the European Respiratory Society (ERS) meeting in September 2015. Further research on the use of this strategy in clinical practice is under way.

References

Jones, P., Harding, G., Berry, P., Wiklund, I., Chen, W. H., & Leidy, N. K. (2009). Development and first validation of the COPD Assessment Test (CAT). *European Respiratory Journal, 34,* 648–654.

Leidy, N. K. (1994). Functional status and the forward progress of merry-go-rounds: Toward a coherent analytical framework. *Nursing Research 43*(4), 196–202.

Leidy, N. K. (1999). Psychometric properties of the Functional Performance Inventory in patients with chronic obstructive pulmonary disease. *Nursing Research, 48*(1), 20–28.

Leidy, N. K., Abbott, R. D., & Fedenko, K. M. (1997). Sensitivity and reproducibility of the dual-mode actigraph under controlled levels of activity intensity. *Nursing Research, 46*(1), 5–11.

Leidy, N. K., Kim, K. K., Bacci, E. J., Yawn, B. P., Mannino, D. M., Thomashow, B. M., . . . Martinez, F. (2015). Identifying cases of undiagnosed clinically significant COPD in primary care: Qualitative insight from patients in the target population. *npj Primary Care Respiratory Medicine, 25.* doi:10.1038/npjpcrm.2015.24

Leidy, N. K., Murray, L. T., Jones, P. W., & Sethi, S. (2014). Performance of the EXAcerbations of Chronic Pulmonary Disease Tool (EXACT) in three randomized controlled trials of COPD. *Annals of the American Thoracic Society, 11*(3), 316–325.

Leidy, N. K., Sexton, C. C., Jones, P., Notte, S. M., Monz, B. U., Nelsen, L., . . . Sethi, S. (2014). Measuring respiratory symptoms in clinical trials of COPD: Reliability and validity of a daily diary. *Thorax, 69*(5), 424–430. doi:10.1136/thoraxjnl-2013-204428

Leidy, N. K., Wilcox, T., Jones, P. W., Roberts, L., Powers, J., Sethi, S., & the EXACT-PRO Study Group. (2011). Standardizing measurement of COPD exacerbations: Reliability and validity of a patient-reported diary. *American Journal of Respiratory and Critical Care Medicine, 183,* 323–329.

Investigating Cardiovascular Risk in a Conflict Zone

Samar Noureddine, PhD, RN, FAAN

My area of clinical specialty is cardiovascular nursing. My research focuses on *health-seeking behaviors*, which I define as "behaviors that people engage in to prevent illness and promote and/or restore their health," and their modification to reduce health risk. I focus on cognitive and psychosocial predictors of health behaviors, as these are amenable to intervention by nurses in both healthy and chronically ill populations. During my doctoral study at the University of Michigan School of Nursing, I developed an interest in studying health behaviors that impact cardiovascular risk. My dissertation work examined cognitive and psychological predictors of healthy eating in a community sample of middle-aged adults in the United States, which showed strong associations among behavior, self-efficacy, and perceived health risk. As I moved back to my home country, Lebanon, it became clear that cardiovascular disease (CVD) is quite prevalent and the leading cause of morbidity and mortality, so my research program centered on secondary prevention of CVD. The first step was investigating health-seeking behaviors of patients with acute coronary syndrome in order to identify their responses to their cardiac events, the underlying mechanisms, and related factors. The findings reflected aspects similar to those reported by investigators from Western countries, such as the nature of symptoms and their perceived threat, in addition to aspects unique to the Lebanese culture—namely, the strong involvement of the family in patients' lives. One finding worth noting was that the mean time from symptom onset to arrival to the emergency hospital (4.5 hours, which is longer than what is reported in the United States) did not differ by whether the event was the first or a recurrent one.

Because the above study suggested misperceptions about heart disease, a community sample of healthy adults was investigated in a survey of beliefs and perceptions about heart disease and the way to respond to it. The findings suggested adequate knowledge of the main symptoms and the main causes of heart disease but inconsistent perceptions about the measures to treat and control it. The response to an acute cardiac event that was solicited using hypothetical scenarios was not adequate when the symptoms were not typical of heart disease, with participants choosing self-help measures rather than seeking health care in response to a heart attack. These findings led to a clinical study that used a mixed method design to explore the decision-making process that underlies the response of cardiac patients to symptoms of acute myocardial infarction (MI) and related factors. The qualitative component addressed the experience of the cardiac event with emphasis on cognitive and emotional aspects, and the quantitative component assessed knowledge of symptoms of MI and the appropriate response to them.

As the data are analyzed, it becomes apparent that there is a need for raising awareness and educating the public about heart disease. Since again in this study the family was shown to have a key role in the decision to seek care for acute coronary events, a community rather than individual intervention might be more appropriate. Another relevant finding was the inappropriate reaction of some general practitioners (GPs) to patients who seek their advice when having a heart attack, as these physicians were asking patients to do blood tests and electrocardiograms and return back to them, adding to the delay in emergency care. This suggests that GPs need more training in how to detect and manage a heart attack.

Another striking finding in all studies was the high rate of tobacco smoking among patients with CVD, regardless of whether their cardiac event was new or recurrent (prevalence rates 40%–60%). Smoking status is significant not only because it increases cardiovascular risk but also because smokers tend to attribute their cardiac symptoms to the lungs, thus further delaying their seeking emergency care. This led to a longitudinal study on smoking patterns of patients admitted with acute coronary syndrome or for elective coronary revascularization (percutaneous intervention and open heart surgery). This current study is investigating smoking cessation and relapse rates and related factors using follow-up interviews at 1, 3, 6, and 12 months following discharge from the hospital. The studied predictors include smoking history and nicotine addiction, self-efficacy, depression, stress, and social support, in addition to clinical and demographic characteristics. Data collection continues and the findings will be used to develop a smoking cessation intervention. Preliminary findings suggest that patients prefer an individual counseling type of intervention, and only few are aware of pharmacotherapy for smoking cessation, so a multidisciplinary team including psychiatry/addiction experts and public health professionals will be sought for planning the next intervention study.

My research at this point remains descriptive but has been disseminated locally, regionally, and internationally. Patient education material on heart disease is being developed based on the findings for use in our affiliated medical center. One of my graduate students developed cardiovascular education material targeting women, and education sessions were provided using the video and educational pamphlet in some primary health care centers. Another use of the findings will be providing education to nurses who work in primary health centers so they can teach their clients behavioral strategies aimed at cardiovascular risk reduction, including responding to symptoms of coronary heart disease, smoking cessation, dietary measures, and physical activity. This initiative was decided upon with the Order of Nurses in Lebanon in collaboration with the Ministry of Public

Health. As a member of the global leadership nursing forum of the Preventive Cardiology Nursing Association, I am involved in the preparation of a tool kit for community
nurses for use in teaching patients cardiovascular risk-reduction strategies through behavior change. This work was started recently following a meeting that we had in New York
in November 2014.

At present there is no national policy in Lebanon on cardiopulmonary resuscitation
and the poor survival rate of OHCA patients. I completed a national online survey of
physicians on resuscitation practices for OHCA patients in emergency departments in
Lebanon. The results showed that the most important factors in the physicians' decision
to initiate or continue resuscitation were the presence of pulse on arrival, the underlying
cardiac rhythm, the physician's ethical duty to resuscitate, and the time from the arrest
to resuscitation. The physicians reported frequent resuscitation in medically futile situations. The most frequently reported challenges during resuscitation decisions related to
the victim's family and lack of policy. These results are being used by a group from the
American University of Beirut Faculty of Medicine, on which I serve; the group is charged
with developing national guidelines for resuscitation of those experiencing out-of-hospital
cardiac arrest (OHCA).

In summary, my program of research is in the area of health behaviors related to cardiovascular health and illness, an area that is significant for Lebanon. I am hoping to
secure funding to advance this research from the descriptive to the intervention level,
especially psychoeducational intervention studies on health behaviors aimed at reducing cardiovascular risk. I continue to collaborate with colleagues in medicine and health
sciences, since my interest overlaps with these disciplines and because I believe that the
best outcomes are achieved when health disciplines join hands in practice, education, and
research. Some of the publications reflecting part of the work described above are provided
in the reference list.

Selected Publications

Noureddine, S. (2009). Patterns of responses to cardiac events over time. *Journal of Cardiovascular Nursing, 24*(5),
    390–397.
Noureddine, S., Adra, M., Arevian, M., Dumit, N., Puzantian, H., Shehab, D., & Abchee, A. (2006). Delay in
    seeking health care for acute coronary syndromes in a Lebanese sample. *Journal of Transcultural Nursing, 17*,
    341–348.
Noureddine, S., Arevian, M., Adra, M., & Puzantian, H. (2008). Response to signs and symptoms of acute coro-
    nary syndrome: Differences between Lebanese men and women. *American Journal of Critical Care, 17*, 26–35.
Noureddine, S., Froelicher, E. S., Sibai, A., & Dakik, H. (2010). Response to a cardiac event in relation to cardiac
    knowledge and risk perception: A descriptive study in a Lebanese sample. *International Journal of Nursing Studies,
    47*(3), 332–347.
Noureddine, S., Massouh, A., & Froelicher, E. S. (2013). Perceptions of heart disease in community-dwelling Leba-
    nese. *European Journal of Cardiovascular Nursing, 12*, 56–63. doi:10.1177/1474515111430899

Noureddine, S., & Metzger, B. (2014). Do health-related feared possible selves motivate healthy eating? *Health Psychology Research, 2*, 25–29. doi:10.4081/hpr.2014.1043

Noureddine, S., & Stein, K. F. (2009). Eating and body weight self-schemas as predictors of dietary behavior in middle aged adults. *Western Journal of Nursing Research, 31*(2), 201–218.

A Program of Research to Improve Memory in Heart Failure

Susan J. Pressler, PhD, RN, FAAN, FAHA

Heart failure (HF) is a major public health problem. In the United States, 5.8 million adults are estimated to have HF, and prevalence is projected to continue increasing as the population ages. Heart failure is associated with high mortality rates, frequent hospitalizations, and poor health-related quality of life.

Health-related quality of life is diminished in HF because of two hallmark symptoms: dyspnea and fatigue. In three separate studies, Pressler and colleagues found that cognitive dysfunction was another common HF-related symptom. Among 63 patients (62 men and 1 woman) with HF, patients with poorer cognitive function had significantly more hospitalizations at 6 months after baseline (Bennett, Pressler, Hays, Firestine, & Huster, 1997). Among 30 women with HF, 12 (40%) reported cognitive dysfunction (Bennett & Baker, 1998). In a focus group study investigating self-care strategies used to manage HF, patients (n = 23) and family members (n = 18) identified cognitive dysfunction (e.g., poor concentration, memory loss) as the third most common symptom after dyspnea and fatigue. These studies were instrumental in highlighting the burden of cognitive losses experienced by patients with HF and in directing future research.

After conducting an extensive review of theoretical and empirical literature, a conceptual framework was developed to guide the study "Cognitive Deficits in Chronic Heart Failure" (THINK study) (R01 NR008147) (Pressler, Subramanian, et al., 2010). The aims, design, sample, and main findings of THINK are summarized in Table 2-a.

Table 2-a. Conceptual Framework for the "Cognitive Deficits in Chronic Heart Failure" Study

Aim	Design and sample	Summary of findings
1. Compare types, frequency, and severity of cognitive deficits among HF patients, age-matched healthy older adults, and adults with major medical conditions but not HF (Pressler, Subramanian, et al., 2010).	Design: Comparative, cross-sectional Sample: 249 HF patients, 63 healthy adults, and 102 patients with major medical conditions but not HF	• Compared with older adults and patients with medical conditions, HF patients had significantly more cognitive deficits. • HF patients most commonly had deficits in memory (23%), psychomotor speed (19%), and executive function (19%). • Of HF patients, 24% had deficits in three or more cognitive domains.
2. Examine variables that explain cognitive deficits, depressive symptoms, and health-related quality of life in HF patients (Pressler, Subramanian, et al., 2010).	Design: Explanatory, cross-sectional Sample: 249 HF patients	• HF severity and age were associated with more cognitive deficits. • Cognitive deficits were not associated with depressive symptoms and health-related quality of life.
3. Explore self-care strategies used to manage HF by HF patients with cognitive deficits (Sloan & Pressler, 2009).	Design: Phenomenology Sample: 12 HF patients with cognitive deficits in three or more domains	Patients recognized vulnerabilities in physical, social, and emotional health and the nearness of death resulting from HF.
4. Evaluate cognitive deficits as predictors of 12-month mortality (Pressler, Kim, Riley, Ronis, & Gradus-Pizlo, 2010).	Design: Prospective Sample: 166 HF patients	Baseline cognitive function (mental status, spatial memory loss) predicted 12-month all-cause mortality.

Impact. Findings from THINK supported the urgent need for intervention studies (Pressler et al., 2011; Pressler et al., 2015) to prevent or delay memory loss and thereby reduce mortality and improve health-related quality of life in HF. National clinical practice guidelines now recommend assessment of cognitive function in HF patients.

Intervention studies. Our teams have conducted two intervention studies to evaluate the efficacy of a novel, computerized cognitive training program: Brain Fitness, developed by PositScience. Brain Fitness was developed based on scientific principles of neuroplasticity. Forty hours of training with Brain Fitness is proposed to improve the biological process of neuroplasticity and thereby improve memory. Efficacy of computerized cognitive training with Brain Fitness was demonstrated among healthy older adults randomized to Brain Fitness or an active control intervention. However, it was unknown whether the intervention program would be efficacious in improving cognitive outcomes among HF patients who have or are at risk for cognitive dysfunction. We conducted two studies among patients with HF, Nurse-Enhanced Memory Intervention in Heart Failure (Pressler et al., 2011) (MEMOIR) (R01 NR008147 and P30 NR009000) and Cognitive Training to Improve Memory in Heart Failure (Pressler et al., 2015) (MEMOIR-2), to evaluate efficacy of computerized cognitive training with Brain Fitness in improving memory and secondary outcomes of working memory, processing speed, executive function, and health care resource use. In MEMOIR-2, we added outcome variables of serum brain-derived neurotropic factor (BDNF), mobility, depressive symptoms, and health-related quality of life and examined the BDNF gene as a potential variable that might explain response to outcomes.

In MEMOIR and MEMOIR-2, HF patients were randomized to Brain Fitness or a health education intervention. Both interventions were delivered in patients' homes over an 8-week period to minimize the travel burden for patients and caregivers. In addition, a home-based intervention can be more easily "scaled up" to larger groups of HF patients. Both studies included a nurse enhancement to monitor intervention adherence and assess HF-related symptoms that might interfere with adherence. In MEMOIR, advanced practice nurses made weekly home visits to patients in both groups for 8 weeks during intervention delivery. In MEMOIR-2, advanced practice nurses made weekly telephone calls to patients in both groups for 8 weeks during intervention delivery. Data were collected at baseline and at 8 and 12 weeks after baseline.

In MEMOIR (Pressler et al., 2011), 40 HF patients were enrolled and randomized; 34 patients completed the study. Using a linear mixed models analysis, we found that compared with patients in the active control group, patients in the Brain Fitness group had improved delayed recall memory ($p = .032$) at 12 weeks. Patients in both groups had improved recall ($p < .001$) and delayed recall ($p = .015$) memory, psychomotor speed ($p = .029$), and instrumental activities of daily living ($p = .006$) over the 12 weeks of the study. Health care resource use was 49% higher for patients in the control group compared with the computerized cognitive training group, but this difference did not reach significance (Pressler et al., 2013).

In MEMOIR-2, 30 HF patients were enrolled and randomized; 27 patients completed the study. In a linear mixed models analysis, we found that compared with patients in the active control group, patients in the cognitive training Brain Fitness group had increased serum BDNF ($p = .011$) and improved working memory ($p = .046$) over time. Further analyses of this study are ongoing at the time of this writing.

Impact. To our knowledge, MEMOIR was the first study to evaluate efficacy of a computerized cognitive training intervention in HF patients, and MEMOIR-2 was the first to examine BDNF as a variable that might influence outcomes in cognitive training studies.

These studies documented that HF patients benefit from nurse-enhanced computerized cognitive training with Brain Fitness.

Future directions. Our team continues to test interventions to improve memory, understand mechanisms that underlie memory improvements, and enhance the quality of life of HF patients.

References

Bennett, S. J., & Baker, S. L. (1998). Quality of life of women with heart failure. *Health Care for Women International, 19,* 217–229.

Bennett, S. J., Pressler, M. L., Hays, L., Firestine, L. A., & Huster, G. A. (1997). Psychosocial variables as predictors of hospitalization in persons with chronic heart failure. *Progress in Cardiovascular Nursing, 12,* 4–11.

Pressler, S. J., Kim, J., Riley, P., Ronis, D. L., & Gradus-Pizlo, I. (2010). Memory dysfunction, psychomotor slowing, and decreased executive function predict mortality in heart failure patients with low ejection fraction. *Journal of Cardiac Failure, 16*(9), 750–760.

Pressler, S. J., Martineau, A., Grossi, J., Giordani, B., Koelling, T. M., Ronis, D. L., . . . Smith, D. G. (2013). Healthcare resource use among heart failure patients in a randomized pilot study of a cognitive training intervention. *Heart & Lung, 42*(5), 332–338.

Pressler, S. J., Subramanian, U., Kareken, D., Perkins, S. M., Gradus-Pizlo, I., Sauve, M. J., . . . Shaw, R. M. (2010). Cognitive deficits in chronic heart failure. *Nursing Research, 59*(2), 127–139.

Pressler, S. J., Therrien, B., Riley, P. L., Chou, C. C., Ronis, D. L., Koelling, T. M., . . . Giordani, B. (2011). Nurse enhanced memory intervention in heart failure: The MEMOIR Study. *Journal of Cardiac Failure, 17*(10), 832–843.

Pressler, S. J., Titler, M., Koelling, T. M., Riley, P. L., Jung, M., Hoyland-Domenico, L., . . . Dorsey, S. G. (2015). Nurse-enhanced computerized cognitive training increases serum brain-derived neurotropic factor levels and improves working memory in heart failure. *Journal of Cardiac Failure, 21*(8), 630–641.

Sloan, R. S., & Pressler, S. J. (2009). Cognitive deficits and chronic heart failure: Re-cognition of vulnerability as a strange new world. *Journal of Cardiovascular Nursing, 24,* 241–248.

Challenges in Contemporary Pediatric Pain Management

Terri Voepel-Lewis, PhD, RN

I received my master's degree from the school of nursing in 1988 with a focus in advanced medical-surgical practice and my PhD in nursing in 2013. Broadly speaking, my research over the past two decades has focused on developing and improving our methods of assessment to study, model, predict, diagnose, and manage the care of children during and following surgery. This work has been extremely important because, historically, valid, reliable, and sensitive outcome measures have been lacking in the pediatric setting.

Most notably, I have conducted several prospective studies to improve our understanding of and ability to measure pain in the research and clinical settings (Voepel-Lewis, Burke, Jeffreys, Malviya, & Tait, 2011; Voepel-Lewis, Malviya, et al., 2008; Voepel-Lewis, Merkel, Tait, Trzcinka, & Malviya, 2002). These studies were aimed at tool development, refinement, and utility in the clinical and research settings. These studies not only have led to national and international clinical use of our pain measures in hospital and ambulatory settings but have provided sensitive measures that have facilitated innumerable prospective clinical trials both institutionally and nationally. Additionally, providers and pain experts at large pediatric hospital settings found our instrument to have greater clinical utility compared to other pain assessment instruments (Voepel-Lewis, Malviya, et al., 2008). I have also conducted several prospective studies to examine, develop, and test measures to assess sedation, perioperative risk, and pain outcomes in children (Voepel-Lewis, Malviya, & Tait, 2003; Voepel-Lewis, Marinkovic, Kostrzewa, Tait, & Malviya, 2008). These studies have improved our understanding of risk and safety outcomes in children.

Currently, my research activities are concentrated on assessing and improving parents' knowledge and decision making to safely and effectively manage their children's pain in the home setting and testing the hypothesized role that baseline pain sensitivity plays in the postoperative pain experience in children.

Effective pain management requires analgesic decisions that balance the need to maximize pain relief and safety. Past research has demonstrated widespread analgesic use in our communities, yet very little is known about factors that influence at-home analgesic decision making. Furthermore, recent reports of unrelieved childhood pain, analgesic misuse, and substantial increases in the number of deaths as a result of analgesic-related adverse drug effects suggest that analgesic trade-off decisions in the home are often inadequate. My recent and novel work grounded in decision theory has thus prospectively examined parents' complex analgesic decisions and explored factors that influence their responsiveness to varying pain and analgesic adverse-effect signals. Our ongoing studies have examined and tested several of the hypothesized relationships among knowledge, preferences, patient education, and parents' decisions to treat their children's pain (see Figure 2-b), using both hypothetical and real postdischarge decisions.

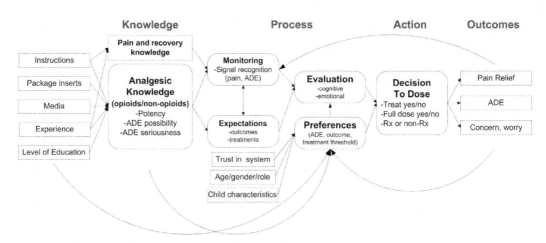

Figure 2-b. Conceptual model of analgesic decisions.

Our most recent analyses and publications have shown that many parents lack a critical understanding of serious analgesic-related adverse events and that strong parent preferences for pain relief interfere with analgesic knowledge and decision making, potentially leading to poor or unsafe opioid decisions (Voepel-Lewis et al., 2014; Voepel-Lewis, Zikmund-Fisher, Smith, Zyzanski, & Tait, 2015a; Voepel-Lewis, Zikmund-Fisher, Smith, Zyzanski, & Tait, 2015b). This work has enabled me to identify specific knowledge deficits that contribute to unsafe use and that might lead to poor pain outcomes in children. These data have, furthermore, informed our planned research aimed at developing and testing strategies to improve parents' use of analgesics, with an overall goal to improve pain outcomes in children.

References

Voepel-Lewis, T., Burke, C. N., Jeffreys, N., Malviya, S., & Tait, A. R. (2011). Do 0–10 numeric rating scores translate into clinically meaningful pain measures for children? *Anesthesia & Analgesia, 112*(2), 415–421. doi:10.1213/ANE.0b013e318203f495

Voepel-Lewis, T., Malviya, S., & Tait, A. R. (2003). A prospective cohort study of emergence agitation in the pediatric postanesthesia care unit. *Anesthesia & Analgesia, 96*(6), 1625–1630.

Voepel-Lewis, T., Malviya, S., Tait, A. R., Merkel, S., Foster, R., Krane, E. J., & Davis, P. J. (2008). A comparison of the clinical utility of pain assessment tools for children with cognitive impairment. *Anesthesia & Analgesia, 106*(1), 72–78.

Voepel-Lewis, T., Marinkovic, A., Kostrzewa, A., Tait, A. R., & Malviya, S. (2008). The prevalence of and risk factors for adverse events in children receiving patient-controlled analgesia by proxy or patient-controlled analgesia after surgery. *Anesthesia & Analgesia, 107*(1), 70–75. doi:10.1213/01ane.0000287680.21212.d0.

Voepel-Lewis, T., Merkel, S., Tait, A. R., Trzcinka, A., & Malviya, S. (2002). The reliability and validity of the Face, Legs, Activity, Cry, Consolability observational tool as a measure of pain in children with cognitive impairment. *Anesthesia & Analgesia, 95*(5), 1224–1229.

Voepel-Lewis, T., Zikmund-Fisher, B. J., Smith, E., Redman, R., Zyzanski, S., & Tait, A. R. (2014). Parents' analgesic trade-off dilemmas: How analgesic knowledge influences their decisions to give opioids. *Clinical Journal of
Pain, 32*(3), 187–195. doi:10.1097/AJP.0000000000000137. PMID: 25232863

Voepel-Lewis, T., Zikmund-Fisher, B. J., Smith, E. L., Zyzanski, S., & Tait, A. R. (2015a). Opioid-related adverse
events: Do parents recognize the signals? *Clinical Journal of Pain, 31*(3), 198–205. PMID: 24810650

Voepel-Lewis, T., Zikmund-Fisher, B. J., Smith, E. L., Zyzanski, S., & Tait, A. R. (2015b). Parents' preferences
strongly influence their decisions to withhold prescribed opioids when faced with analgesic trade-off dilemmas
for children: A prospective observational study. *International Journal of Nursing Studies, 52*(8), 1343–1353.
doi:10.1016/j.ijnurstu.2015.05.003.

SHORT PAPERS SUBMITTED FOR CHAPTER 3

Elizabeth R. A. Beattie
Gwi-Ryung Son Hong
Ann Kolanowski
Margaret Scisney-Matlock
Jun-Ah Song
Ann L. Whall
Reg A. Williams and Bonnie M. Hagerty

A Journey With Nursing Science

Australia to Michigan and Back Again

Elizabeth R. A. Beattie, PhD, RN, FGSA, MCNA, FAAN

I came to the University of Michigan School of Nursing (UMSN) for the first time in
1993 on a sabbatical visit from my academic position in the School of Nursing at James
Cook University in Townsville, Queensland, Australia. My clinical and scholarly interest
was in understanding the negative functional and emotional outcomes of behavioral and
psychological symptoms in people living with dementia (BPSD), specifically wandering
behavior. Donna Algase was undertaking pioneering research in that area, and we had
a rare intellectual fit. I returned to Australia, won the Centaur Memorial Fellowship to

study in the United States, and began my PhD work under her mentorship in 1994, graduating in 1997 from James Cook University (in Australia, the PhD is generally based on research only, and coursework is not required).

In 2008, after more than a decade as a research scientist working on major grants within the Center on Frail and Vulnerable Elders (COFVE) led by Donna Algase and Ann Whall, I accepted a 100% research professorship in the School of Nursing at Queensland University of Technology, a top-ranked Australian school. Also in that year, I was appointed as the only nurse director of a Dementia Collaborative Research Centre (DCRC; http://www.dementiaresearch.org.au/). The DCRC: Carers and Consumers (DCRC: CC) is a Commonwealth-funded collaborative of universities, nursing home providers, and Alzheimer's Australia (the leading national advocacy body representing those living with dementia and their families). The DCRC: CC investigators are predominantly nurse scientists, and the broad focus of the center is improving the quality of life of people living with dementia and their caregivers. I also serve as director of the Queensland Dementia Training Study Center (DTSC), one of five in a national Australian consortium with a mandate of dementia-focused knowledge translation for health professionals (http://dtsc.com.au/).

In Australia, the equivalent of the National Institutes of Health is the National Health and Medical Research Council (NHMRC). Other competitive funding is provided by the Australian Research Council, the Department of Social Services, and a small philanthropic sector including, for example, Alzheimer's Australia. There is no specific research funding body akin to the National Institute of Nursing Research (NINR), focused on nursing science, or the National Institute on Aging, focused on aging. The cadre of nurse scientists prepared at a level to be competitive is small overall, and within my specialty of geropsychiatric nursing, even smaller (fewer than 10 in academic positions). To be successful as a nurse scientist, it is necessary for individuals to maintain a broader scope and focus in their research than that typically expected of nurse scientists in the United States. Further, within the national dementia initiative in Australia, the identified research priorities of people living with dementia and their caregivers contribute significantly to the determination of the national priority research funding foci enacted by the DCRCs and NHMRC. For some time, research funding opportunities have been disproportionately skewed toward cure and prevention research. In this climate, it has been very challenging to develop and maintain a program of nurse-led research focused on care.

Program of Research

My collaborative research has involved a number of streams addressing the broader theme of quality of life in dementia, including (a) the first national descriptive exploratory study of the quality of life of residents with dementia living in Australian nursing homes (Beattie et al., 2015), (b) a series of studies focused on respite care, and (c) a set of knowledge-translation activities via the DTSCs focused on supporting staff working with people experiencing dementia-related BPSD that impact quality of life. My recent individual work, using a biobehavioral approach informed by the need-driven behavior model (Algase et al., 1996), has focused on (a) the development and testing of interventions designed to ameliorate BPSD, specifically agitation and wandering, and to enhance engagement in meaningful activities and (b) knowledge translation. One large funded study (Moyle, Fetherstonhaugh, et al., 2015) of a harp seal companion robot (PARO) and two pilot studies focused on the impact of daily structured walking and preferred music, respectively, on wandering are in progress (with MacAndrew). A recent PhD student of mine undertook a descriptive exploratory study of wandering-related boundary transgression in nursing home residents with dementia, the first analysis chapter of which has just been published in *The Gerontologist* (MacAndrew, Beattie, O'Reilly, Kolanowski, & Windsor, 2015).

Quality of life of people living with dementia in Australian nursing homes. This study, completed in 2014, is the first of its kind in Australia and one of very few country-level studies conducted internationally (Beattie et al., 2015a). It represents an unprecedented collaboration among six of Australia's leading geropsychiatric nurse scientists. The study took several approaches that distinguish it from others in the field. First, we used a sophisticated stratified random sampling method, recruiting from all six states and one territory (Fielding, Beattie, O'Reilly, McMaster, & the AusQoL Group, 2015). Second, we examined quality of life from three perspectives (person with dementia, family caregivers, and staff) using multiple tools and qualitative techniques (Moyle, Fetherstonhaugh, Greben, Beattie, & the AusQoL Group, 2015). Most other studies have included only health-related quality-of-life measures and have not included self-reports by people with dementia. Third, we used a brief decisional capacity assessment tool to determine whether participants with dementia were able to provide their own self-reports (after their proxies had agreed that we could do so), an approach not generally taken in the international literature. This approach increased the number of participants capable of providing their own informed consent by more than a third from the number who were deemed able to provide informed consent by proxy opinion alone and thus supported the dignity and autonomy of participants. Fourth, we included tools focused on aspects of the physical and social environment and person-centered care (the primary philosophy guiding dementia care), allowing us to better understand the complex interaction of staff- and facility-level factors that impact perceived quality of life. Data analysis is in progress, and several papers are in review. Our findings are broadly consistent with international findings about self-reported quality of life in dementia—people living with dementia consistently rate their quality of life higher and their depression lower than do either staff or family members, and these differences are statistically significant.

Collaborative work with consumers to improve dementia-specific respite care. In consultation with the Consumer Dementia Research Network, a Commonwealth-funded national group of consumer dementia advocates, we conducted a literature review of respite care services and issues in Australia (Neville, Beattie, Fielding, & MacAndrew, 2015) and a national survey of caregivers of people with dementia focused on their experiences of the respite system (Fielding, Beattie, Readford, Neville, & Gresham, 2012). From the results of that survey, and utilizing consumers' own words and preferences, a consumer guide to respite care was recently launched and is now available across the nation (O'Reilly, Fielding, & Beattie, 2015). This work is a powerful example of a collaborative approach between researchers and consumers leading to a much-needed community resource about respite support. An evaluation of the impact of the resource on respite service use and patterns is planned, and two funded pilot studies are in progress, designed to support caregivers in making respite care decisions and staff in caring for respite residents in nursing homes, respectively.

Translational work to support registered nurses and allied health staff working in dementia care. Since 2001, major funding has been made available in Australia for applied research and knowledge translation activities focused on improving dementia care. Via our DTSC, I have led extensive national resource development about pressing dementia issues—for example, the BPSD Core Skills Quick Reference Cards (Dementia Training Study Centers, n.d.), a clinical resource providing evidence-based fundamentals of BPSD recognition, assessment, and management. This resource has been nationally distributed to more than 2,500 facilities in Australia; supported by urban and regional seminars; and requested from Canada, the United States, the United Kingdom, Singapore, New Zealand, and Denmark.

References

Algase, D., Beck, C., Kolanowski, A., Whall, A., Berent, S., Richards, K., & Beattie, E. (1996). Need-driven dementia-compromised behavior: An alternative view of disruptive behavior. *American Journal of Alzheimer's Disease and Other Dementias, 11*(6), 10–19.

Beattie, E., O'Reilly, M., Moyle, W., Chenoweth, L., Fetherstonhaugh, D., Horner, B., . . . Fielding, E. (2015). Multiple perspectives on quality of life for residents with dementia in long-term care facilities: Protocol for a comprehensive Australian study. *International Psychogeriatrics, 27*(10), 1739–1747. doi:10.1017/S1041610215000435

Dementia Training Study Centers. (n.d.). Have you seen the new BPSD Quick Reference Cards? Retrieved from http://dtsc.com.au/2015/06/18/have-you-seen-the-new-bpsd-quick-reference-cards

Fielding, E., Beattie, E., O'Reilly, M., McMaster, M., & the AusQoL Group. (2015). Achieving a national sample of nursing homes: Balancing probability techniques with practicalities. *Research in Gerontological Nursing, 28,* 1–8. doi:10.3928/19404921-20151019-03

Fielding, E., Beattie, E., Readford, M., Neville, C., & Gresham, M. (2012). *Summary of "Respite Care in Dementia: Carer Perspectives": Report on Full Study.* Retrieved from http://www.dementiaresearch.org.au/images/dcrc/output-files/316-respite_care_summary_report.pdf

MacAndrew, M., Beattie, E., O'Reilly, M., Kolanowski, A., & Windsor, C. (2015). The trajectory of tolerance for wandering-related boundary transgression: An exploration of care staff and family perceptions. *Gerontologist.* Epub ahead of print. doi:10.1093/geront/gnv136

Moyle, W., Beattie, E., Draper, B., Shum, D., Thalib, L., Jones, C., . . . Mervinet, C. (2015a). Effect of an interactive therapeutic robotic animal on engagement, mood states, agitation and psychotropic drug use in people with dementia: A cluster-randomised controlled trial protocol. *BMJ Open, 5*(8). doi:10.1136/bmjopen-2015-009097

Moyle, W., Fetherstonhaugh, D., Greben, M., Beattie, E., & the AusQoL Group. (2015b). Influencers on quality of life as reported by people living with dementia in long-term care: A descriptive exploratory approach. *BMC Geriatrics, 15*(50). doi:10.1186/s12877-015-0050-z

Neville, C., Beattie, E., Fielding, E., & MacAndrew, M. (2015). Literature review: Use of respite by carers of people with dementia. *Health and Social Care in the Community, 23*(1), 51–63.

O'Reilly, M., Fielding, E., & Beattie, E. (2015). *Getting the most out of respite care: A guide for carers of people with dementia*. Retrieved from http://www.dementiaresearch.org.au/images/2077_DCRC_respite_guide_6web.pdf

Improving Quality of Life

Culturally Sensitive Nursing Interventions Using the Concept of Familiarity in Korean Elders With Dementia

Gwi-Ryung Son Hong, PhD, RN

I joined the biobehavioral program of the Center for Enhancement and Restoration of Cognitive Function at the University of Michigan School of Nursing (UMSN) in 1998 as a postdoctoral fellow to extend my study of dementia caregivers begun at Case Western Reserve University. My findings showed that the most significant predictors of burden and satisfaction among Korean caregivers of elders with dementia were memory and behavioral problems of persons with dementia (burden) and social support (satisfaction) (Son, Wykle, & Zauszniewski, 2003). These findings are consistent with other studies of U.S. and Korean caregivers, despite the cultural differences existing between these two groups. Thus I was encouraged to consider a new theoretical focus for my work—that of "implicit memory and familiarity in dementia" (Son, Therrien, & Whall, 2002)—as an eventual basis for nursing intervention for elders with dementia to decrease behavioral problems such as aggressive behavior and wandering and to increase functions such as cognition and mood (Hong, 2011). Two years of postdoctoral training helped enlighten my overall research focus on the improvement of overall quality of life among older adults.

With the guidance of Drs. Whall and Therrien, I conducted projects toward developing theory-based interventions for caregivers of elders with dementia. These included instrument development to examine burdens of dementia care in a Korean American population as well as two complementary components of the theory: culturally specific cognitive familiarity and implicit memory. A sense of familiarity is thought to support and access enduring memory structures; therefore, culturally relevant triggers may improve cognition and behavior. Similarly, considerable evidence shows that implicit memory is spared in Alzheimer's disease. Both constructs offer a powerful therapeutic framework to influence dementia behaviors as well as caregiver burden (Son, Therrien, & Whall, 2002). The concept of familiarity was intended to apply as a possible intervention tool.

After the postdoctoral fellowship, I had an opportunity to get involved in the Interactive Research Project Grants (IRPGs) of principal investigators Drs. D. Algase, A. Whall, and C. Beck as a member of the research faculty at UMSN. This opportunity expanded the breadth and depth of my knowledge in the research areas of dementia care, especially in reliability and validity issues of instruments and observation methods used in persons with dementia (Algase et al., 2008; Whall et al., 2008).

In the context of this work, I met a great mentor, Dr. Algase, who significantly influenced me to become a nurse researcher; I learned from Dr. Algase's example in teaching, managing, conducting, and developing nursing research and came to have a deep interest in improving the quality of life of persons with dementia. In conducting research on those areas, it is critical to use valid and reliable instruments and methods to examine behaviors of persons with dementia. Collaborating within Dr. Algase's research team provided important experiences in developing and refining instruments of wandering behavior, way-finding effectiveness, and ambience (Algase et al., 2007). Consequently, I also translated several instruments from English into Korean versions and engaged in the evaluation of their psychometric properties of the Caregiving Satisfaction Scale, Revised Algase Wandering Scale, Way-Finding Effectiveness Scale, and Perceived Stress Scale. I also developed the Familiar Environmental Scale, which is still undergoing psychometric testing among Korean older adults. Based on those experiences, I am currently teaching a course on instrument development in social science offered in the doctoral-level curriculum at Hanyang University.

In addition to my methodological work, I was awarded grants from the Korean National Research Foundation to support a study testing the effect of the multisensory stimulation, utilizing the concept of familiarity, on functions in older adults with dementia who are residing in nursing homes. Results demonstrated that the intervention was marginally effective in improving patients' cognition, depression, wandering, and aggression (Hong, 2011). In another 3-year funded project to examine the effect of digital reminiscence therapy, dementia patients living in nursing homes are being studied using observational methods learned from my mentors to code behaviors and affection. This work is guided by my framework of implicit memory and familiarity.

While at UMSN, I also teamed up with Dr. Janis Miller's research team, giving me the opportunity to learn about urinary incontinence in older adults, such as the effect of pelvic exercises on women with stress urinary incontinence. I also gained research experience in urodynamic testing, paper towel testing, and other tools to study urinary incontinence. Thanks to the success of that project, Dr. Miller and I received funding from the Society of Urological Nurses and Associates to support a project examining urinary incontinence among Asian women. That experience also led me to Dr. Mary Palmer at the University of North Carolina at Chapel Hill while I was on sabbatical. We are currently collaborating on international research about the urinary incontinence of older adults (Hong, Park, Kang, & Palmer, 2014).

Also while at UMSN, I received the New Investigator Research Award from the Center on Frail and Vulnerable Elders (COFVE). Frailty is an important concept for both older adults and for those who study problems affecting these individuals; it was an unfamiliar but intriguing concept to me. In 2008, Dr. Hong and Dr. J. A. Song jointly conducted a national survey of older adults to examine the prevalence rate of frail older adults in the Republic of Korea. In addition to that study, I received a grant to develop a Korean frailty index in nursing homes, which is currently being refined to better explicate the measurable constructs.

The invitation to author a brief paper for this volume brought me back to 1998, when I began my career there as a postdoctoral fellow, and to the following 6 years as a member of the research faculty. As a then novice PhD, I knew little about where to start toward becoming an independent nurse researcher. Seven years later, I had confidence about where in the world of nursing science I wanted to be. Thus, in the summer of 2006, I began my new career journey as a faculty member at Hanyang University in Seoul, Korea. Nine years of tenure at Hanyang University and a continuing dedication to nursing research have given me expertise on the nursing issues of older adults with dementia. I owe much of my career success to the support of UMSN and great mentors such as Dr. Whall and Dr. Algase. In particular, I still love Dr. Whall's saying: "You learn by doing." Dr. Algase gave an impressive speech at the international conference held at Hanyang University in 2010; here is an excerpt: "For 30 years, I was wandering around to find out about the wandering behavior of persons with dementia." Indeed, Dr. Algase perseveres as a prominent figure in nursing research. I deeply appreciate the wonderful time and the greatly talented scientists with whom I associated at UMSN, where a solid foundation was formed upon which I could build a successful career.

References

Algase, D., Son, G.-R., Beel-Bates, C., Song, J., Yao, L., Beattie, E., & Leitsch, S. (2007). Initial psychometric evaluation of the wayfinding effectiveness scale. *Western Journal of Nursing Research, 29*(8), 1015–1032.

Algase, D. L., Antonakos, C., Yao, L., Beattie, E., Hong, G. R. S., & Beeal-Bates, C. (2008). Are wandering and physically nonaggressive agitation equivalent? *American Journal of Geriatric Psychiatry, 16*, 293–299.

Hong, G. R. S. (2011). Effects of multisensory stimulation using familiarity: Persons with dementia in long-term care facility in Korea. *Journal of Korean Academy of Nursing, 41*(4), 528–538.

Hong, G. R. S., Park, J. O., Kang, H. K., & Palmer, M. (2014). Activities of daily living and cognitive status: Associations with urinary incontinence in Korea. *International Journal of Urological Nursing, 8*(3), 130–136. doi:10.1111/ijun.12050

Son, G.-R., Therrien, B., & Whall, A. (2002). Implicit memory and familiarity among elders with dementia. *Journal of Nursing Scholarship, 34*(3), 263–267.

Son, G.-R., Wykle, M. L., & Zauszniewski, J. A. (2003). Korean adult child caregivers of older adults with dementia: Predictors of burden and satisfaction. *Journal of Gerontological Nursing, 29*(1), 19–28.

Whall, A. L., Colling, K. B., Kolanowski, A., Kim, H. J., Hong, G. R. S., DeCicco, B., . . . Beck, C. (2008). Factors associated with aggressive behavior among nursing home residents with dementia. *The Gerontologist, 48*(6), 721–731.

Theory-Based Nonpharmacological Interventions for Persons Living With Dementia

Ann Kolanowski, PhD, RN, FAAN

My program of research centers on the development of theory-based nonpharmacological interventions for the behavioral and cognitive symptoms of persons living with dementia.

In 1990, we knew very little about the causes of and interventions for the behavioral and psychological symptoms of dementia (BPSD). My early publications reflect the work I did with colleagues at the Universities of Michigan and Arkansas to identify factors related to these behaviors and to incorporate these factors into a model: the need-driven dementia-compromised behavior (NDB) model. This model was one of the first to reframe the view of behavioral symptoms from "disturbing" to behaviors that communicate unmet needs. My contribution to the model was the importance of premorbid personality as a risk factor for BPSD and as an expression of individual needs. In two large studies funded by the National Institute of Nursing Research (NINR), we found that premorbid personality traits were related to aggression and problematic vocalizations in persons living with dementia.

By 2000, there was some clinical evidence that recreational activities could reduce BPSD in nursing home residents with dementia, but we did not have a systematic method for prescribing these activities in an individualized manner or strong empirical evidence supporting their use. I used the NDB model to design an innovative, theory-based method for identifying the style of interest (activity preferences) of people with dementia vis-à-vis an assessment of their personality traits. This approach gave "voice" to people living with dementia who have difficulty expressing their activity preferences. Activities that match style of interest are more therapeutic because they meet individual needs expressed by personality. We tested this hypothesis in two NINR-funded clinical trials. In both trials, we found that personality style of interest was the activity component that produced the most efficacious results for improving engagement, attention, and alertness while reducing BPSD. Activities matched to both function and style of interest improved pleasure.

My current work builds on earlier research and addresses the cognitive symptoms of delirium in persons living with dementia. We learned that interest-capturing activities engage people with dementia, and we are now using this approach to improve inattention, the most prominent cognitive feature in delirium. In our NINR-funded clinical trial, we are testing the efficacy of interest-tailored cognitive activities for focusing attention and restoring disrupted cognitive function—a problem that is found in delirium regardless of precipitating cause. As such, this nondrug intervention has the potential to complement other well-targeted medical treatments for delirium. I lead the interdisciplinary team that refined the theoretical framework that guides the testing of this innovative intervention.

My current research also includes work on the Centers for Medicare and Medicaid Services' National Partnership to Improve Dementia Care and Reduce Antipsychotic Use in Nursing Homes. This work entails translating into clinical practice earlier findings about the efficacy of nondrug behavioral and cognitive interventions for BPSD. Supported by a grant from the Commonwealth Foundation, I co-led an expert interdisciplinary team in the development of a free, web-based tool kit that helps staff implement nondrug interventions for BPSD (http://www.nursinghometoolkit.com). Additionally, I am a member of the Dementia Action Alliance, a grassroots organization dedicated to the promotion of person-centered care for people living with dementia. I am cochair of their Education, Health, and Well-Being Committee.

Selected Publications

Algase, D. L., Beck, C., Kolanowski, A. M., Whall, A., Berent, S., Richards, K., & Beattie, E. (1996). Need-driven dementia-compromised behavior: An alternative view of disruptive behavior. *American Journal of Alzheimer's Disease, 11*(6), 10, 12–19.

Beck, C., Richards, K., Lambert, C., Doan, R., Landes, A., Whall, A., . . . Feldman, S. (2011). Factors associated with problematic vocalizations in nursing home residents with dementia. *Gerontologist, 51*(3), 389–405.

Kolanowski, A. M., Bossen, A., Hill, N., Guzman-Velez, E., & Litaker, M. (2012). Factors related to sustained attention during an activity intervention in nursing home residents with dementia. *Dementia and Geriatric Cognitive Disorders, 33*(4), 233–239.

Kolanowski, A. M., Litaker, M., & Buettner, L. (2005). Efficacy of theory-based activities for behavioral symptoms of dementia. *Nursing Research, 54*(4), 219–228.

Kolanowski, A. M., Litaker, M., Buettner, L., Moeller, J., & Costa, P. (2011). A randomized clinical trial of theory-based activities for the behavioral symptoms of dementia in nursing home residents. *Journal of the American Geriatrics Society, 59*(6), 1032–1041.

Kolanowski, A. M., Mogle, J. A., Fick, D. M., Hill, N., Mulhall, P., Nadler, J., . . . Behrens, L. (2015). Pain, delirium and physical function in skilled nursing home patients with dementia. *JAMDA, 16*(1), 37–40.

Kolanowski, A. M., Van Haitsma, K., Penrod, J., Hill, N., & Yevchak, A. (2015). "Wish we would have known that!": Communication breakdown impedes person-centered care. *The Gerontologist, 55*(Suppl. 1), 50–60.

Kolanowski, A. M., Van Haitsma, K., Resnick, B., & Boltz, M. (2014). A new toolkit for behavioral health. *JAMDA, 15*(4), 298–299.

Whall, A., Colling, K., Kolanowski, A. M., Kim, H., Son Hong, G., DeCicco, B., . . . Beck, C. (2008). Factors associated with aggressive behavior among nursing home residents with dementia. *Gerontologist, 48*(6), 721–731.

Cognitive Representations Assessment to Guide Medication Taking and Dietary Interventions to Improve Blood Pressure in Diverse Women

Margaret Scisney-Matlock, PhD, RN, FAAN

In the United States, one in three adults, or 67 million, has the clinical diagnosis of essential hypertension (HTN) or high blood pressure (HBP), and in 2013, more than 360,000 American deaths included HBP as a primary or contributing cause—almost 1,000 deaths each day. In reality, the cause of HTN is unknown. Among all adults with HTN, 84% of African Americans aged between 20 and 75 will have HTN compared to 68% of Caucasians or White Americans. The HTN health disparity is complex and might be linked to a lack of access to quality health care and chronic nonadherence to medical regimens, including prescription medications, and recommendations regarding dietary and lifestyle modifications (Scisney-Matlock et al., 2009). This reality suggests the significance of the national health agenda on HTN and the need to improve the scientific understanding of how people with different cultural-ethnic perspectives think about and behave about HTN, as well as how they follow self-care regimens.

My research goal is to clarify what and how people think about disease/diagnosis (i.e., how declarative and procedural knowledge is cognitively represented in their minds) and how this thinking is linked to resulting health behaviors toward managing HTN. The objective is to build cognitive representations for the purposes of knowledge integration and to discover what role cognitive processes such as appraisal, coping, adaptation, and continuous learning play in sustaining daily self-care regimes. Social cognitive theory posits that the brain functions to organize information into neural networking systems for "enduring" or "working" memories or cognitive representations that function to guide decision-making behavior. Cognitive representations are influenced by an individual's social, cultural, environmental, psychological, and physiological experiences. Cognitive representation assessment is critical for identifying knowledge needs or information deficits for control of the condition before providing information to the patient for effective

HTN management. Thus, for more than 25 years, my research program has been, and continues to be, structured to determine how best to measure, understand, and modify (if necessary) one's cognitive representations of illness (HTN) and related health behaviors (medication-taking and dietary choices) to improve blood pressure and reduce cardiovascular disease risk.

Since completing my postdoctoral studies at the University of Michigan, I have been the principal investigator for more than 15 studies focused on hypertension-related cognitive representations, including instrument development, concept development and measurement, and cognitive-behavioral interventions to address two major theoretical questions.

Question 1. Is the underlying structure of the measurement of cognitive representations reliable and valid to predict hypertension-related self-care knowledge deficits? Qualitative and quantitative methodological studies addressed this question. The survey instrument development and testing procedures established psychometric properties of cognitive representations of hypertension scales to document valid 21-item, three-dimensional cognitive representations of hypertension scales (Scisney-Matlock & Watkins, 2003).

Question 2. To what extent do limited cognitive representations predispose a person with essential HTN to be at risk for developing cardiovascular disease? In 1996, I developed and pilot tested the Manage Associated Perceptions (MAP) Program from an emerging conceptual framework adapted from Leventhal's self-regulation cognition theory. The major hypothesis was to test whether cognitive representations could be shaped to guide long-term behavior to affect compliance to lower blood pressure toward therapeutic levels in diverse hypertensive women. The research application, titled "Shaping Cognitive Representations in Hypertensive Women," was funded by the National Institutes of Health, National Institute of Nursing Research. The MAP incorporates a self-directed 30-day program for all participants to take blood pressure medication from an electronic monitoring system; perform self blood pressure measures; and for the cognitive behavioral intervention (CBI) experimental group, read daily printed, tailored messages for building a cognitive representation of medication-taking behavior or memories of beliefs, attitudes, and intentions for behavior. Repeated measures analysis of variance showed significant blood pressure reductions and greater medication compliance in the experimental group as compared to the control group. African American women in the CBI group showed greater blood pressure improvement and compliance compared to White American women.

In 1998, to emphasize the importance of therapeutic lifestyle modifications and strategies for controlling HBP, the article: "Reliability and Validity of the Lifestyle Cognitive Representations Scales" was published (Scisney-Matlock, 1998). This research offers new insight into the role of cognitive representations for predicting the extent of knowledge deficits and health behavior—that is, healthy eating habits. This discovery led to the development and evaluation of tailored messages designed to fit the cognitive representations or knowledge needs of patients using the Dietary Approaches to Stop Hypertension (DASH) diet. The National Institute on Aging Research funded my project, "A Lifestyle Intervention for Hypertensive Women."

Testing the experimental CBI, named Women's and Men's Hypertension Experiences and Emerging Lifestyles Intervention (WHEELS), compared to controls revealed results that supported the claim that the CBI provides critical knowledge needed for enhancing compliance with dietary modifications. The main article published from this research (Scisney-Matlock, Kachorek, McClerking, & Glazewski, 2006), titled "Development and Evaluation of DASH Diet Tailored Messages for Hypertension Treatment," led to recognition in *Science Direct* as 1 of the 25 hottest, most read, or most downloaded articles in 2007.

The impact of WHEELS research is indicated by the American Dietetic Association's Evidence Analysis Library (now the Academy of Nutrition and Dietetics; http://www.andeal.org) to address the question, "Which nutrition intervention methods have been shown to be effective in improving nutrition outcomes among adults with cardiovascular diseases with varying socio-economic status, racial/ethnic groups or geographic locations?" Moreover, a Cochrane Systematic Review article included the WHEELS study as one of the evidence-based interventions found to enhance adherence to dietary advice for preventing and managing chronic diseases in adults.

The final phase of my research agenda was to determine its usefulness and effectiveness for diverse populations at the greatest risk for morbidity and premature death from HBP. In 2009, a Blue Cross Blue Shield of Michigan Foundation grant provided major support for a series of four studies to specifically develop, test, and evaluate the efficacy of a computerized CBI: the WHEELS-I program for improving blood pressure and unhealthy eating habits. The major research hypothesis was to test if there are significant differences between experimental and control groups on outcome measures for blood pressures, DASH diet cognitive representations, and DASH diet adherence in women from diverse ethnic backgrounds with hypertension.

The WHEELS-I program is a technological innovation that provides unique mechanisms and algorithms for assessing DASH diet cognitive representations, providing DASH diet information, and tracking behavior with daily morning and evening messages linked to web-based rapid response surveys. The intervention processes were to capture momentary assessment (close in actual time to the behavior) of self-efficacy to set goals for DASH diet recommendations, DASH diet cognitive representations, DASH diet adherence, and self blood pressure status evaluation. The data analysis, using repeated measures procedures to compare intervention with control groups, revealed compelling evidence of the effectiveness of the WHEELS-I program for reducing blood pressure, enhancing DASH diet adherence, and positively shaping DASH diet cognitive representations in women recruited at the point of care and treatment (Scisney-Matlock et al., 2015).

My science has benefited from being a part of the University of Michigan's community of faculty researchers in and outside of the School of Nursing and from sustained collaborations with national (Scisney-Matlock et al., 2009) and international professional research networks (Flack et al., 2010) on this topic. National and international recognition of the significant impact of this research occurred on several fronts, including an invited presentation at the American Society of Hypertension press conference leading to a CNN.com story by medical writers headlined as "one of three top health stories" by *Yahoo* and *Reuters*. The story, archived by WebMD News, emphasized the motivation women needed to keep their high blood pressure under control and to take their medication as recommended.

To date, covering more than 25 years, my research program has provided the only compelling evidence of a theory-based CBI via a computer-mediated, lifestyle evidence–based information program with women from diverse backgrounds. In 2010, the University of Michigan Office of Technology Transfer evaluated the WHEELS-I program for "proof of concept," granting a license for a commercial product.

References

Flack, J. M., Sica, D. A., Bakris, G., Brown, A. L., Ferdinand, K. C., Grimm, R. H., Jr., . . . Scisney-Matlock, M. (2010). On behalf of the International Society on Hypertension in Blacks. Management of high blood pressure in Blacks: An update of the *International Society on Hypertension in Blacks Consensus Statement. Hypertension, 56,* 780–800.

Scisney-Matlock, M. (1998). Reliability and validity of the lifestyle cognitive representations scales. *Journal of Association of Black Faculty in Higher Education, 2,* 28–34.

Scisney-Matlock, M., Batts-Turner, M. L., Bosworth, H. B., Coverson, D., Dennison, C. R., Dunbar-Jacob, J. M., & Strickland, O. L. (2009). Strategies for sustained behavioral modification as part of hypertension management. *Post Graduate Medicine, 121,* 147–157.

Scisney-Matlock, M., Brough, E., Daramola, O., Jones, M., Jones, L., & Holmes, S. (2015). A non-pharmacological approach to decrease unhealthy eating patterns and improve blood pressure in African Americans. In K. C. Ferdinand (Ed.), *Hypertension in high risk African Americans: Current concepts, evidence-based therapeutics and future considerations* (pp. 35–58). New York, NY: Springer.

Scisney-Matlock, M., Kachorek, L., McClerking, C., & Glazewski, C. (2006). Development and evaluation of DASH diet tailored messages for hypertension treatment. *Applied Nursing Research, 19,* 78–87.

Scisney-Matlock, M., & Watkins, K. (2003). Validity of the cognitive representations of hypertension scales. *Journal of Applied Social Psychology, 33,* 1–19.

Managing Behavioral and Psychological Symptoms of Elders With Dementia

Jun-Ah Song, PhD, RN

I have been interested in elders with dementia (EWD) and their caregivers ever since I was a student in the MS program at the University of Michigan School of Nursing (UMSN). In particular, I was interested in the behavioral and psychological symptoms of dementia (BPSD) in elders and how to effectively manage those symptoms without the use of medications. My experiences in the MS and PhD programs at UMSN—especially with the wandering research team of Interactive Research Project Grants of Drs. Algase, Beck, and Whall—have led to my involvement in various studies that explore the causes and outcomes of BPSD, establish effective BPSD management strategies, and determine effective methods to deliver such knowledge to caregivers of EWD.

As in other international countries, South Korea is faced with an aging society wherein the number of EWD is increasing rapidly. This has resulted in the increased demand for long-term care (LTC). However, the availability of informal or family caregivers has diminished due to changes in family structure, increased women's labor participation, and decreased willingness to provide care. Accordingly, the need for LTC facilities for elders has grown. In response to these challenges, the South Korean government passed a law in 2008 establishing a public LTC insurance program for elders. Since then, there has been a surplus of LTC facilities (i.e., nursing homes and housing programs where seniors congregate). In 2012, there were a reported 4,352 LTC facilities in South Korea (Korean Statistical Information Service, 2013). Despite such a rapid increase in the number of LTC facilities, caregivers working in these LTC facilities are not well equipped to take care of EWD. This implies that appropriate education programs are necessary to train caregivers of EWD.

My program of research reflects the needs of the current Korean society and consists of mainly three parts: (a) exploration of BPSD of Korean EWD, (b) development of appropriate management approaches for BPSD, and (c) development of effective educational methods to train caregivers in managing BPSD. Detailed explanations of the three research areas follow.

BPSD of Korean Elders With Dementia

Among various BPSD, my earlier research focused more on the wandering behavior of Korean EWD. Wandering is one of the most difficult symptoms to manage not only for family caregivers but also for formal professional caregivers. Accordingly, it was necessary to explore characteristics of wandering in Korean EWD using a reliable and valid instrument. Therefore, the Revised Algase Wandering Scale (RAWS) for community- and nursing home–dwelling EWD was translated and implemented in my research. It was confirmed that the RAWS is reliable and valid in Korean culture as well (Son, Song, & Lim, 2006). Using the RAWS, I was able to explore characteristics of wandering behavior of Korean EWD (Song, Lim, & Hong Son, 2008), similarities and differences of wandering in different environments or cultures, related factors of wandering, and negative outcomes of wandering for EWD themselves and for their caregivers. Currently, through qualitative research methods, I am studying the experiences of family caregivers who deal with the wandering behavior of EWD. The findings of this study will provide useful information to develop an evidence-based guideline for managing wandering of community-dwelling EWD.

I have also studied the eating behavior of EWD in nursing homes, including characteristics of eating behavior and related influencing factors and outcomes (Lee & Song, 2015). The findings have implications for the staffing levels in LTC facilities and LTC insurance in Korea. In addition, based on the findings of the research and additional qualitative data, the next step is to develop an instrument to measure the needs of EWD in managing their mealtime behavior, which is one of my ongoing studies.

Finally, I have also studied the frequency and severity of BPSD in nursing home residents and its relationship with caregiver distress based on their job category (registered nurses vs. care workers) (Song & Oh, 2015). The findings provide useful evidence for determining appropriate staffing levels and thus contribute to improving the quality of care in nursing homes.

Management and Educational Approaches for BPSD

The second and third parts of my program of research are interrelated. Based on the need-driven dementia-compromised behavior model, which was developed by Algase et al. in 1996, my intervention research has focused on how to understand and interpret the needs of EWD and, in turn, how to use this comprehension to better manage their BPSD. In the study (Song & Park, 2011) that examined the effect of an institution-based group walking program to prevent and/or decrease wandering, it was found that the group walking program with social interactions was effective in increasing sleep efficiency, improving affect, and decreasing night-time walking of EWD. Other studies focus on how to effectively deliver management skills of BPSD to formal (Song, Kim, Kim, & Park, 2013) and informal (Song, Park, Cheon, & Park, 2015) caregivers. With support from the research fund of the National Institute of Dementia, web-based educational programs for caregivers were developed and evaluated for their usefulness. Further studies are needed to examine their short-term and long-term effects on the decrease of BPSD and the burden of caregivers, as well as the increase in caregivers' self-efficacy when managing BPSD.

My research will continue to be related to various phenomena in dementia care, and I believe it will be able to contribute to the scientific nursing knowledge base and promote the quality of life of EWD and their caregivers.

References

Korean Statistical Information Service. (2013). Home page. Retrieved from http://kosis.kr

Lee, K. M., & Song, J. (2015). Factors influencing the degree of eating ability among people with dementia. *Journal of Clinical Nursing, 24*(11–12), 1707–1717.

Son, G.-R., Song, J., & Lim, Y. M. (2006). Translation and validation of the Revised-Algase Wandering Scale (community version) among Korean elders with dementia. *Aging & Mental Health, 10*(2), 143–150.

Song, J., Kim, H., Kim, T., & Park, J. (2013). Effects of a web-based education program designed for nursing home caregivers to enhance the management of behavioral psychological symptoms of dementia (BPSD). *Journal of Korean Gerontological Nursing, 15*(3), 192–204.

Song, J., Lim, Y. M., & Hong Son, G.-R. (2008). Wandering behavior in Korean elders with dementia residing in nursing homes. *Journal of Korean Academy of Nursing, 38*(1), 29–38.

Song, J., & Oh, Y. (2015). The association between the burden of formal caregivers and behavioral and psychological symptoms of dementia (BPSD) in Korean elderly in nursing homes. *Archives of Psychiatric Nursing, 29*, 346–354. doi:10.1016/j.apnu.2015.06.004

Song, J., & Park, J. (2011). Effects of an institution-based group walking program (IGWP) to manage wandering behavior of persons with dementia residing in nursing homes: A pilot study. *Journal of Korean Gerontological Nursing, 13*(1), 37–47.

Song, J., Park, J., Cheon, H., & Park, M. (2015). Development of web-based education program for family caregivers in managing behavioral and psychological symptoms of dementia. *Journal of the Korean Gerontological Society, 35*(2), 411–432.

Care of Chronically Mentally Ill and Late-Stage Dementia Patients

A Scientific Journey Embedded Within Philosophy of Science

Ann L. Whall, PhD, MSN, FAAN, FGSA

The Beginnings

My interest in and thus research into two areas—care for persons with mental illness and late-stage dementia—began as fieldwork in the late 1960s during my first graduate degree in public health nursing at Wayne State University and continued throughout my later graduate degrees in psychiatric and gerontological nursing. In the 1980s, these interests served as the basis for my two Fulbright Scholar awards in the United Kingdom and Ireland and for National Institutes of Health (NIH) visiting professorships in Asia (Japan and Korea) and at multiple U.S. universities.

As large state mental hospitals across the nation started to close, I began working with graduate students in psychiatric mental health nursing (1960s and 1970s) to assess the needs of patients as they moved into new community homes. One of the health problems we repeatedly identified was a repetitive muscular movement (sometimes irreversible) known as tardive dyskinesia (TD), related to usage of psychotropic drugs. I contacted the Michigan Department of Public Health, which had funds newly available for research into TD. I applied for and received funding at the state level and carried out research on identification of TD via improved screening; the resultant publications led to 10 Michigan state-wide presentations across many sites. Years later, personnel at the National Institute of Nursing Research (NINR) have continued to report these publications regarding "early identification of TD" as part of the NIH packet for early detection of TD.

These studies helped change the goals for TD from "impossible to avoid" to "possible to decrease and avoid," making "normalcy" possible for these persons. We related this research to the philosophic ideals of nursing identified in Carper's work (1978) as focused on the ethical, experiential, artistic, and scientific aspects of care situations.

Addressing the Care of Persons With Dementia

In 1985, I was invited to join the faculty of the University of Michigan (UM), Ann Arbor, as they began a major thrust into gerontological nursing. Moreover, my work with persons with late-stage dementia had not yet begun. I collaborated with interdisciplinary colleagues on the NIH-funded cross-national Alzheimer's Disease Research Project that had been awarded to UM.

An excellent group of scholars was on the faculty of the UM School of Nursing, which is essential to successful joint investigations; there were colleagues such as Thelma Wells, Donna Algase, and others, who were well funded for their research. Because of these environmental features, we were able to attract NIH-funded postdoctoral scholars to work with us on a new joint research project. We began monthly meetings with this group to provide feedback on the interlocking research proposals we were all developing that addressed the three most troubling behaviors of dementia—that is, aggression, wandering, and constant screaming.

We also presented our investigative progress at the annual meetings of the Gerontological Society of America (GSA) and met Cornelia Beck's research team from the University of Arkansas at these meetings, and thus we began our joint collaborations. Our work has helped change care into a more open model for people with the three most troubling behaviors.

Our collaboration expanded across five universities, tapping persons with research interests to change the care of persons with dementia with behavioral problems. Our Interactive Research Project Grant (IRPG) across collaborating universities was submitted to NINR and the National Institute on Aging (NIA), which jointly funded research projects totaling more than $7 million and would run for more than 10 years to completion. This was, and is, a win-win situation for each university and the scientists within our group, as we received funding separately but were jointly responsible for the success of the overall intellectual outcome.

All three investigations on aggression, wandering, and constant screaming were successfully completed on time, within all requirements, and all have been published and presented across the nation. One of the final conclusions/lessons of the IRPG experience is that it is possible to accomplish much more through cooperative efforts than through individual studies; most importantly, we were able to change the care for persons with Alzheimer's disease.

Endings and New Beginnings

As our work was winding down, I was invited by Oakland University (OU) to occupy an endowed professorship, the Maggie Allesee Professorship in Geriatric Nursing Research. I thus left UM as professor emerita and accepted this appointment at OU, which has opened new opportunities for me to make explicit the philosophy of science content that undergirds the discipline of nursing.

Philosophy of Science Undergirding the Discipline of Nursing

Philosophy of science uses argumentation via philosophic analyses, and data are items such as publications and papers found in the theoretic area of interest. This paper is not the forum to describe the content needed in graduate nursing programs to fulfill these requirements, but we emphatically state the importance of philosophy of science in the guidance of theory and research within every discipline. The work of philosophic analysis must continue today and into the future, as the guidance it gives to future research and care is incalculable.

In summary, my programs of research have had and will continue to have positive impacts on the quality of nursing care. The work is relevant for both nursing and allied health practitioners, as the clarity, quality, and targeting of best practices for each of the targeted and vulnerable populations has been positively affected. Recognition has extended across the world, as I have worked and continue to work as an invited scholar in the countries of Japan, Korea, the United Kingdom, and Ireland.

Selected Publications

Tardive Dyskinesia

Whall, A. L., Engle, V., Edwards, A., Bobel, L., & Haberland, C. (1983). Development of a screening program for tardive dyskinesia: Feasibility issues. *Nursing Research, 32*, 151–156.

Alzheimer's Disease

Algase, D.L., Beck, C., Kolanowski, A., Whall, A., Berent, S., Richards, K. & Beattie, E. (1996). Need-driven dementia-compromised behavior: an alternative view of disruptive behavior. *American Journal of Alzheimer's Disease, 11*(6), 10, 12–19.

Whall, A., Colling, K., Kolanowski, A., Kim, H., Hong, G., DeCicco, B., . . . Beck, C. (2008). Factors associated with aggressive behavior among nursing home residents with dementia. *The Gerontologist, 48*(6), 721–731.

Philosophic Analysis

Carper, B. (1978). Fundamental patterns of knowing in nursing. *Advances in Nursing Science, 1*(1), 13–23.

Whall, A. L. (2005). Lest we forget: An issue concerning the doctor of nursing practice. *Nursing Outlook, 53*(1), 1.

Whall, A. L., Sinclair, M., & Parahoo, K. (2006). Philosophical analysis of evidence-based nursing. *Nursing Outlook, 54*(1), 30–35.

Depression and Stress

Research to Practice and Practice to Research

Reg A. Williams, PhD, RN, FAAN
Bonnie M. Hagerty, PhD, RN

In 1991, Bonnie received a National Institute of Mental Health (NIMH) Faculty Scholar Award to study a concept she had developed: the sense of belonging as it relates to depression. Reg had collected data on nursing students, so Bonnie talked with him about looking at the work through the lens of depression. Because both of us had degrees in higher education and nursing, it was logical to sample a student population, which we did. We published the results, and most striking was the depressive symptoms that the nursing students expressed (Williams, Hagerty, Murphy-Weinberg, & Wan, 1995). This essentially opened the door to our work in depression. In addition, Bonnie was developing a conceptual model and a measure of sense of belonging (Hagerty, Lynch-Sauer, Patusky, Bourwsema, & Collier, 1992). This instrument, the *Sense of Belonging Instrument* (SOBI), with excellent validity and reliability, is now used internationally. We used the SOBI in a number of studies, and it proved to be an important predictor of depressive symptoms. Sense of belonging is the experience of personal involvement in a system or environment so that persons feel themselves to be an integral part of their environment (Hagerty et al., 1992).

Our work in depression led to a program of research: We examined sense of belonging and indicators of social and psychological functioning, and we investigated prodromal symptoms of depression using qualitative analysis. Our results demonstrated that many patients diagnosed with recurrent major depressive disorder did not recognize when their depression was reoccurring, preventing them from seeking treatment early. We also examined the effects of sense of belonging, social support, conflict, and loneliness on depression and found that sense of belonging was the most important predictor of depressive symptoms. As we were conducting these studies, we submitted a grant application to the TriService Nursing Research Program, Department of Defense, and were funded to examine the factors associated with depressive symptoms in navy recruits. This study was conducted at the Naval Training Center in Great Lakes, Illinois. A group of 443 navy recruits participated, and we were able to determine the cut-off scores for those "at risk" for stress and depression. This led into our intervention study that we called the BOOT STRAP, an acronym for "Boot Camp Survival Training for Navy Recruits—A Prescription." Recruits at risk for stress and depression were randomly assigned to the intervention and nonintervention groups, and the remaining recruits served as the comparison group. A total of 801 recruits participated. The recruits at risk significantly increased their sense of belonging, experienced less loneliness, used more problem-solving and coping skills, and decreased insecure attachment by the end of recruit training. Percentages of recruits in the study successfully completing basic training were 84% of the comparison group, 86% of the at-risk intervention group, and only 74% of the at-risk nonintervention group. This had serious implications, since the results provided evidence that the intervention improved recruit functioning, strengthened trainee performance, and helped reduce attrition.

Our next study, titled STARS (Strategies to Assist Navy Recruits' Success), involved biobehavioral intervention. This was a prospective study to describe hypothalamic-pituitary-adrenal axis (HPA) functioning using salivary cortisol levels (considered a measure of stress response) and to investigate the effects of the BOOT STRAP intervention. Instead of randomly selecting at-risk recruits, we randomly selected divisions (approximately 80 recruits at a time) that were assigned for the intervention or nonintervention groups. A total of 1,199 recruits participated over the duration of the grant. We found that the recruits in the division receiving the intervention developed significantly greater group cohesion, greater problem-solving skills, and better perceived social support while reporting less anger than the control group. There were significant differences in the cortisol levels between the intervention and nonintervention groups. Most significant was the fact that we were able to show that the intervention had the potential of cost savings for the navy and, in turn, the taxpayers. Cost-effectiveness analysis showed that if the intervention were fully implemented by the navy with all recruits in basic training, cost savings per year would be an estimated $18.6 million. The cost to train facilitators and run the groups would be $1.5 million, still leaving a cost savings of $17.1 million (Williams et al., 2007). The navy consequently changed its training plan to include helping recruits manage and cope with stressful conditions. The series of studies we conducted at Great Lakes brought about policy changes for the betterment of young men and women in the navy.

In our next study, we broadened our perspective to consider the larger navy. We did a 2-year follow-up of sailors who had participated in the studies at Great Lakes and were now in the fleet, and we tested the feasibility of developing a web-based program about stress. Specifically, we translated a group-facilitated intervention into a web-based format and assessed the qualitative experiences of those in the active-duty military who were offered the opportunity to use Stress Gym, an online cognitive/behavioral self-help intervention. We examined the pre and post differences in stress among those who tried Stress Gym and identified differential responses to Stress Gym. There were 142 officers/enlisted sailors at a naval medical center who completed the program. Users evaluated Stress Gym positively for its user interface, content, feasibility, and satisfaction. Positive evaluation was not influenced by rank/status, sex, or previous deployment. Stress ratings also decreased significantly while using the program. We were able to show that Stress Gym was feasible to deploy, was accepted by the intended end users, and demonstrated the intended goal of reducing stress (Williams, Hagerty, Brasington, Clem, & Williams, 2010).

At the request of the TriService Nursing Research Program, we developed a proposal to specifically address the needs of military nurses and combat-wounded patients. Therefore, we were funded to (a) explore the lived experience of combat-wounded patients and the military nurses who care for them and (b) examine military nurses and combat-wounded patients' evaluation of Stress Gym adapted specifically for combat patients in the air force, army, marines, and navy. In the first part of the study, we used a qualitative/phenomenological approach; focus groups were conducted with 20 nurses and 8 combat-wounded patients. Themes common to nurses and patients were coping, shared experiences, finding meaning, psychosocial nursing care, families, and bureaucratic structure. Differences between the two groups were that the patients' perspectives "changed self," while nurses described "professional boundaries" (Hagerty, Williams, Bingham, & Richard, 2010). As a result of the outcomes of this study, we modified Stress Gym to address the needs of the combat-wounded patients and the nurses who cared for them in the air force, army, marines, and navy.

In the second part of the study, we examined the responses of 129 military nurses and combat-wounded patients in treatment facilities. The nurses and patients logged on to Stress Gym, reviewed the nine modules available, and completed a short evaluation of the website. There were no significant differences in the evaluation based on military services, sex, deployment, or education levels (Williams et al., 2013). The strength of Stress Gym was that it enabled all military members to learn about and get help with problems such as stress, anxiety, anger, and depressive symptoms anonymously and in private. Stress Gym was a versatile tool that could help nurses address the psychosocial needs of their patients by encouraging its use and including it in treatment protocols. We also adapted Stress Gym for a general population, and it is used as a web-based intervention in the University of Michigan Depression Center's Depression Toolkit (http://www.depressiontoolkit.org/stressgym/).

It is of note that in our research studies we included master's and doctoral students, and they were included in many of our research publications. Likewise, we gave students the opportunity to be the first authors in works they completed for their theses and dissertations. An example is Kaesornsamut et al. (2012).

Another outcome was the number of newspapers, lay publications, and radio interviews that highlighted our work. Some examples include *The Detroit News*, *Ladies Home Journal*, *Glamour*, and *Navy Times*. Also, we were interviewed on radio stations such as *WJR News Radio* and *Veterans Radio*. We also published an edited book on global perspectives on depression (Williams & Hagerty, 2005).

Depression is a serious illness, no different from any other physiological illness; therefore, biobehavioral research has consistently run throughout all of our studies. We hope our work has contributed to a better understanding of depression, has reduced the stigma of the illness, and has contributed to the science.

References

Hagerty, B. M., Lynch-Sauer, J., Patusky, K., Bourwsema, M., & Collier, P. (1992). Sense of belonging: A vital mental health concept. *Archives in Psychiatric Nursing, 6*, 172–177.

Hagerty, B. M., Williams, R. A., Bingham, M., & Richard, M. (2010). Military nurses and combat wounded patients: A qualitative analysis of psychosocial care. *Perspectives in Psychiatric Care, 47*, 84–92. doi:10.1111/j.1744-6163.2010.00275.x

Kaesornsamut, P., Sitthimongkol, Y., Williams, R. A., Sangon, S., Rohitsuk, W., & Vorapongsathorn, T. (2012). Effectiveness of the BAND intervention program on Thai adolescents' sense of belonging, negative thinking, and depressive symptoms. *Pacific Rim International Journal of Nursing Research, 16*, 29–47.

Williams, R. A., Gatien, G., Hagerty, B. M., Kane, M., Otto, L., Wilson, C., & Throop, M. (2013). Addressing psychosocial care using an interactive website for combat wounded patients. *Perspectives in Psychiatric Care, 49*, 152–161. doi:10.1111/j.1744-6163.2012.00344

Williams, R. A., & Hagerty, B. M. (Eds.). (2005). *Depression research in nursing: Global perspectives.* New York, NY: Springer.

Williams, R. A., Hagerty, B. M., Andrei, A.-C., Yousha, S. M., Hirth, R. A., & Hoyle, K. S. (2007). STARS: Strategies to assist Navy recruits' success. *Military Medicine, 72*, 942–949.

Williams, R. A., Hagerty, B. M., Brasington, S., Clem, J., & Williams, D. A. (2010). Stress gym: Feasibility of deploying a web-enhanced behavioral self-management program for stress in a military setting. *Military Medicine, 175*, 487–493.

Williams, R. A., Hagerty, B. M., Murphy-Weinberg, V., & Wan, J.-Y. (1995). Symptoms of depression among female nursing students. *Archives of Psychiatric Nursing, 9*(5), 269–278.

SHORT PAPERS SUBMITTED FOR CHAPTER 4

Bernadine Cimprich
Sonia A. Duffy
Ellen M. Lavoie Smith

Cognitive Dysfunction in Breast Cancer

Bernadine Cimprich, PhD, RN, FAAN

Altered cognitive function associated with cancer diagnosis and treatment is a distressing clinical problem with detrimental effects on daily functioning and the quality of cancer survivorship. Since 1990, Dr. Cimprich's research program has focused on identifying and treating altered cognitive function, particularly the loss of the ability to attend, in women treated for breast cancer. Since the early 1990s, she conducted a series of studies that documented for the first time (a) the pattern of early loss in attentional function in women newly diagnosed with breast cancer; (b) the problem of cognitive or attentional fatigue with loss of attention following diagnosis of breast cancer; (c) the efficacy of a theoretically based environmental intervention to maintain and restore cognitive function; and (d) risk factors associated with cognitive impairment in women with breast cancer. In addition, a cognitive self-report measure, the Attentional Function Index, was developed to assess perceived effectiveness in daily activities requiring attention and executive function (Cimprich, Visovatti, & Ronis, 2011). This instrument has been widely used with healthy and ill populations. In her most recent research, she led a multidisciplinary team in a prospective study examining cognitive impairment over time using functional magnetic resonance imaging (fMRI) in women treated with adjuvant chemotherapy for breast cancer.

The early program of research focused on the unexplained clinical problem of loss of concentration in women newly diagnosed with breast cancer. In the first longitudinal prospective study, changes in attention were assessed prior to any treatment and again at 3 weeks (before any adjuvant treatment), 2 months, and 3 months after primary surgery for breast cancer (Conducted with National Institutes of Health [NIH] funding, via a National Research Service Award, CA08390). The findings demonstrated a pattern of significant loss of the capacity to attend in women newly diagnosed with breast cancer, which was not related to extent of surgery, pain medications, or depressed mood state (Cimprich, 1992) and which appeared amenable to a new natural environmental intervention designed to reduce attentional fatigue (Cimprich, 1993). These findings demonstrated for the first time (a) the detrimental impact of attentional fatigue on cognitive function, (b) the presence of cognitive problems before any treatment that persisted and impaired daily function over time, and (c) the benefits of therapeutic intervention with regular exposure to the natural environment to counteract attentional fatigue and decline in cognitive function. This initial work indicated that early therapeutic application of the newly discovered environmental intervention based on attention restoration theory held promise for preserving cognitive function over the course of treatment.

In a prospective randomized clinical trial (National Institute of Nursing Research, NIH, R29 NR04132), the efficacy of the natural restorative environmental intervention aimed at counteracting attentional fatigue was tested in women newly diagnosed with breast cancer with five repeated measures from pretreatment to 1 year after diagnosis. Compared with the nonintervention control group, early restorative benefits in improved attention were manifested in response to regular exposure to nature ranging from walking or sitting in nature, gardening, and engaging in activities such bird-watching (Cimprich & Ronis, 2003). The benefits for improved cognitive function persisted over the course of the 1-year interval regardless of treatment type. These findings indicated that cognitive problems due to fatigue-related decline in ability to focus or direct attention could be ameliorated by a theoretically based, low-cost, nonpharmacological intervention. This intervention has been widely adapted by others for use in various healthy and ill populations and was incorporated into a broader intervention developed to aid transition to breast cancer survivorship called Taking CHARGE (Cimprich, Janz, et al., 2005).

No previous research had been done to determine factors that might predispose women newly diagnosed with breast cancer to impairments of attention. Thus several studies were done to identify possible risk factors for cognitive decline in women newly diagnosed with breast cancer. Taken together, the findings showed that (a) older women (46 to 64 years) who underwent more extensive surgery (mastectomy) for breast cancer had worse attentional performance postsurgery than younger women and those treated with breast conservation; and (b) in women 55 years or older, those with breast cancer had worse cognitive performance prior to any treatment compared with healthy controls of similar age, and higher levels of symptom severity predicted poorer cognitive performance over the 3 months following surgery (NIH, NIA PO-AG 13094; Cimprich & Ronis, 2001). Further study of risk factors prior to any treatment in women newly diagnosed with breast cancer (27 to 86 years) showed that older age, lower education, presence of chronic health problems, and postmenopausal status were each related to poorer performance on the battery of neuropsychological measures. However, only age and education remained significant predictors when controlling for all covariates. In contrast, greater symptom severity and mood distress were associated with self-reports or complaints of lowered effectiveness in cognitive functioning. Importantly, the findings indicated that different predictive factors were associated with measured test performance versus self-reports of cognitive functioning prior to any breast cancer treatment (Cimprich, So, Ronis, & Trask, 2005).

In summary, the studies in this program of research using neuropsychological measures and self-reported complaints consistently found a lowered capacity to attend prior to any treatment that persisted without intervention. While the exact sources of pretreatment cognitive problems remain unclear, it is likely that the stress and fatigue associated with the mental and emotional demands of a new diagnosis of breast cancer are contributory factors. Such early cognitive alterations could further compound any toxic effects of chemotherapy, contributing to the patients' complaints of "chemo brain." To better understand the nature, source, and trajectory of "chemo brain," more advanced brain assessment methods such as fMRI were needed. Use of fMRI involves a noninvasive brain scan that permits examination of pathophysiologic cerebral blood flow changes during testing in executive function networks that support attention and working memory (Reuter-Lorenz & Cimprich, 2013).

Since fMRI had not been used previously to assess attention and working memory in women treated for breast cancer, a preliminary study was conducted in collaboration with an interdisciplinary team of investigators. The findings of this first published pretreatment fMRI study showed that patients were less accurate and had a pattern of altered bilateral brain activation in higher task demand conditions in prefrontal and parietal regions that suggested compensatory activity. This suggested early cognitive compromise that could not be explained by treatment with adjuvant chemotherapy (Cimprich et al., 2009).

A prospective longitudinal study (R01, NIH, NR01039) was then done in women newly diagnosed with breast cancer to examine the trajectory of changes in neurocognitive function and self-reported complaints and possible contributory factors, including worry, fatigue, and overall symptom burden. The study assessed neuropsychological task performance and executive network function during fMRI with three repeated measures over a 1-year period in breast cancer patients treated with and without adjuvant chemotherapy and healthy controls without breast cancer. To date, the major findings have shown that (a) worry is a significant contributor to neurocognitive dysfunction before any adjuvant treatment and might contribute to reports of "chemo brain" over the course of treatment (Berman et al., 2014); (b) pretreatment neural inefficiency or compromise in the executive network was a better predictor of posttreatment cognitive and fatigue complaints than exposure to chemotherapy per se (Askren et al., 2014); (c) pretreatment executive network inefficiency and performance deficits predicted executive dysfunction at 1 year, particularly in chemotherapy patients (Jung et al., 2015); and (d) persistent cognitive complaints over time were linked with overall symptom severity and worry regardless of chemotherapy or other adjuvant treatment.

Taken together, these findings indicate that multiple factors, both physical and psychological, contribute to cognitive dysfunction in patients with breast cancer. Early alterations in cognitive function may compound any toxic effects of adjuvant chemotherapy. Overall, the findings signal the need for future research to continue to delineate the sources of cognitive dysfunction in cancer. One area of priority research is the need for development of pretreatment interventions that target both cognitive performance deficits and symptom burdens of worry, fatigue, and other sources of distress to improve cognitive outcomes for breast cancer survivors.

References

Askren, M., Jung, M., Berman, M., Zhang, M., Therrien, B., Peltier, S., . . . Cimprich, B. (2014). Neuromarkers of fatigue and cognitive complaints following chemotherapy for breast cancer: A prospective fMRI investigation. *Breast Cancer Research and Treatment, 147*(2), 445–455.

Berman, M., Askren, M., Jung, M. S., Therrien, B., Peltier, S., Noll, D. C., . . . Cimprich, B. (2014). Pretreatment worry and neurocognitive responses in women with breast cancer. *Healthy Psychology, 33*(3), 222–231.

Cimprich, B. (1992). Attentional fatigue following breast cancer surgery. *Research in Nursing & Health, 15*, 199–207.

Cimprich, B. (1993). Development of an intervention to restore attention in persons with cancer. *Cancer Nursing, 16*(2), 83–92.

Cimprich, B., Janz, N. K., Northouse, L., Wren, P. A., Given, B., & Given, C. W. (2005). Taking CHARGE: A self-management program for women following breast cancer treatment. *Psycho-Oncology, 14*, 704–717.

Cimprich, B., Reuter-Lorenz, P., Nelson, J., Clark, P. M., Therrien, B., Normolle, D., . . . Welsh, R. C. (2009). Pre-chemotherapy alterations in brain function in women with breast cancer. *Journal of Clinical and Experimental Neuropsychology, 29*, 1–8.

Cimprich, B., & Ronis, D. (2001). Attention and symptom distress in women with and without breast cancer. *Nursing Research, 50*(2), 86–94.

Cimprich, B., & Ronis, D. (2003). An environmental intervention to restore attention in women newly diagnosed with breast cancer. *Cancer Nursing, 26*(4), 284–292.

Cimprich, B., So, H., Ronis, D. L., & Trask, C. (2005). Pretreatment factors related to cognitive functioning in women newly diagnosed with breast cancer. *Psycho-Oncology, 14*(1), 70–78.

Cimprich, B., Visovatti, M., & Ronis, D. (2011). The Attentional Function Index: A self-report measure of cognitive function. *Psycho-Oncology, 20*, 194–202.

Jung, M., Zhang, M., Askren, M., Berman, M., Peltier, S., Hayes, D. F., . . . Cimprich, B. (2015). *Cognitive dysfunction and symptom burden in women treated for breast cancer: A prospective behavioral and fMRI analysis.* Work in progress.

Reuter-Lorenz, P. A., & Cimprich, B. (2013). Cognitive function and breast cancer: Promise and potential insights from functional brain imaging. *Breast Cancer Research and Treatment, 137*(1), 33–43.

The Case for Nurse-Delivered Health Behavior Interventions

Sonia A. Duffy, PhD, RN, FAAN

Directly out of my undergraduate program, I worked as a public health nurse in the Detroit Cass Corridor. While there was generally a "diagnostic" reason for the visit (i.e., wound care or a premature baby), it was not too long before I realized that the diagnosis was only the tip of the iceberg, as there were a host of biobehavioral problems that contributed to the disease. Moreover, health behaviors such as some poor lifestyle choices are the leading cause of death, and they are rarely addressed by the health care system. That began my interest in biobehavioral medicine.

After working for 5 years as a public health nurse, I came to the University of Michigan and received my master's degree in community health nursing. Using my new knowledge and prior work experience, I taught undergraduate community health nursing for 10 years. Because I wanted to remain in academia and do research on health behaviors, I returned to school to obtain my PhD in public health from the University of Illinois at Chicago with an emphasis in health behavior. Finally, I was returning to my passion.

Although my dissertation was related to adolescent smoking, I took a postdoc and continued to work as a research scientist at the Ann Arbor Veterans Affairs (VA) hospital, where I have conducted health behavior research. Working with head and neck cancer patients, I published papers on how smoking, problem drinking, and depression were highly correlated and wondered if it would be easier for people to quit smoking if their alcohol and depression were addressed. Hence, my first randomized controlled trial (RCT) was to test a nurse-delivered combined smoking, alcohol, and depression intervention among head and neck cancer patients. This led to a large National Cancer Institute–supported, Specialized Programs of Research Excellence (SPOREs) grant conducted at the University of Michigan, which was a longitudinal study of head and neck cancer patients. This study showed that even after a diagnosis of head and neck cancer, poor health behaviors could adversely affect biomarkers, cancer recurrence, and survival. What was alarming was that health behaviors were rarely addressed among this population.

At this point, there are enough RCTs that have showed that health behavior change improves health outcomes, and efficacious interventions are available. However, the challenge remains to integrate health behavior change into routine clinical practice. Hence, my current research focuses on implementation research designed to integrate evidence-based health behavior change interventions in busy clinical practices. And who better to implement those interventions than nurses!

When I came to the University of Michigan School of Nursing as faculty member with a joint appointment with the VA, I had just received a large VA Service Directed Research (SDR) grant to implement the inpatient, nurse-administered Tobacco Tactics intervention, an intervention that I developed. Then I was awarded a VA-funded Rapid Response Proposal to further evaluate the use of volunteers to provide peer support to inpatients to quit smoking upon discharge. At about the time the larger grant was ending, there was a call for proposals from the National Institutes of Health (NIH) for inpatient tobacco cessation dissemination U01 grants. With the help of others from the School of Nursing, I submitted and obtained funding to further disseminate the Tobacco Tactics intervention in the Trinity health care system. As a result, I was one of six researchers across the country to be funded and hence was a part of this national consortium to disseminate inpatient smoking cessation interventions, and it was the only grant with a nurse-based intervention.

At the School of Nursing, I was approached by another faculty member to consider implementing tobacco cessation interventions among operating engineers, a population that she had worked with on hearing protection. To thoroughly assess the health behaviors of this population, I received a small grant, which lead to a Blue Cross Blue Shield of Michigan Foundation grant to pilot test a web-based Tobacco Tactics intervention among operating engineers. This Blue Cross Blue Shield grant led to a R21 to further implement the web-based Tobacco Tactics intervention among operating engineers.

Melanoma rates are on the rise, and since operating engineers are outdoor workers, I assessed their sunburn behaviors. Many of them sunburn every summer and rarely use protective clothing or sunscreen. This led to a small grant to develop the Sun Solutions intervention for operating engineers, which I hope to develop further.

As my career continues at Ohio State University, where I received an endowed chair to continue this work, I intend to expand my work in health behavior interventions delivered by nurses. Yet I must acknowledge that my years at the University of Michigan (where I once screamed, "Go blue!") were instrumental in shaping my career in health behavior change. It was during my master's program that I was turned on to research. Working on the head and neck cancer SPORE grant, I published biomarker papers. At the School of Nursing, I was able to achieve associate and full professor ranks, was inducted into the American Academy of Nursing, and developed my skills in implementation research. Many of these things could never have been accomplished without the support of my fine colleagues at the School of Nursing. Thank you for all your support in my career and also for this opportunity to reminisce about my years at Michigan.

Selected Publications

Choi, S. H., Waltje, A. H., Ronis, D. L., Noonan, D., Hong, O., Richardson, C. R., . . . Duffy, S. A. (2014). Web-enhanced Tobacco Tactics with telephone support versus 1-800-QUIT-NOW telephone line intervention for operating engineers: Randomized controlled trial. *Journal of Medical Internet Research, 16*(11), e255.

Duffy, S., Terrell, J., Valenstein, M., Ronis, D., Copeland, L., & Connors, M. (2002). Effect of smoking, alcohol, and depression on the quality of life of head and neck cancer patients. *General Hospital Psychiatry, 24*(3), 140–147.

Duffy, S. A., Ronis, D. L., Karvonen-Gutierrez, C. A., Ewing, L. A., Dalack, G. W., Smith, P. M., . . . White, R. (2014). Effectiveness of the Tobacco Tactics program in the Department of Veterans Affairs. *Annals of Behavioral Medicine, 48*, 265–274.

Duffy, S. A., Ronis, D. L., Valenstein, M., Lambert, M., Fowler, K. E., Gregory, L., . . . Terrell, J. E. (2006). A tailored smoking, alcohol, and depression intervention for head and neck cancer patients. *Cancer Epidemiology, Biomarkers and Prevention, 15*(11), 2203–2208.

Duffy, S. A., Taylor, J. M. G., Terrell, J. E., Islam, M., Li, Y., Fowler, K. E., . . . Teknos, T. (2008). Interleukin-6 predicts recurrence and survival among head and neck cancer patients. *Cancer, 113*(4), 750–757.

Duffy, S. A., Teknos, T., Taylor, J. M., Fowler, K. E., Islam, M., Wolf, G. T., . . . the University of Michigan Head and Neck Cancer SPORE Team. (2013). Health behaviors predict higher interleukin-6 levels among patients newly diagnosed with head and neck squamous cell carcinoma. *Cancer Epidemiology, Biomarkers & Prevention, 22*(3), 374–381.

Lee, C., Duffy, S. A., Louzon, S., Waltje, A. H., Ronis, D., Redmond, R. W., & Kao, T. A. (2014). The impact of Sun Solutions educational intervention on selected health belief model constructs among Operating Engineers. *Workplace Health & Safety, 62*(2), 70–79.

Measuring and Managing Chronic Pain in Cancer Survivors

Ellen M. Lavoie Smith, PhD, ANP-BC, FAAN, AOCN

Most of the nearly 14 million cancer survivors living in the United States today receive chemotherapy, a mainstay cancer treatment. Many chemotherapy drugs are neurotoxic, and a common side effect of neurotoxic chemotherapy is painful chemotherapy-induced peripheral neuropathy (CIPN). Unfortunately, there are few effective treatments for painful CIPN and no widely accepted method of clinical assessment. The real-life impact of this distressing chemotherapy side effect became apparent to me after many years of clinical practice as an oncology nurse practitioner. I witnessed how patients suffered from painful CIPN. I noticed that in many cases, the patient's suffering was not obvious because oncology clinicians seldom asked about it, and patients were reluctant to report their symptoms due to fear that their life-prolonging chemotherapy treatments would be discontinued. Thus my research program is informed by burning questions arising from my clinical practice.

Program of Research

There are three cogs of my CIPN-focused research program: I have led or co-led five studies focused on discovering better ways to assess, treat, and prevent CIPN and associated neuropathic pain in adults and children. My research studies have employed descriptive, correlational, quasi-experimental, and experimental designs, and my program of research has been shaped by my strong clinical background, collaborative interdisciplinary relationships, and funding opportunities. Furthermore, my science has benefited from being a part of extensive national (Cancer and Leukemia Group B [CALGB] and ALLIANCE Cancer Cooperative Research Groups) and international research networks (CI-PeriNomS–European CIPN Research Consortium). I received intramural or extramural support for each of the studies described below, and the findings have been broadly disseminated.

The first cog of my research program is focused on improving CIPN and associated pain assessment. I have advanced the field by refining, developing, and testing new CIPN assessment methods. Two of my publications (Lavoie Smith, Cohen, Pett, & Beck, 2011; Lavoie Smith, Barton, et al., 2013) report the results of psychometric research designed to test and revise two established instruments previously developed for use in non-CIPN populations. Specifically, I revised the Total Neuropathy Score (TNS) into two short-form versions: a 2- and 5-item TNS for use in busy adult and pediatric oncology settings. My paper on TNS-based pediatric assessment—one of only three known papers focused on CIPN measurement in pediatric populations—makes a significant scientific contribution to the field by establishing psychometrically sound and feasible CIPN assessment approaches for use in young children. I also devised and tested a 6-item version of the Neuropathic Pain Scale (NPS) that can be used to quantify CIPN-related pain (NPS for chemotherapy-induced neuropathy) (Lavoie Smith, Barton, et al., 2013). My work, published in *Quality of Life Research*, further advances the field by documenting the psychometric properties of the European Organisation for Research and Treatment of Cancer (EORTC) CIPN-20, a patient-reported CIPN outcome measure (Lavoie Smith, Barton, et al., 2013). I am currently expanding this work via a National Cancer Institute–funded study that delves deeply into the psychometric properties of the CIPN-20. The anticipated outcome will be an improved instrument version that can serve as a gold-standard CIPN measure.

I have partnered with physicians, geneticists, and pharmacologists at Indiana University and the University of Michigan, serving as a coinvestigator or consultant on several grants funded by the National Institutes of Health (NIH) (Challenge, Clinical and Translational Science Awards [CTSA] Administrative Supplement, R01) designed to explore pharmacogenetic predictors of CIPN in adults and children. My unique contribution to this work has been to design the assessment methods used to quantify the phenotype (Lavoie Smith et al., 2013; Lavoie Smith et al., 2015). Lastly, I have partnered with researchers to develop and test a measure of pain-focused quality care: the Pain Care Quality (PainCQ) survey tool.

My psychometric research has led to the development of better CIPN measures. However, it takes more than a good measurement tool to improve clinical outcomes. Clinicians must actually use these measures when providing routine care. In an effort to take an entrepreneurial approach to translating my research findings into practice, I have partnered with industry to explore new and innovative ways to bring the best measurement approaches to the bedside. I have recently received industry funding from On Q Inc. and Genentech to pilot test a web-based electronic platform for obtaining reliable and valid patient-reported CIPN and pain severity data that can be eventually integrated into the electronic medical record. This research is designed to test whether the On Q platform fosters patient and provider engagement in CIPN assessment and provider adherence to quality care metrics, specifically CIPN symptom assessment (numbness, tingling, and neuropathic pain) and CIPN-associated pain management behaviors. Consistent with this theme, I published two papers reporting pilot study results whereby a similar electronic, web-based platform was used to engage patients and their families in symptom assessment.

The second cog of my research program is focused on discovering new treatments for painful CIPN. My research addresses an urgent need to identify interventions for a common, life-altering complication of neurotoxic chemotherapy for which no known treatments have been discovered. I conducted two important intervention studies to examine pharmacologic interventions for painful CIPN. In the first study, I tested an evidence-based CIPN treatment algorithm. Study findings provided preliminary evidence that the algorithm might be effective in decreasing CIPN pain while improving patient function and satisfaction. Results were published in the *Journal of Pain and Symptom Management* and the *Journal of Cancer Education* (Smith et al., 2009; Smith et al., 2011). My second intervention study was a national, multisite, randomized, placebo-controlled trial testing duloxetine as a treatment for painful CIPN. This study was funded by the National Cancer Institute and conducted via the CALGB Cancer Cooperative Research Group. This practice-changing study was the first large phase III trial to reveal an effective intervention that decreases CIPN pain severity while also improving functional capacity and quality of life. This study attracted significant national and international attention after the results were published in the *Journal of the American Medical Association (JAMA)* on April 3, 2013 (Smith et al., 2013). *JAMA* produced a video clip highlighting the study results. The video was distributed to television stations and website producers worldwide. According to *JAMA*'s estimates, the video was viewed by nearly 100 million people. This research garnered additional exposure through highlights in the *New York Times*, *US News and World Report*, WebMD, and three lay journals: *Coping, Scientific American Mind*, and *CURE Magazine*. The study results have been defined as "practice-changing" in two publications describing the National Cancer Institute's symptom management research portfolio. Based on this work, a systematic review paper published in the *Journal of Clinical Oncology* recommends duloxetine as the only evidence-based treatment for painful CIPN.

The third cog of my research program is focused on identifying individuals at high risk for developing painful, chronic CIPN pain. I am currently conducting a pilot study to explore whether a physiologic and biobehavioral phenotype predicts the development of chronic CIPN pain following breast cancer treatment. This work is funded by a competitive KL2 training grant awarded through the University of Michigan's NIH-funded CTSA and through pilot funds awarded by the School of Nursing. Study findings will lead to a greater understanding of chronic pain mechanisms in patients with painful CIPN and mechanism-based treatments to prevent and treat chronic pain in high-risk, pain-prone individuals.

References

Lavoie Smith, E. M., Barton, D. L., Qin, R., Steen, P. D., Aaronson, N. K., & Loprinzi, C. L. (2013). Assessing patient-reported peripheral neuropathy: The reliability and validity of the European organization for research and treatment of cancer QLQ-CIPN20 questionnaire. *Quality of Life Research: An International Journal of Quality of Life Aspects of Treatment, Care and Rehabilitation, 22*(10), 2787–2799. doi:10.1007/s11136-013-0379-8

Lavoie Smith, E. M., Cohen, J. A., Pett, M. A., & Beck, S. L. (2011). The validity of neuropathy and neuropathic pain measures in patients with cancer receiving taxanes and platinums. *Oncology Nursing Forum, 38*(2), 133–142.

Lavoie Smith, E. M., Li, L., Chiang, C., Thomas, K., Hutchinson, R. J., Wells, E. M., & Renbarger, J. (2015). Patterns and severity of vincristine-induced peripheral neuropathy in children with acute lymphoblastic leukemia. *Journal of the Peripheral Nervous System, 20*(1), 37–46. doi:10.1111/jns.12114

Lavoie Smith, E. M., Li, L., Hutchinson, R. J., Ho, R., Burnette, W. B., Wells, E., & Renbarger, J. (2013). Measuring vincristine-induced peripheral neuropathy in children with acute lymphoblastic leukemia. *Cancer Nursing, 36*(5), E49–60.

Smith, E., Bakitas, M. A., Homel, P., Fadul, C., Meyer, L., Skalla, K., & Bookbinder, M. (2009). Using quality improvement methodology to improve neuropathic pain screening and assessment in patients with cancer. *Journal of Cancer Education, 24*(2), 135–140.

Smith, E. M. L., Bakitas, M. A., Homel, P., Piehl, M., Kingman, L., Fadul, C. E., & Bookbinder, M. (2011). Preliminary assessment of a neuropathic pain treatment and referral algorithm for patients with cancer. *Journal of Pain and Symptom Management, 42*(6), 822–838.

Smith, E. M., Pang, H., Cirrincione, C., Fleishman, S., Paskett, E. D., Ahles, T., . . . Alliance for Clinical Trials in Oncology. (2013). Effect of duloxetine on pain, function, and quality of life among patients with chemotherapy-induced painful peripheral neuropathy: A randomized clinical trial. *Journal of American Medical Association, 309*(13), 1359–1367. doi:10.1001/jama.2013.2813; 10.1001/jama.2013.2813.

SHORT PAPERS SUBMITTED FOR CHAPTER 5

Kristy K. Martyn
Lorraine B. Robbins
Antonia M. Villarruel
JoAnne M. Youngblut

Event History Calendars

A Clinical Intervention Innovation

Kristy K. Martyn, PhD, RN, FAAN

While working at the University of Michigan from 1999 to 2013, I developed and tested the first clinical intervention event history calendar (EHC) that improved assessment and communication to reduce adolescent risk behavior and childhood obesity and improved adolescent mental health and other research. EHC methods were originally developed for retrospective demographic data collection at the University of Michigan's Survey Research Center. I was introduced to EHC methods by Dr. Deborah Oakley and adapted them to increase adolescent risk data collection in qualitative studies.

Pilot studies I conducted using the EHC with adolescent patients and providers revealed increased patient recall, report, reflection, and patient-provider communication. These studies were funded by the Rackham Faculty Fellowship, in National Institutes of Health (NIH) / National Institute of Nursing Research (NINR) P20 MESA (2003) and P30 MICHIN (2007) grants, and provided preliminary data for an adolescent EHC clinical intervention randomized controlled trial (RCT) funded by the NIH / National Institute of Mental Health (NIMH). The RCT results showed the EHC improved adolescent-provider assessment and communication (Martyn, Munro, et al., 2013) and adolescent awareness of sexual risk behaviors and intentions to use condoms, now in progress. This research was conducted with a highly collaborative team, including the University of Michigan School of Nursing faculty researchers Cindy Darling-Fisher, Antonia Villarruel, David Ronis, Michelle Pardee, and Michelle Munro.

My research on clinical use of EHCs for adolescents has focused on feasibility, type of data collected, gender differences in use, and patient-provider communication (Martyn et al., 2012; Martyn, Reifsnider, & Murray, 2006; Martyn, Saftner, Darling-Fisher, & Schell, 2013). Foundational to this research has been engagement of patients, providers, and other stakeholders (e.g., clinic staff and social workers) in developing the EHC assessment and communication intervention and conducting the research in real-world clinic settings. As a result, our clinical intervention EHC research has led to improved adolescent patient-centered assessment and communication (Martyn, Munro, et al., 2013).

My EHC research has also influenced the work of a number of colleagues at the University of Michigan, including PhD students (e.g., Melissa Saftner, Laura Gultekin), postdoctoral fellows (e.g., Cynthia Danford) and faculty (e.g., Darling-Fisher, Pardee, Kao, Brush), and interdisciplinary colleagues in the United States and globally. Their research using EHCs and has focused on a variety of population/foci, including the following:

1. Diverse ethnic/racial groups with Michigan doctoral students (e.g., Saftner's sexual risk research with urban American Indian adolescents) and faculty (e.g., Annie Kao's sexual risk research with Asian American adolescents)
2. Younger ages and dyads with Michigan postdoctoral fellows (e.g., Danford's obesity research with parent-child dyads)
3. Health foci with colleagues at Michigan and other universities
4. Other life circumstances, such as work with juvenile justice or with families of incarcerated individuals
5. Global adaptation, such as by investigators in the Netherlands, Canada, Korea, and elsewhere

The University of Michigan School of Nursing collaborations and support (mentoring and funding) described in this brief were instrumental to the development and outcomes of the clinical intervention EHC.

References

Martyn, K. K., Darling-Fisher, C. S., Pardee, M., Ronis, D. L., Felicetti, I. L., & Saftner, M. A. (2012). Improving sexual risk communication with adolescents using event history calendars. *Journal of School Nursing, 28*(2), 108–115. [2013 JOSN/Sage Scholarly Writing Award winning paper].

Martyn, K. K., Munro, M. L., Darling-Fisher, C. S., Ronis, D. L., Villarruel, A. M., Pardee, M., . . . Fava, N. M. (2013). Patient-centered communication and health assessment with youth. *Nursing Research, 62,* 383–393.

Martyn, K. K., Reifsnider, E., & Murray, A. (2006). Improving adolescent sexual risk assessment with event history calendars: A feasibility study. *Journal of Pediatric Health Care, 20*(1), 19–26.

Martyn, K. K., Saftner, M. A., Darling-Fisher, C. S., & Schell, M. (2013). Sexual risk assessment using event history calendars with male and female adolescents. *Journal of Pediatric Health Care, 27*(6), 460–469. doi:10.1016/j.pedhc.2012.05.002

Promoting Physical Activity of Children and Adolescents in Diverse Populations

Lorraine B. Robbins, PhD, RN, FAAN, FNP-BC

After obtaining my PhD in nursing in 1998, I completed a 2-year institutional post-doctoral fellowship (T32 NR07073), followed in 2000 by a 1-year National Research Service Award individual postdoctoral fellowship (F32 NR007509). My research focused on the cognitive and affective responses of adolescent girls to physical activity. During the 3-year postdoctoral fellowship at the University of Michigan School of Nursing (UMSN) in health promotion/risk reduction, I was mentored by Dr. Nola Pender to enhance my expertise in adolescent health research. I developed a commitment to increasing the physical activity of youth in order to decrease the prevalence of adolescent obesity. In 1999, I received the UMSN Award for New Investigators.

Following the postdoctoral experience, I served as coinvestigator and assistant research scientist for a study testing the efficacy of a computer-based physical activity counseling intervention for adolescent girls funded by the Robert Wood Johnson Foundation (N. J. Pender, PI). In 2004, to further strengthen my understanding of children and adolescents, I successfully completed a 2-year postmaster's pediatric nurse practitioner program at

UMSN. From 2005 to the present, I have held the position of associate professor at Michigan State University (MSU) College of Nursing, where I continue my research career.

My research efforts have been continuously funded by the National Institutes of Health (NIH), to test first the feasibility (R21HL090705; 2009–2011; Robbins, PI) and then the efficacy (R01HL109101; 2011–2016; Robbins, PI) of a multicomponent school-based "Girls on the Move" intervention with fifth- to eighth-grade girls to increase their physical activity. More than 1,500 underserved urban girls have participated in the "Girls on the Move" intervention, providing them with an opportunity to engage in various physical activities to promote their health and well-being. As a result of a 2-year research supplement award received from the NIH in 2013 (3R01HL109101-02S1; 2011–2016; Robbins, PI), I served as the primary research mentor for a student pursuing a master's degree in kinesiology at MSU. My grant awards to date total more than $4 million.

I have authored multiple publications in the area of adolescent physical activity in both nursing and interdisciplinary journals, including several international journals, indicating a sustained contribution to the science of adolescent health. One of my early publications resulting from a preconference on physical activity interventions at the Midwest Nursing Research Society was the first published review of the state of the science of physical activity research in nursing (Robbins et al., 2001).

During the early part of my career, findings from my research provided empirical evidence to support relationships among constructs in theories such as social cognitive theory and the health promotion model (HPM) in adolescent populations (Robbins, Pender, Ronis, & Kazanis, 2004). My research also contributed to the understanding of physical activity self-definition, physical activity self-efficacy, perceived benefits of and barriers to physical activity, social support for physical activity, and gender differences in perceptions of physical activity. This investigative work underscored the importance of personal perceptions of physical activity and demonstrated the low level of physical activity among adolescents. Research results were reported in multiple publications.

As a result of my postdoctoral work with Dr. Pender, I used the HPM as the theoretical foundation for my studies, as the basis for developing instruments to measure cognition and interpersonal influences related to physical activity (Ling, Robbins, Resnicow, & Bakhoya, 2014), and in the identification of variables associated with overweight and obesity among girls (Vanden Bosch, Robbins, Pfeiffer, Kazanis, & Maier, 2014). I developed and tested school-based interventions with underserved boys and girls in urban areas to help increase physical activity (Robbins et al., 2013). The HPM was integrated with motivational interviewing to create a roadmap for counselors to follow to personally encourage adolescents to increase their physical activity. The roadmap was well received by counselors in the "Girls on the Move" intervention. I trained numerous professionals in nursing, public health, education, and other disciplines across the state of Michigan to apply the roadmap and adhere to the motivational interviewing communication style. In 2014, at Michigan's Premier Public Health Conference, I presented the roadmap in a research- and theory-based presentation, "Integrating the Health Promotion Model With Motivational Interviewing to Promote Positive Behavior Change." My work has informed the sciences of process evaluation and treatment fidelity of interventions designed to increase physical activity among boys and girls (Robbins, Pfeiffer, Maier, LaDrig, & Berg-Smith, 2012.)

I have been invited to present my work at local, regional, national, and international conferences, providing evidence of a dissemination record that reflects the impact of my work. I recently completed a 2-year term as a member of the editorial advisory board for the *Journal of School Nursing* and began serving as associate editor for the journal in 2015. In 2013, I gave the keynote address at the first International Conference on Research in Health Promotion and Disease Prevention in Barranquilla, Colombia. I also conducted a workshop for faculty and students at Simón Bolívar University on application of the HPM to nursing practice. In 2014, I presented the "Girls on the Move" intervention, a group randomized trial, at the American Heart Association Scientific Sessions. My research was featured in the MSU President's Report, on an MSU-designed billboard displayed in downtown Lansing, Michigan, and in the publication of the Michigan Society for Adolescent Medicine. Awards I have received include the Midwest Nursing Research Society (MNRS) New Investigator and Senior Researcher Awards for research in adolescent health. My publication on sixth-grade adolescent boys' perceived benefits and barriers to physical activity received the *Journal of School Nursing* SAGE Scholarly Writing Award (Robbins, Talley, Wu, & Wilbur, 2010). I was recently inducted as a fellow of the American Academy of Nursing.

In addition to my research in the area of adolescent health nursing, I have mentored a number of junior faculty, undergraduate students, and graduate students both within the College of Nursing and within other colleges and departments at MSU in regard to scholarship, research, publications, and presentations. I have chaired the MNRS Adolescent Health Research Section. Furthermore, I have translated my research into community settings to impact school health policies relevant to child and adolescent health in school and community settings. Collaboration with the Healthy Schools Initiative Committee for the Lansing School District in the capital city of Michigan is an example of the translation of my research into improved health care for adolescents.

I am passionate about and committed to reducing health disparities and promoting child, adolescent, and family health through positive behavior change in individuals, families, and communities. The problem of adolescent obesity is epidemic; low levels of energy from sedentary lifestyles impair learning, and lack of physical activity predisposes adolescents to a high level of chronic illness as adults. The precursors of chronic disease begin in childhood. Physical inactivity contributes to compromised quality of life throughout the life-span. My goal, as I move ahead in my research career, is to develop efficacious and effective interventions to increase physical activity in adolescent girls and boys of all racial and ethnic backgrounds and socioeconomic levels. Further, public health policies must be transformed based on sound theory and empirical evidence in order to develop effective programs for obesity prevention. Evidence-based approaches to improving child/adolescent health, especially in underserved populations, can have a positive impact on the nation's health, including decreasing health disparities, if the programs are structured for sustainability and integrated into school and community organizations. Thus my future research goals include partnering with state, regional, and national public and private child health entities to conduct large-scale, randomized, controlled trials of child/adolescent physical activity interventions using the latest technologies and strategies to deliver culturally appropriate interventions to increasingly diverse populations.

References

Ling, J., Robbins, L. B., Resnicow, K., & Bakhoya, M. (2014). Social support and peer norms scales for physical activity in adolescents. *American Journal of Health Behavior, 38*(6), 881–889. PMCID: 4349196

Robbins, L. B., Pender, N. J., Conn, V. S., Frenn, M. D., Neuberger, G. B., Nies, M. A., . . . Wilbur, J. (2001). Physical activity research in nursing. *Journal of Nursing Scholarship, 33*(4), 315–321.

Robbins, L. B., Pender, N. J., Ronis, D. L., & Kazanis, A. S. (2004). Physical activity, self-efficacy, and perceived exertion among adolescents. *Research in Nursing and Health, 27*(6), 435–446.

Robbins, L. B., Pfeiffer, K. A., Maier, K. S., LaDrig, S. M., & Berg-Smith, S. M. (2012). Treatment fidelity of motivational interviewing delivered by a school nurse to increase girls' physical activity. *Journal of School Nursing, 28*(1), 70–78. PMCID: 3262065

Robbins, L. B., Pfeiffer, K. A., Vermeesch, A., Resnicow, K., You, Z., An, L., & Wesolek, S. M. (2013). "Girls on the Move" Intervention protocol for increasing physical activity among low-active underserved urban girls: A group randomized trial. *BMC Public Health, 13*, 474. PMCID: 3661346

Robbins, L. B., Talley, H. C., Wu, T. Y., & Wilbur, J. (2010). Sixth-grade boys' perceived benefits of and barriers to physical activity and suggestions for increasing physical activity. *Journal of School Nursing, 26*(1), 65–77.

Vanden Bosch, M. L., Robbins, L. B., Pfeiffer, K. A., Kazanis, A. S., & Maier, K. S. (2014). Demographic, cognitive, affective, and behavioral variables associated with overweight and obesity in low-active girls. *Journal of Pediatric Nursing, 29*(6), 576–585. PMCID: 4252398

Reducing Sexual Risk Among Mexican and Latino Adolescents

Antonia M. Villarruel, PhD, RN, FAAN

Utilizing a community-engaged approach, this program of research focuses on the development, testing, dissemination, and scale-up of interventions designed to reduce sexual risk behavior among Latino and Mexican youth. Studies that comprise this program of research include randomized controlled trials (RCTs) to test an adolescent behavioral intervention (called *¡Cuídate!* [Take care of yourself]) in the United States and Mexico and RCTs to test the efficacy of a parent-adolescent communication intervention (called *¡Cuídalos!* [Take care of them]) in the United States, Mexico, and Puerto Rico using a small-group format and web-based/computer-based formats. Ecodevelopmental theory, the theory of reasoned action/planned behavior, and social cognitive theory served as the basis of the adolescent and parent interventions. Scale-up and dissemination of efficacious interventions have incorporated the use of technology—specifically virtual environments and web-based applications. The following is a summary of major studies.

Adolescent Studies

The broad objective of these studies was to examine the efficacy of a behavioral intervention to reduce sexual risk behavior among Latino adolescents (Villarruel, Jemmott, & Jemmott, 2006). *¡Cuídate!* is a culture- and theory-based HIV sexual risk reduction program designed specifically for Latino youth. The theme of *¡Cuídate!* is woven throughout the program. *¡Cuídate!* incorporates cultural beliefs (i.e., familialism, gender roles, respeto) that are common among Mexican, Puerto Rican, and Latino subgroups and associated with sexual risk behavior (Villarruel, Jemmott, & Jemmott, 2005). These beliefs frame abstinence and condom use as culturally accepted and effective ways to prevent unwanted pregnancy and sexually transmitted diseases, including HIV/AIDS.

¡Cuídate! was tested in two separate RCTs using similar designs (e.g., follow-up periods, interventions, measures). In Philadelphia, adolescents (n = 642) recruited from community and school settings were randomly assigned to a 6-hour sexual risk reduction intervention or a health promotion control intervention. Data were collected preintervention; immediately postintervention; and at 3-, 6-, and 12-month follow-ups with excellent retention rates (87%–97%) for the postintervention follow-ups. GEE analyses revealed that adolescents in the sexual risk reduction intervention group were less likely to report sexual intercourse, multiple partners, or days of unprotected intercourse and more likely to report consistently using condoms. Nearly all theoretical variables (attitudes, norms, control beliefs) mediated the intervention's effects on sexual behavior and condom use intentions.

In a subsequent RCT in Monterrey, Mexico (Gallegos, Villarruel, Loveland-Cherry, Ronis, & Zhou, 2008), adolescents (n = 829) 14 to 17 years of age and one of their parents (n = 791) were recruited from school and community settings and randomly assigned to a sexual risk reduction intervention or a general health promotion control condition. Data were collected preintervention; immediately postintervention; and at 3- (adolescent only), 6-, and 12-month follow-ups, again with excellent retention rates (83%–97%). GEE multivariate linear regression models indicated there were no significant intervention effects on consistent condom use, condom use at last sex, and number of sexual partners. However, adolescents in the sexual risk reduction intervention group were more likely to be older at first sex, more likely to use contraception at first sex, and more likely to use condoms at first sex than those in the health promotion group.

Parent Studies

In the study in Monterrey, parents who participated in the sexual risk reduction intervention—*¡Cuídalos!*—received an intervention focused on sexual risk communication with their adolescents. Results of GEE analysis revealed more general communication, sexual risk communication, and comfort with communication than those in the control group. Mediation analyses indicated that prevention beliefs, reaction beliefs, and communication efficacy about communication significantly mediated the effect of the intervention on general communication, sexual communication, and comfort with sexual communication (all p-value < .001). Familialism mediated intervention effects on all communication outcomes—general communication, sexual risk communication, and comfort with communication. Additional analyses indicate that parent reports of parent-child sexual risk communication were shown to mediate the effect of the intervention on adolescent intentions to use condoms (Villarruel, Loveland-Cherry, Gallegos, Ronis, & Zhou, 2008).

In a subsequent study, we converted the effective small-group intervention program to a computer-based format that would be feasible and acceptable, especially for parents with limited education and low literacy. In the study, dominant Spanish-speaking parents (n = 130) and adolescents (n = 130) were recruited from community-based organizations and schools in Detroit, Michigan. Parents (and therefore dyads) were randomly assigned by the computer to the experimental group or to a 3-month wait list control group; retention was excellent (93%–99%). Results indicated that among parents who used the computer-based intervention, general communication and sexual risk communication were significantly increased (p < .01, .0001, respectively) from pretest to 3-month follow-up and also significantly higher compared with the wait list control group at the 3-month follow-up (p < .05; p < .001). The theoretical variables of attitudes, perceived behavioral control, and intentions to communicate with adolescents about sex and contraceptives and condoms were significantly higher in the experimental group (p < .05). Further, perceived behavioral control was a partial mediator of the intervention in relation to all communication outcomes (Villarruel, Loveland-Cherry, & Ronis, 2010).

Results from these studies formed the basis of another RCT, which is currently in progress, designed to test a web-based version of *¡Cuídalos!* with Puerto Rican parents (Varas-Diaz and Villarruel, 2012). This version incorporates many of the suggestions from parents in this study to improve the program (e.g., increased flexibility in viewing modules, ability to share materials/program with other family and friends).

Dissemination

The impact of this program of research on practice is evident in the scale-up of *¡Cuídate!* This program has been disseminated by the Centers for Disease Control and Prevention (CDC) as part of their Diffusion of Evidence-Based Intervention Programs. Extensive work was undertaken during this process to develop materials that could be used and disseminated by community members (Villarruel, Gal, et al., 2010). In addition, we have completed a study examining the efficacy of providing facilitator training in a virtual environment, thus reducing the cost of facilitator training (Valladares, Aebersold, Tschannen, & Villarruel, 2014).

Because it is recognized as an effective, evidenced-based program by the CDC and the Office of Adolescent Health, it is part of a compendium of interventions that must be used in conjunction with federal funding. Currently, more than 30 U.S. states and Puerto Rico are actively implementing *¡Cuídate!*

Impact on Policy

This program of research is part of a body of evidence that changed federal policy from an abstinence only approach to a safer sex approach. These studies, as well as the work of others, demonstrated that a sexual risk reduction approach was effective in reducing sexual risk behavior (e.g., multiple partners, unprotected sex, early initiation) and supporting sexual protective behaviors (e.g., delayed sexual debut, condom use, abstinence).

In summary, this program of research is one of the few extensive programs of research that has focused on Latino adolescents and families. *¡Cuídate!* and *¡Cuídalos!* contribute to allaying the scarcity of rigorously evaluated, evidence-based programs that are available and accessible to families and communities to reduce sexual risk behavior and help promote adolescent health and well-being.

References

Gallegos, E. C., Villarruel, A. M., Loveland-Cherry, C., Ronis, D. L., & Zhou, Y. (2008). Intervention to reduce sexual risk behavior in adolescents. Results of a randomized controlled trial. *Salud Pública de México, 50*, 1–10.

Valladares, A., Aebersold, M., Tschannen, D., & Villarruel, A. (2014). Preparing facilitators from community-based organizations for evidence-based intervention training in second life. *Journal of Medical Internet Research, 16*(9), e220.

Varas-Diaz, N., & Villarruel, A. M. (2012). Testing a Latino web-based parent-adolescent sexual communication intervention. Co-PI. NINR, NIH. R01 NR013505

Villarruel, A. M., Gal, T., Eakin, B. L., Wilkes, A., & Herbst, J. H. (2010). From research to practice: The importance of community collaboration in the translation process. *Research and Theory in Nursing Practice, 24*, 25–34.

Villarruel, A. M., Jemmott, J. B., III, & Jemmott, L. S. (2006). A randomized controlled trial testing an HIV pre-vention intervention for Latino youth. *Archives of Pediatrics & Adolescent Medicine, 160*(8), 772–777.

Villarruel, A. M., Jemmott, L. S., & Jemmott, J. B., III. (2005). Designing a culturally based intervention to reduce HIV sexual risk for Latino adolescents. *Journal of the Association of Nurses in AIDS Care, 16*(2), 23–31.

Villarruel, A. M., Loveland-Cherry, C., Gallegos Cabriales, E. C., Ronis, D., & Zhou, Y. (2008). A parent-adolescent intervention to increase sexual risk communication: Results of a randomized controlled trial. *AIDS Education and Prevention, 20*(5), 371–383.

Villarruel, A. M., Loveland-Cherry, C., & Ronis, D. (2010). Testing of a Latino parent adolescent computerized sexual communication intervention. *Journal of Family Relations, 59*(5), 533–543.

Critically Ill Children and Their Families

JoAnne M. Youngblut, PhD, RN, FAAN

My program of research is focused on critically ill children and their families after the child's hospital discharge or death; its aim is to identify individual family members at risk for adverse physical and mental/emotional health and the functioning of the parent dyad and the family system. These data laid the foundation for tailored interventions to promote health and decrease risk for adverse parent, child, and family outcomes. I have been the principal investigator of four R01s funded by the National Institute of Nursing Research (NINR) (two with multiple principal investigator Brooten) and a research sub-project funded by the National Institute of General Medical Sciences (NIGMS) through one of their programs for minority-serving institutions. Florida International University is a federally designated Hispanic-serving institution with a student body of 53,000 students that is approximately 61% Hispanic, 15% White non-Hispanic, 13% Black non-Hispanic, 4% Asian/Pacific Islander, and 7% other.

Contributions to Science

The impact of a child's intensive care unit (ICU) death on family members. Most stud-ies of parents experiencing a child's death have been limited to those dying from cancer. However, the milieu of an ICU death is very different from that of a death due to cancer, which often occurs in the family's home with hospice care. Visits to the child in the ICU are often limited in time and in who can visit; parents may not be able to be present when the child dies in the ICU or the operating room if organs are being donated. The ICU predeath period includes unfamiliar equipment and people; intubation and ventilation hampering parent-child communication; and the child's overall appearance as pale and/ or cyanotic, puffy or emaciated, comatose and/or agitated, with tubes coming from many places (e.g., pressure monitoring device in the head) and use of arm and sometimes leg restraints. Most studies on parent grief and bereavement have recruited participants through support groups and advertisements, with the age of the deceased ranging from a fetus through 40 years old and the time since death ranging from 1 month to 30 years when parent outcome data are obtained. Most do not measure effects on parents' physical health. The very few studies of grandparents after a grandchild's death are mostly qualitative, focused on grief and mental health, and have wide variations in age at death and time since death. Interventions for parents are rarely based on empirical evidence from the first 13 months postdeath.

Our sample of parents (NR R01 009120) was recruited in South Florida through the neonatal intensive care units (NICUs) and pediatric intensive care units (PICUs) where the child died. Some parents and all of the grandparents were recruited through official state death records. The age of the deceased and the time since death were controlled by design. In our parent study, the deceased's age ranged from newborn through 18 years, and data collection occurred at 1, 3, 6, and 13 months postdeath. In our grandparent study (S06 GM 008205), the deceased's age ranged from newborn through 6 years, and data collection occurred between 1 and 6 months postdeath for 95% of grandparents; the remaining 5% occurred between 6 and 12 months postdeath. In our sample of 249 parents, ages 18 to 40, the number of chronic health conditions more than doubled after the child's death, and management of preexisting chronic conditions required changes in medications (Youngblut, Brooten, Cantwell, del Moral, & Totapally, 2013). The proportion of parents (Youngblut, Brooten, Cantwell, del Moral, & Totapally, 2013) and grandparents (Youngblut, Brooten, Blais, Kilgore, & Yoo, 2015) with moderate to severe depression was 3 times higher than the national rate. Employed fathers returned to their jobs by 2 weeks and employed mothers by 4 weeks, but they reported having difficulty concentrating on their work. The parent findings were covered by national print media and nursing newsletters.

In their qualitative interviews at 7 and 13 months postdeath, many parents talked about their other children's responses to the sibling's death (Youngblut & Brooten, 2013). Content analysis yielded six themes: *not understanding what was going on* and *believing the sibling is in a good place*, primarily about preschoolers; *changed behaviors* and *maintaining a connection with the deceased*, primarily about school-age children and adolescents; and *not having enough time with their siblings before death and/or to say goodbye* and *not believing the sibling would die*, primarily about adolescents. White parents made few comments about their children compared with Black and Hispanic parents. All comments about the sibling being in a good place were made by Black parents. Children, regardless of age, recognized their parents' grief and tried to comfort them. Children also needed "alone" time as a respite from their parents' overwhelming grief and for their own grief.

The purpose of our current study (NR R01 012675) is to describe children's responses to the death of a sibling (newborn through 18 years) in the NICU/PICU, the emergency department (ED), or at the scene. Hispanic, Black non-Hispanic, and White non-Hispanic school-age children and adolescents throughout Florida are being recruited through NICU/PICU/ED clinical partners and through public websites with obituary notices and funeral or memorial notices, among others. Quantitative data on grief, depression, anxiety, and relationships with parents, siblings, and friends are collected from all eligible children in a family who agree to participate at 2, 4, 6, and 13 months postdeath. Qualitative data are obtained from a subset of these children through semistructured interviews at 7 and 13 months postdeath. The study is in progress.

Effects of children's critical illness and PICU hospitalization on parents. When this work began in the 1980s, research on parents' responses to their child's PICU hospitalization was almost nonexistent. Most research was focused on parents of critically ill neonates during and after their NICU stay. Research was needed on the more heterogeneous group of PICU patients, from newborn through 18 years old with a variety of critical health conditions. When a child is admitted to the PICU, parents are often unable to voice their concerns/fears about their child, information that is important for the clinical care of parents. Youngblut and Jay (1991) found that parents were most concerned about their child's survival and potential future disabilities. In another study of a small sample of parents after their child's PICU hospitalization, the longer the child was intubated, the less satisfied mothers were with their families and the less cohesive they perceived their families to be. Conversely, the longer the child's hospital stay, the more satisfied fathers were with their families in terms of family cohesion. (Youngblut & Shiao, 1993). In a study of preschool children hospitalized for head trauma and their families (NR R01 04430), mothers (but not fathers) had more stress if their child was in the PICU versus the general care units. Mother-father couples rated their child's injury severity similarly, but mothers had more stress than fathers (Youngblut, Brooten, & Kuluz, 2005). Parents' perceptions of their child's injury severity were negatively related to quality of family functioning at 2 weeks postdischarge (Youngblut & Brooten, 2006) and to mothers' mental health at 3 months postdischarge (Youngblut & Brooten, 2008). Mothers' baseline mental health and ongoing social support, but not injury severity, had positive effects on the mother-child relationship and family adaptability at 3 months postdischarge. This research found that mothers with greater stress and poorer mental health during their child's hospitalization might be at risk for negative mother-child and family outcomes.

Effects of maternal employment on child outcomes pre–welfare reform. When this research began in the 1990s, the large research base was focused on effects of maternal employment on healthy children, and the results of these studies varied considerably. I posited that studying children and families already at risk would more clearly demonstrate any negative effects of maternal employment. I conducted one of the first studies of maternal employment effects for preterm infants (F31 NR 06152) in two-parent families (as part of a larger study [Youngblut, Loveland-Cherry, & Horan, 1994; R01 NR 01390, 1986–1989]) and later preschoolers born preterm in female-headed, single-parent families (R01 NR 02707). In the study of preterm infants in two-parent families, child development outcomes at 3, 9, 12, and 18 months postbirth were the same for preterm infants with employed mothers and those with nonemployed mothers (Youngblut, Loveland-Cherry, & Horan, 1994). In a study of preschoolers in female-headed, single-parent families (66% African American, 75% not employed), the preschoolers' outcomes (achievement, mental processing, language) were better if their single mothers were employed (Youngblut et al., 2001). Forty percent of this sample of primarily low-income, single, African American mothers of preschoolers (half born preterm) used alternate child care for more than 75% of their children's lives; 20% used alternate child care when not employed. Preschool children born preterm were more likely to receive child care from nonrelatives throughout their lives than children born at term. Children with health problems used a greater number of different child care arrangements, controlling for chronologic age (Youngblut, Brooten, Lobar, Hernandez, & McKenry, 2005). These findings were highlighted in parenting magazines, on television, and in print news media. The news media were especially interested in these findings when welfare reform was being discussed and implemented. Specifically, my work influenced legislation by addressing concerns about the impact that welfare reform provisions would have on the children and about the availability of sufficient alternate child care arrangements.

References

Youngblut, J. M., & Brooten, D. (2006). Pediatric head trauma: Parent, parent-child and family functioning 2 weeks after hospital discharge. *Journal of Pediatric Psychology, 31*, 608–618. doi:10.1093/jpepsy/jsj066. PMCID: 2424404

Youngblut, J. M., & Brooten, D. (2008). Mothers' mental health, mother-child relationship, and family functioning 3 months after a preschooler's head injury. *Journal of Head Trauma Rehabilitation, 23*, 92–102. doi:10.1097/01.HTR.0000314528.85758.30. PMCID: 2442865

Youngblut, J. M., & Brooten, D. (2013). Parent report of child response to sibling death in a neonatal or pediatric ICU. *American Journal of Critical Care, 13*, 474–481. doi:10.4037/ajcc2013790. PMCID: 3881261

Youngblut, J. M., Brooten, D., Blais, K., Kilgore, C., & Yoo, C. (2015). Health and functioning in grandparents after a young grandchild's death. *Journal of Community Health, 40*(5), 956–966. doi:10.1007/s10900-015-0018-0. PMCID: 4556739

Youngblut, J. M., Brooten, D., Cantwell, G. P., del Moral, T., & Totapally, B. (2013). Parent health and functioning 13 months after infant or child NICU/PICU death. *Pediatrics, 132*(5), e1295–301. doi:10.1542/peds.2013-1194. PMCID: 3813397

Youngblut, J. M., Brooten, D., & Kuluz, J. (2005). Parent reactions at 24–48 hrs after a preschool child's head injury. *Pediatric Critical Care Medicine, 6*, 550–556. PMCID: 2614927

Youngblut, J. M., Brooten, D., Lobar, S., Hernandez, L., & McKenry, M. (2005). Child care use by low-income single mothers of preschoolers born preterm vs those of preschoolers born full term. *Journal of Pediatric Nursing, 20*, 246–257. doi:10.1016/j.pedn.2005.02.013. PMCID: 2753406

Youngblut, J. M., Brooten, D., Singer, L. T., Standing, T., Lee, H., & Rodgers, W. L. (2001). Effects of maternal employment and prematurity on child outcomes in single parent families. *Nursing Research, 50,* 346–355. PMCID: 2792577

Youngblut, J. M., & Jay, S. S. (1991). Emergency admission to the pediatric ICU: Parental concerns. *AACN Clinical Issues in Critical Care Nursing, 2,* 329–337.

Youngblut, J. M., Loveland-Cherry, C. J., & Horan, M. (1994). Maternal employment effects on families and preterm infants at 18 months. *Nursing Research, 43,* 331–337.

Youngblut, J. M., & Shiao, S.-Y. P. (1993). Child and family reactions during and after pediatric ICU hospitalization: A pilot study. *Heart & Lung, 22,* 46–54.

See my bibliography for a complete list of published work:

http://www.ncbi.nlm.nih.gov/sites/myncbi/joanne.youngblut.1/bibliography/10259945/public/?sort=date& direction=ascending

SHORT PAPERS SUBMITTED FOR CHAPTER 6

OiSaeng Hong
Madeline J. Kerr
Marjorie McCullagh

Reducing Auditory Problems Due to Harmful Noise and Chemical Exposure

OiSaeng Hong, PhD, RN, FAAN

Dr. OiSaeng Hong is a professor at University of California San Francisco (UCSF) and the director of the Occupational and Environmental Health Nursing Graduate Program within the Northern California Education and Research Center, funded by the National Institute of Occupational Safety and Health. She was formerly a postdoctoral fellow working with Dr. Sally Lusk's mentorship and was on the faculty of University of Michigan School of Nursing until she transitioned to UCSF in 2007. Dr. Hong is a recognized nurse scientist who is highly respected for her expertise in auditory impairment (hearing loss and tinnitus) due to environmental and occupational exposure to noise and other ototoxicants.

Through an innovative approach that applies information technology and the concept of tailoring, Dr. Hong and her multidisciplinary team conduct hearing loss prevention intervention studies for at-risk populations, such as firefighters and construction workers. The following are the short reports of five selected papers.

- Hong, O. (2005). Hearing loss among operating engineers in American construction industry. *International Archives of Occupational and Environmental Health, 78*(7), 565–574.

This paper described the prevalence and characteristics of noise-induced hearing loss (NIHL) among operating engineers in the United States. The study was a collaboration among committed team members representing a university, a worker labor union, and workers. In particular, through both worker and union involvement in the development and implementation of the program, this study provided a model for worker/union participatory safety and health training.

This is considered one of the first reports on the prevalence rates and characteristic patterns of NIHL among American operating engineers in the construction industry. The study also demonstrated the protective effect of hearing protection use on workers' audiometric test results. Findings from this study have added insights about the seriousness of the NIHL problem and the importance of the interventions to promote the use of hearing protection in the study population. This study revealed the prevalence of hearing loss in American construction workers.

- Hong, O., Ronis, D. L., Lusk, S. L, & Kee, K. S. (2006). Effectiveness of a computer-based hearing test and tailored hearing protection intervention. *International Journal of Behavioral Medicine, 13*(4), 304–314.

The purpose of this research was to test the efficacy of a computer-based hearing test and a tailored intervention to increase workers' attention to hearing ability and hearing protection. The computer-based program was developed by a multidisciplinary team and then implemented for operating engineers in a partnered labor union training center in a Midwestern state. This is one of a few intervention studies that applied behavioral theories to guide intervention research to promote workers' hearing protection behaviors and that used a sophisticated randomized experimental research design to test the effectiveness of the intervention. The study was one of the first to use the novel approach of combining a computer-based self-administered hearing test with highly individualized hearing protection training to prevent NIHL. Taking the hearing test makes workers think about their hearing status and creates a teachable moment.

This work makes an important contribution in the occupational health field by addressing a significant occupational health problem as well as advancing the science related to delivery vehicles for health screening and health education to change workers' health behaviors; thus it improves their health and safety. In recognition of its innovative approach and its broad implication for reducing NIHL in working populations, this study earned the 2006 Blue Cross Blue Shield of Michigan Foundation's Excellence in Research Award in the area of health services.

- Hong, O., Samo, D., Hulea, R., & Eakin, B. (2008). Perception and attitudes of firefighters on noise exposure and hearing loss. *Journal of Occupational & Environmental Hygiene, 5*(3), 210–215.

This paper represents research funded by the National Institute of Nursing Research. This is a rare qualitative study conducted with firefighters to assess their attitudes and beliefs concerning occupational noise exposure, hearing loss, the use of hearing protection, and the importance of their hearing for firefighting service. Firefighters acknowledged the significance of good hearing in firefighting, but they perceived NIHL as an unavoidable part of their work and viewed it as a small risk they were willing to take, compared to other hazards.

Firefighters are routinely exposed to high levels of intermittent noise on the job, particularly during emergency responses, when sirens, air horns, and vehicle engines are running. Noise exposure for firefighters is usually high in intensity and short in duration, unlike the steady, constant noise exposure that workers in manufacturing industries experience. This qualitative study identified various sources of noise exposure and noisy work activities related to firefighting. The findings of the study provide critical information for designing training programs concerning NIHL that are specific to firefighters. This study provided important supporting evidence for securing R01 grant funding from the Department of Homeland Security to conduct a hearing protection intervention for firefighters.

Based on these identified sources, we conducted noise measurement to estimate firefighting noise exposure potentials using Task-Based Exposure Assessment Modeling in collaboration with fire departments in Michigan and Northern California. The results of noise exposure assessment showed that, on any given day, firefighters have a risk of exposure to harmful levels (time-weighted average of 85 decibels over an 8-hour work day). Sounds that are louder than 85 decibels can cause permanent hearing damage if proper protection is not used. Firefighters also have a distinctive noise exposure pattern, wherein a fraction of their occupational time is spent in high-noise emergency environments, while the remaining time is spent in a semi-nonoccupational environment (the fire station) with exposures likely similar to those of typical U.S. residents.

- Hong. O, Eakin, B., Chin, D., Feld, J., & Vogel, S. (2013). An Internet-based tailored hearing protection intervention for firefighters: Development process and users' feedback. *Health Promotion Practice, 14*(4), 572–579.

With funding from the Department of Homeland Security/Federal Emergency Management Agency, a novel Internet-based, tailored hearing protection training program called S.I.R.E.N. (Safety Instruction to Reduce Exposure of Noise and Hearing Loss) was developed and widely implemented through the Internet to educate firefighters about the harmful auditory effects of noise exposure and prevention of NIHL by promoting hearing protection behaviors. Internet-based programs are easily accessible, time efficient, and flexible—attributes that are particularly important to firefighters, who often face unpredictable work hours and environments. The S.I.R.E.N. program was created as a self-directed, self-study, web-based intervention to specifically address the unique needs of firefighters and their profession. The benefit of web-based learning is that the firefighters have the flexibility to log in from anywhere at the time most convenient for them. This study demonstrated that multimedia computer technology using the Internet is a feasible method of delivering information to firefighters from 35 fire departments in several states. The research team has established excellent collaborative arrangements with partnered fire departments and firefighter unions, occupational and primary health clinicians, and national organizations in fire services from the development to the successful implementation of the program. This S.I.R.E.N. project provided a much-needed service to firefighters, and it was also recognized for being the first nursing intervention project to ever receive funding from the Department of Homeland Security.

- Hong, O., Chin, D., & Kerr, M. (2015). Lifelong occupational exposures and hearing loss among Latino American elderly. *International Journal of Audiology, 54*(Suppl. 1), S57–64.

The purpose of the study was to investigate the relationship between lifelong occupational exposures and hearing loss among older populations of Latino Americans, using data from the Sacramento Area Latino Study of Aging (SALSA) (an R01 study funded by the National Institutes of Health) with a longitudinal cohort study of 1,789 Latino American older adults aged 60 or older residing in rural and urban areas of Sacramento County, California, between 1998 and 1999.

This study demonstrated that lifelong occupational exposure to ototoxic hazards at work, such as loud noise and ototoxic chemicals (pesticides, lead, cadmium, solvents, other heavy metal), after controlling for aging effect, was significantly associated with hearing loss among older populations of Latino Americans. Hearing loss due to loud noise exposure remains a major public health problem and creates enormous economic burden and human suffering. While occupational noise exposure has long been recognized as one of the most prevalent causes of adult onset hearing loss, the impact of chemical-induced hearing loss on workers should not be underestimated. The study's finding on the significant linkage between exposure to ototoxicants and hearing loss validates that hearing loss prevention programs for workers, as well as for the general public, should obtain data regarding exposures to ototoxic chemicals in standardized hearing assessments. Further, surveillance programs should assess both noise and ototixicant exposures in order to develop appropriate interventions.

Occupational Health

Hearing Health Behavior Research and Public Health Informatics

Madeleine J. Kerr, PhD, RN

Dr. Madeline Kerr's program of research in occupational hearing loss prevention addresses several themes in health promotion and risk reduction. In addition, she has contributed to new research methods in the field of public health informatics defined as "the systematic application of information and computer science and technology to public health practice, research and learning" (Yasnoff, O'Carroll, Koo, Linkins, & Kilbourne, 2000).

Understanding Factors That Influence Hearing Protection Behavior

Building on the research of her mentor, Dr. Sally Lusk, Dr. Kerr identified the predictors of use of hearing protection devices (HPDs) among two different populations of workers, Mexican American factory workers and construction workers.

Mexican American Factory Workers

Dr. Kerr identified predictors of Mexican American workers' use of HPDs using a descriptive design (Kerr, Lusk, & Ronis, 2002). Mexican American garment workers (n = 119) completed a questionnaire. Factors that directly influenced the use of HPDs were benefits of minus barriers to HPD use, a clinical conception of health, self-efficacy in the use of HPDs, and perceived health status (R^2 = .25, Adj. R^2= .19). In an exploratory analysis, the required use of HPDs and plant site, along with three cognitive-perceptual factors (benefits of minus barriers to HPD use, a clinical conception of health, and perceived health status), were directly related to the use of HPDs (R^2 =.55, Adj. R^2=.45). These results suggested that Mexican American workers' use of hearing protection could be supported by promoting benefits of use, decreasing perceived or actual barriers to use, promoting a sense of self-efficacy in using HPDs, and relating a clinical conception of health to using HPDs.

Construction Workers

As part of her intervention study with construction workers, Dr. Kerr examined the factors influencing use of hearing protection (Kerr, Savik, Monsen, & Lusk, 2007). She found that the predictors of use of hearing protection model (PUHPM) was useful in explaining the changes in use of HPDs. Using multiple regression, 58% of the variance in postintervention use of hearing protection was explained by three variables representing four model factors: baseline use of hearing protection, social models of use of HPD, and benefits minus barriers—that is, participants who improved their use of hearing protection were more likely to experience social models of use of HPDs (e.g., supervisors, coworkers) and to perceive that the benefits of using HPDs outweigh the barriers.

Describing the Problem of Occupational Hearing Loss

Dr. Kerr has engaged in two projects using secondary data analysis to describe hearing loss prevalence and compare it to self-reporting of hearing ability. High levels of hearing loss were not surprising in the relatively unprotected populations of construction laborers (53%) and farmers (67%) (Kerr, McCullagh, Savik, & Dvorak, 2003). A similar study described the prevalence of hearing loss among factory workers (n = 2691) (McCullagh, Raymond, Kerr, & Lusk, 2011). The high rate of hearing loss (42%) was surprising to discover in a population that is served by an Occupational Health and Safety Administration–compliant hearing conservation program. Both studies found low sensitivity of a single-item measure of hearing ability, therefore the researchers concluded that perceived hearing loss is not an adequate screening tool.

Designing and Testing an Intervention to Promote Hearing Protection Behavior

Dr. Kerr's intervention study with construction workers used an experimental design to contrast the effect of a tailored intervention and a nontailored intervention on construction workers' use of HPDs and tested the effect of a booster intervention on workers' HPD use (Kerr, Savik, Monsen, & Lusk, 2007). The computer-based intervention was theory-based, using concepts from PUHPM. For example, health messages were designed to increase perceptions of self-efficacy and the benefits and value of using HPDs while decreasing perceptions of barriers to use. A video game–style format used an espionage story line, in which participants were engaged in the mission of foiling Dr. Noise by using their hearing protection devices (the voice of Peter Graves helped set the scene). The non-tailored version gave a standard, generic message incorporating these concepts, whereas the tailored intervention individualized these health messages based on worker responses to model-related questions and the reported use of HPDs.

Overall, participants reported improved use of HPDs at Time 2 ($p < .001$; Wilcoxon matched-pairs signed-rank test); the median reported use of HPDs was 42% at Time 1, improving to 50% at Time 2—an increase over the baseline of 19%. Both tailored and nontailored computer-based interventions appeared to be effective in improving construction workers' hearing health behavior. On average, tailored participants improved their use of HPDs by 8.3 % ($SD = 30.2$), while those receiving nontailored messages improved their use of HPDs by 6.1% ($SD = 29.8$) ($p = .51$). Those that received a booster improved 9.5% ($SD = 28.9$), whereas those who did not improved 5.6% ($SD = 30.6$), ($p = .24$). Tailoring plus booster yielded the greatest improvement of 12.6% ($SD = 28.7$, $p= .48$), an increase of 30% over baseline.

Public Health Informatics Methods for Occupational Health

Dr. Kerr and colleagues have developed a method to incorporate occupational health data into electronic health records. This is relevant and timely because the National Institute for Occupational Safety and Health is leading a charge to "ensure meaningful use of occupational information in electronic health records by 2015" (National Academy of Sciences, 2011). Using hearing health data from 346 firefighters, the team completed a successful demonstration project using standardized language to represent occupational health assessment, interventions, and outcomes in the electronic health record (Hong et al., 2012).

References

Hong, O., Monsen, K. A., Kerr, M. J., Chin, D. L., Lytton, A. B., & Martin, K. S. (2012). Firefighter hearing health: An informatics approach to screening, measurement, and research. *International Journal of Audiology, 51*(10), 765–770.

Kerr, M. J., Lusk, S. L., & Ronis, D. L. (2002). Explaining Mexican American workers' hearing protection use with the health promotion model. *Nursing Research, 51*(2), 100–109.

Kerr, M. J., McCullagh, M., Savik, K., & Dvorak, L. A. (2003). Perceived and measured hearing ability in construction laborers and farmers. *American Journal of Industrial Medicine, 44*(4), 431–437.

Kerr, M. J., Savik, K., Monsen, K. A., & Lusk, S. L. (2007). Effectiveness of computer-based tailoring versus targeting to promote use of hearing protection. *Canadian Journal of Nursing Research, 39*(1), 80–97.

McCullagh, M. C., Raymond, D., Kerr, M. J., & Lusk, S. L. (2011). Prevalence of hearing loss and accuracy of self-report among factory workers. *Noise & Health, 13*(54), 340–347.

National Academy of Sciences. (2011). *Incorporating Occupational Information in Electronic Health Records: Letter Report*. Washington, DC: National Academies Press.

Yasnoff, W. A., O'Carroll, P. W., Koo, D., Linkins, R. W., & Kilbourne, E. M. (2000). Public health informatics: Improving and transforming public health in the information age. *Journal of Public Health Management and Practice, 6*(6), 67–75.

Cultivating Hearing Health Among Farm Operators

Marjorie McCullagh, PhD, RN, FAAN

My research program focuses on promoting the health and safety of farm operators through the development of hearing conservation policy and practice. My primary focus has been in the development and testing of prevention programs. Specifically, this research is aimed at (a) the development of conceptual models of hearing protector use behavior, (b) the development and testing of model-based interventions for adults and youth, and (c) the development of public and agricultural organization policies that support the provision of hearing conservation services and the elimination of noise-induced physical, psychological, and social health problems, including hearing loss, tinnitus, communication difficulties, and increased risk for injury among agricultural workers. This research is expected to reduce rates of noise-induced hearing loss and tinnitus and improve the hearing health and quality of life of farm operators, their families, and communities. There are an estimated 3 million agricultural workers who are at high risk for hearing loss primarily because they work in high-noise environments and are not served by policies and programs designed to limit the health risks associated with workplace noise exposure enjoyed by most other industrial sectors (i.e., Occupational Health and Safety Administration regulations).

Research Trajectory

The trajectory of my studies illustrates the progression of my research program from prevalence, descriptive instrument development and pilot studies to large-scale randomized controlled trials of interventions. My research also illustrates my use of diverse funding sources (e.g., foundation and government grants, in-kind support) and interdisciplinary teamwork to advance my research aims. The projects also demonstrate the evolution of my long-standing relationship as research partner with the agricultural sector, including government agencies, farm advocacy groups, and commodity groups. This work was also made possible through work with scientists from multiple disciplines representing nursing, applied statistics, rural sociology, safety engineering, agronomy, and many others.

Development of research methods for use with a unique population. My research in the promotion of health of farm operators has been in development since 1985, when I explored the ammonia-handling safety knowledge, practices, and information sources of farmers (McCullagh, Green, & Fanning, 1988). In this and subsequent studies, I (a) developed and tested research methods for use with this unique worker population, (b) developed an interdisciplinary team of scientists, (c) developed long-standing research partnerships with farm organizations, (d) developed funding sources, and (e) mentored colleagues and students in nursing and other disciplines.

Development of validated instruments and a conceptual model of hearing protector use behavior among farmers. In a cross-sectional study of farm operators, I established prevalence of farm noise exposure and hearing protector use and developed and validated instruments to measure hearing-related behavior and attitudes (McCullagh, Lusk, & Ronis, 2002). In a subsequent predictors study (McCullagh, Ronis, & Lusk, 2010), I developed and tested a conceptual model in a random sample, which was successful in predicting hearing protector use in 74% of cases. Study findings also included a large distribution of farm operators who were trying to increase their use of hearing protection; this finding suggested receptivity to behavior change, lending support for an intervention to increase hearing protector use.

Development of informational brochures targeting farm operators. I assisted the Centers for Disease Control and Prevention/National Institute for Occupational Safety and Health (CDC/NIOSH) with the development of two informational brochures for farm operators (NIOSH, 2007a; NIOSH, 2007b). Although these brochures were based on the best science available at the time, they served as the control intervention for a later study that compared the effectiveness of various interventions on promoting the use of hearing protection among farmers (McCullagh & Ronis, 2015).

Development and testing of model-based interventions aimed at increasing hearing protector use among farm operators. The farmers' use of hearing protection model informed the development of interventions that address significant predictors of hearing protector use specific to farm operators. Results of an earlier pilot intervention and farmer interviews were combined to create a set of three distinct interventions for a randomized controlled trial. The interventions were delivered alone and in various combinations to compare their effectiveness in promoting hearing protector use and use-related attitudes and beliefs. The study found that the information-based interventions were not as effective as a simple mailed supply of assorted hearing protectors (McCullagh, Banerjee, Cohen, & Yang, 2016).

Identification of methods of screening workers for noise-induced hearing loss. A cross-sectional survey compared a functional ability questionnaire to audiometric screening and demonstrated the need for the development of self-reported measures of hearing ability (Kerr, McCullagh, Savik, & Dvorak, 2003). A subsequent comparison of the perceived and measured hearing ability of workers (McCullagh, Kerr, Raymond, & Lusk, 2011) showed hearing loss was highly prevalent and that self-reported hearing ability was poorly related to audiometry, suggesting the need for the development of alternative methods of screening for special populations such as farmers.

Establishment of feasibility and methods of hearing protector use among farm operators. A qualitative analysis of video-recorded interviews with farm operators (McCullagh & Robinson, 2009) determined the feasibility of consistent hearing protector use among farm operators and the identification of specific methods for overcoming the most significant obstacles to use.

Development of an intervention designed to increase the use of hearing conservation strategies among farm and rural youth. Because noise-induced hearing loss begins in childhood among farm youth, initiation of prevention from a young age could avoid the disease. However, most farm youth do not receive the benefit of hearing health education, and existing programs have not been tested. A randomized controlled trial of a community-based intervention designed to compare the effectiveness and sustainability of approaches to increase youths' use of hearing conservation strategies is currently under way (funded by the National Institutes of Health for the 2015–2018 period).

Impact

My program of research has provided a significant knowledge base from which to develop policies and programs that promote the conservation of hearing. Under my leadership, my interdisciplinary team of researchers was the first to scientifically measure selected hazards to agricultural workers (i.e., anhydrous ammonia, farm noise) and protective behavior (i.e., hearing protector use) and established the prevalence of health disparities among farmers and the need for services. Among the outcomes of these studies was the development of print- and web-based educational products used by hundreds of thousands of farm operators to protect their health. For example, I assisted CDC/NIOSH with the development of informational literature for farm operators. With more than 800,000 requests, these materials were the most frequently requested of all CDC/NIOSH publications in 2008 and 2009. I also led the development of an educational bulletin on anhydrous ammonia safety that is one of the most popular on the subject.

My publications on the subject of farmer health and safety have advanced the awareness of hearing loss as a health problem among farmers. For example, my model test published in *Nursing Research* was recognized by Lippincott as one of their most-requested works for 2002 across all disciplines. These efforts also resulted in contributions to scientific methods, including the development of instruments and a conceptual model to guide the development and evaluation of the impact of programs to serve at-risk agricultural workers. I have served as consultant and educator to farmer political action groups, helping increase awareness of hearing and other health hazards and collaborating with them to develop policies and other strategies to protect hearing health.

My program of research has been supported by foundations, the NIH, and the CDC since 1998. Through their support, I developed innovative model-based interventions targeted to increase hearing protector use among farm operators. I served as principal investigator of a randomized controlled trial comparing the effectiveness of these interventions that has been used by hundreds of farmers nationwide. Furthermore, I have advocated for the acquisition of resources and access to health programs through engaging the highest level of leaders in major farm organizations and supporting the health and safety missions of these organizations.

My work has contributed to the understanding of the effectiveness of hearing conservation programs in general industry and the feasibility of alternative, lower-cost, more accessible methods of screening for hearing problems for at-risk populations.

My research has established the health risks of noise exposure among farm and rural youth, calling attention to the need for delivery of services to this group. Collaborations with leading international farm safety and hearing conservation organizations have resulted in the development of a novel program designed to meet needs of this high-risk group.

It has been a privilege to work alongside those who grow our food, fiber, and fuel to promote better health and quality of life.

References

McCullagh, M. C., Banerjee, T., Cohen, M. A., & Yang, J. J. (2016). Effects of interventions on use of hearing protectors among farm operators: A randomized controlled trial. *International Journal of Audiology, 55*(Suppl 1) S3–S12. doi:10.3109/14992027.2015. 1122239. PMID: 26766172.

McCullagh, M., Green, J., & Fanning, C. (1988). *How to reduce your risk of exposure to anhydrous ammonia* (No. SF 962). Fargo, ND: North Dakota Agricultural Extension Service, NDSU.

McCullagh, M. C., Kerr, M. J., Raymond, D. M., & Lusk, S. L. (2011). Prevalence of hearing loss and accuracy of self-report among factory workers. *Noise & Health, 13*(54), 340–347. doi:10.4103/1463-1741.85504

McCullagh, M. C., Lusk, S. L., & Ronis, D. L. (2002). Factors influencing use of hearing protection among farmers: A test of the Pender health promotion model. *Nursing Research, 51*(1), 33–39.

McCullagh, M. C., & Robinson, C. (2009). Too late smart: Farmers' adoption of self-protective behavior in response to exposure to hazardous noise. *AAOHN Journal, 57*(3), 99–105.

McCullagh, M. C., & Ronis, D. L. (2015). Protocol of a randomized controlled trial of interventions to increase hearing protector use among farm operators. *BMC Public Health, 15*, 399. doi:10.1186/s12889-015-1743-0

McCullagh, M. C., Ronis, D. L., & Lusk, S. L. (2010). Predictors of use of hearing protection among a representative sample of farmers. *Research in Nursing & Health, 33*(6), 528–538. doi:10.1002/nur.20410

National Institute for Occupational Safety and Health (NIOSH). (2007a). Have you heard? Hearing loss caused by noise is preventable. Retrieved from http://www.cdc.gov/niosh/docs/2007-176

National Institute for Occupational Safety and Health (NIOSH). (2007b). They're your ears: Protect them. Retrieved from http://www.cdc.gov/niosh/docs/2007-175